AF783288

Investigative Urology 4

Edited by
D. Jocham · J. W. Thüroff · H. Rübben

With 124 Figures and 30 Tables

Springer-Verlag
Berlin Heidelberg New York
London Paris Tokyo
Hong Kong Barcelona
Budapest

Volume 1 of the series "Investigative Urology" is "Experimentelle Urologie" edited by R. Harzmann, G.H. Jacobi, L. Weißbach, 1985

Professor Dr. DIETER JOCHAM
Klinik und Poliklinik für Urologie
Medizinische Universität Lübeck
Ratzeburger Allee 160, W-2400 Lübeck 1

Professor Dr. J. W. THÜROFF
Urologische Klinik
Klinikum Barmen
Heusnerstraße 40, W-5600 Wuppertal-Barmen

Professor Dr. HERBERT RÜBBEN
Urologische Klinik und Poliklinik
Medizinische Einrichtungen der Universität – GHS-Essen
Hufelandstraße 55, W-4300 Essen 1

ISBN-13: 978-3-642-75974-1 e-ISBN-13: 978-3-642-75972-7
DOI: 10.1007/ 978-3-642-75972-7

This work is subject to copyright. All rights are reserved, whether the whole or part of the material is concerned, specifically the rights of translation, reprinting, reuse of illustrations, recitation, broadcasting, reproduction on microfilms or in other ways, and storage in data banks. Duplication of this publication or parts thereof is only permitted under the provisions of the German Copyright Law of September 9, 1965, in its current version, and a copyright fee must always be paid. Violations fall under the prosecution act of the German Copyright Law.

© Springer-Verlag Berlin Heidelberg 1991
Softcover reprint of the hardcover 1st edition 1991

The use of registered names, trademarks, etc. in this publication does not imply, even in the absence of a specific statement, that such names are exempt from the relevant protective laws and regulations and therefore free for general use.

Product Liability: The publisher can give no guarantee for information about drug dosage and application thereof contained in this book. In every individual case the respective user must check its accuracy by consulting other pharmaceutical literature.

Typesetting: K+V Fotosatz, Beerfelden

2122/3130-543210 – Printed on acid-free paper

Contents

I. Renal Cancer

^{31}P MRI In Vivo Studies of Human Renal Cell and Transitional Cell Carcinomas Xeno-grafted into Nude Mice
S. POMER, A.C. KÜSEL, G. STAEHLER, and W.E. HULL
(With 5 Figures) 3

Characterization of a Differentiation Antigen Defined by Monoclonal Antibody Due ABC 3
K. DECKEN, P. SIETH, S. SCHLICHTHERLE, T. EBERT, and B.J. SCHMITZ-DRÄGER (With 2 Figures) 10

Lymphocyte Subpopulations and Tumor Necrosis Factor During Interferon-α 2b and Interleukin-2 Therapy in Patients with Metastasized Renal Cell Cancer
A. MANSECK, B. MANSOURI TALEGHANI, and M. WIRTH
(With 4 Figures) 15

Effects of Buthionine Sulfoximine Mediated Glutathione Depletioin in Chemoresistant Human Renal Cell Carcinomas
G. MICKISCH, H. BIER, R. TSCHADA, and P. ALKEN
(With 5 Figures) 21

Renin-Producing Renal Cell Carcinoma – Clinical and Experimental Investigation of a Special Form of Renal Hypertension
J. STEFFENS, R. BOCK, H.U. BRAEDEL, E. ISENBERG, C.P. BÜHRLE, and M. ZIEGLER (With 3 Figures) 30

II. Andrology and Testicular Cancer

Experimental Approach for Assessment of Tumor Biology in Clinical Stage I Nonseminomatous Germ Cell Tumors (NSGCT)
E.P. ALLHOFF, S. LIEDKE, C. WITTEKIND, C. STIEF, H.-J. SCHMOLL, W. DE RIESE, and B. SCHNEIDER
(With 1 Figure) 39

Turbidimetrical Determination of Inflammatory Parameters in Seminal Plasma
M. ZELLNER, P. FORNARA, A. DICHTL, K. EDER, and A.G. HOFSTETTER (With 6 Figures) 43

The Arteries of the Spermatic Cord and Testis: A Dynamic Angiographic Study and its Clinical Relevance
M. SCHARDT, M. MEYER-SCHWICKERATH, and H. RÜBBEN (With 4 Figures) 49

Comparison of Duplex Sonography and Color-Coded-Flow Duplex Sonography for Evaluation of Erectile Dysfunction
K. LANG, W. SCHANTZEN, B.M. CRAMER, and J.W. THÜROFF (With 2 Figures) 54

Registration of Cavernous Electrical Activity and its Interpretation
C.G. STIEF, M. DJAMILIAN, W. DE RIESE, E.P. ALLHOFF, A. KRAMER, and U. JONAS (With 5 Figures) 58

III. BPH, Prostate Cancer

Imprint and Scrape Cytology: Advantages and Possible Uses in Urology
H. AL-ABADI, R. FRIEDRICHS, V. BORGMANN, I. ROTTER, and R. NAGEL (With 5 Figures) 67

^{31}P-NMR Spectroscopy and ^{1}H Imaging of the Prostate – Differences between Benign Hyperplasia and Cancers
F. HERING and S. MÜLLER (With 5 Figures) 72

IV. Bladder, Bladder Cancer

Evaluation of Acute-Phase Proteins for Clinical Monitoring of Urinary Tract Infections and Postoperatively
D.M. WILBERT, C. SCHAERFE, W.L. STROHMAIER, and K.-H. BICHLER (With 2 Figures) 81

Lysosomal Enzymuria in the Diagnosis of Upper Versus Lower Urinary Tract Inflections
C. SKREZEK, H. BERTERMANN, and H. WAND (With 6 Figures) 86

The Caeco-appendiceal Junction: A Urologically Applicable Sphincter Mechanism?
W. HÜBNER and R. HARTUNG (With 4 Figures) 92

DNA/Cytokeration Flow Cytometry in Bladder Lavage:
An Improvement in the Diagnosis of Bladder Tumors?
T. LIEDL, M. PROSINGER, B. GANZMANN, and D. JOCHAM
(With 4 Figures) 100

First Clinical Experiences with Photodynamic Fluorescence
Diagnosis in Urology
R. BAUMGARTNER, A. BUSER, M. KRIEGMAIR, H. LENZ,
H. STEPP, E. UNSÖLD, and D. JOCHAM (With 4 Figures) 107

Analysis of Tumor Heterogeneity in Monolayers and Tumor
Spheroids of a Transitional Cell Carcinoma Cell Line
F.A. OFFNER, G. OTT, L. FÜZESI, V. PREISLER, J. HUNDECK,
B. KLOSTERHALFEN, F. HOFSTÄDTER, S. HAUPTMANN,
H. RÜBBEN, and C.J. KIRKPATRICK (With 2 Figures) 113

Tumour Induction at Ureterosigmoid Anastomosis without
Faecal Stream: An Experimental Study
W.-D.E. MIERSCH and J. VOGEL (With 6 Figures) 119

Endogenous Nitrosation and Induction of Sigmoid Carcinoma
Following Ureterosigmoidostomy in a Rat Model
T. KÄLBLE, A.R. TRICKER, W. SCHREIBER, K. MÖHRING,
and G. STAEHLER (With 1 Figure) 126

In Vitro Cellular Cytotoxicity Against Human Bladder
Carcinoma Cell Lines
A. BÖHLE, A.J. ULMER, M.-H. WANG, and H.-D. FLAD
(With 7 Figures) 131

Ultrastructural Phototoxic Effects of Sulfonated Chlorine-
Aluminum-Phthalocyanine on Bladder Cancer Cell Spheroids
K. MILLER, T. GRAU, and E. REICH (With 3 Figures) 140

Video-Fluorescence Microscopic Studies of Microcirculation
in Urothelial Tumors of the Rat
M. BEER, A. GÖTZ, R. RIEDL, and L. DERVISHI 145

V. Urodynamics

Effects of Isoprenaline, Papaverine and Verapamil
on Rat Isolated Bladder Muscle
W. DIEDERICHS, L. HERTLE, and H. NAWRATH
(With 3 Figures) 153

Effect of Trospium Chloride, Oxybutynin and Propiverine on
the Interaction of Acetylcholine with Isolated Preparations of
the Human Urinary Bladder
S. ALLOUSSI, J. BALDAUF, H. DEROUET, U. ZWERGEL,
and S. MEESSEN (With 3 Figures) 157

Intrathecal Administration of Substance P in the Rat: Effect on Bladder and Urethral Sphincteric Activity
A. MERSDORF, E.A. TANAGHO, and D. JONAS (With 2 Figures) ... 162

Topographic-Anatomical Basis of the Sacral Application of Electro-Neurostimulation: Neuroanatomical Variations
A. MERSDORF, T. MERSDORF, E.A. TANAGHO, and D. JONAS (With 5 Figures) ... 169

Prostaglandin Production by Human Renal Pelvis and Ureter
U. ZWERGEL, T. ZWERGEL, S. ALLOUSSI, H.J. LEIS, and H. GLEISPACH (With 1 Figure) ... 176

VI. Urolithiasis, Lithotripsy, Kidney-Pathophysiology

Electrophoretic Studies on Proteinuria on Calcium Oxalate Stone Patients
O. SCHARREL and A. HESSE (With 4 Figures) ... 183

Creation of an Animal Model to Investigate the Bioeffects of Extracorporeal Shock Wave Lithotripsy and Alternative Treatment Techniques for Renal Stones
G.J. FUCHS, B.A. WOLFSON, R.D. DAVID, and Z.L. BARBARIC (With 3 Figures) ... 189

The Value of Various In Vitro Stone Models for Characterization of Different Shock Wave Sources
J. RASSWEILER, K.U. KÖHRMANN, E. MARLINGHAUS, S. FRÖHNER, M. RAAB, B. BERLE, and P. ALKEN (With 3 Figures) ... 197

Evaluation of Ureteral Tissue Damage Caused by Laser-induced Shock Waves: A Comparison of Laser Systems of Different Wavelengths
R. MUSCHTER, R. ENGELHARDT, R. BRINKMANN, M. SCHEU, P. RENNER, St. THOMAS, and G. BARETTON (With 4 Figures) . 205

Stone Fragmentation Capacities of Different Lasers and EHL in Monohydrate, Cystine and Struvite Urinary Calculi
N. SCHMELLER (With 3 Figures) ... 212

Experimental and First Clinical Results with the Alexandrite Laser Lithotripter
H.M. WEBER, K. MILLER, J. RÜSCHOFF, J. GSCHWEND, and R.E. HAUTMANN (With 2 Figures) ... 216

Effects of Extracorporal Shock Wave Lithotripsy on the Female Reproduction Tract
F. RECKER, P. JAEGER, P. DIENER, and H. KNOENAGEL (With 1 Figure) ... 224

Antitumor Effects of High-Energy Shock Waves are Potentiated by Doxorubicin and Biological Response Modifiers
G. A. H. J. SMITS, G. O. N. OOSTERHOF, A. E. DE RUYTER, J. A. SCHALKEN, and F. J. M. DEBRUYNE (With 2 Figures) 228

A New Method for Renal Perfusion Fixation
M. KALLERHOFF, H. J. GRÖNE, G. KEHRER, T. KNIESS, U. HELMCHEN, H. J. BRETSCHNEIDER, and R. H. RINGERT (With 5 Figures) 238

Investigations into the Medicinal Protection from Acute Kidney Failure of Ischemic Origin in Animal Experiments
B. LANGKOPF, U. REBMANN, H.-J. FORTH, and J. SCHABEL (With 2 Figures) 246

List of Contributors

The addresses are given at the beginning of each contribution

Al-Abadi, H. 67
Alken, P. 21, 197
Allhoff, E.P. 39, 58
Alloussi, S. 157, 176
Baldauf, J. 157
Barbaric, Z.L. 189
Barreton, G. 205
Baumgartner, R. 107
Beer, M. 145
Berle, B. 197
Bertermann, H. 86
Bichler, K.-H. 81
Bier, H. 21
Bock, R. 30
Böhle, A. 131
Borgmann, V. 67
Braedel, H.U. 30
Bretschneider, H.J. 238
Brinkmann, R. 205
Bührle, C.P. 30
Buser, A. 107
Cramer, B.M. 54
David, R.D. 189
Debruyne, F.J.M. 228
Decken, K. 10
Derouet, H. 157
Dervishi, L. 145
Dichtl, A. 43
Diederichs, W. 153
Diener, P. 224
Djamilian, M. 58
Ebert, T. 10
Eder, K. 43
Engelhardt, R. 205
Flad, H.-D. 131
Fornara, P. 43
Forth, H.-J. 246
Friedrichs, R. 67
Fröhner, S. 197
Fuchs, G.J. 189
Füzesi, L. 113
Ganzmann, B. 100
Gleispach, H. 176
Götz, A. 145
Grau, T. 140
Gröne, H.J. 238
Gschwend, J. 216
Hartung, R. 92
Hauptmann, S. 113
Hautmann, R.-E. 216
Helmchen, U. 238
Hering, F. 72
Hertle, L. 153
Hesse, A. 183
Hofstädter, F. 113
Hofstetter, A.G. 43
Hübner, W.A. 92
Hull, W.E. 3
Hundeck, J. 113
Isenberg, E. 30
Jäger, P. 224
Jocham, D. 100, 107
Jonas, D. 162, 169
Jonas, U. 58
Kälble, T. 126
Kallerhoff, M. 238
Kehrer, G. 238
Kirkpatrick, C.J. 113
Klosterhalfen, B. 113
Knieß, T. 238
Knönagel, H. 224
Köhrmann, K.U. 197
Kramer, A. 58
Kriegmair, M. 207

Küsel, A.C. 3
Lang, K. 54
Langkopf, B. 246
Leis, H.J. 176
Lenz, H. 107
Liedke, S. 39
Liedl, Th.M. 100
Manseck, A. 15
Mansouri-Taleghani, B. 15
Marlinghaus, E. 197
Meessen, S. 157
Mersdorf, A. 162, 169
Mersdorf, T. 169
Meyer-Schwickerath, M. 49
Mickisch, G. 21
Miersch, W.-D.E. 119
Miller, K. 140, 216
Möhring, K. 126
Müller, S. 72
Muschter, R. 205
Nagel, R. 67
Nawrath, H. 153
Offner, F.A. 113
Oosterhof, G.O.N. 228
Ott, G. 113
Pomer, S. 3
Preisler, V. 113
Prosinger, M. 100
Raab, R. 197
Rassweiler, J. 197
Rebmann, U. 246
Recker, F. 224
Reich, E. 140
Renner, P. 205
Riedl, R. 145
Riese, W. de 39, 58
Ringert, R.H. 238
Rotter, I. 67
Rübben, H. 49, 113
Rüschoff, J. 216
Ruyter, A.E. de 228
Schabel, J. 246
Schalken, J.A. 228
Schantzen, W. 54
Schardt, M. 49
Schärfe, C. 81
Scharrel, O. 183
Scheu, M. 205
Schlichtherle, S. 10
Schmeller, N. 212
Schmitz-Dräger, B.J. 10
Schmoll, H.-J. 39
Schneider, B. 39
Schreiber, W. 126
Sieth, P. 10
Skrezek, C. 86
Smits, G.A.H.J. 228
Staehler, G. 3, 126
Steffens, J. 30
Stepp, H. 107
Stief, C.G. 39, 58
Strohmaier, W.L. 81
Tanagho, E.A. 162, 169
Thomas, St. 205
Thüroff, J.W. 54
Tricker, A.R. 126
Tschada, R. 21
Ulmer, A.J. 131
Unsöld, E. 107
Vogel, J. 119
Wand, H. 86
Wang, M.-H. 131
Weber, H.M. 216
Wilbert, D.M. 81
Wirth, M. 15
Wittekind, C. 39
Wolfson, B.A. 189
Zellner, M. 43
Ziegler, M. 30
Zwergel, T. 176
Zwergel, U. 157, 176

I. Renal Cancer

^{31}NMR In Vivo Studies of Human Renal Cell and Transitional Cell Carcinomas Xenografted into Nude Mice

S. POMER[1], A.C. KÜSEL[2], G. STAEHLER[1], and W.E. HULL[2]

Introduction

^{31}P NMR is of particular interest for tumor investigations, since various neoplasms can differ from normal cells in pH, energy metabolism, and phospholipid turnover (proliferation rate). Human tumor cells can be studied as cultures in an appropriate matrix or as solid tumors (xenografts) in the nude mouse.

The feasibility of using ^{31}P NMR clinically for monitoring tumor growth and therapy response in vivo is being actively tested in numerous centers (Daly 1989; Hull 1990; Steen 1989). These research and clinical studies have shown that the levels of phosphomonoesters and -diesters (PME, PDE), primarily phospholipid metabolites, are altered in tumor cells and can be influenced by tumor growth.

The interpretation of ^{31}P spectra obtained at low fields (<2.4 T) is generally limited by low resolution and uncertain localization. Our efforts were concentrated on obtaining high quality, high resolution spectra at 7 T of human tumors as xenografts in nude mice and in parallel studies at 11.7 T of tumor cell cultures. This would contribute to a better understanding of phospholipid metabolism in tumors and the associated effects that are detectable in ^{31}P NMR spectra.

Materials and Methods

Human renal cell carcinomas (KT CTL 26A, $n = 3$) and transitional cell carcinomas (EJ 28, $n = 3$) were investigated. Tumors were transplanted subcutaneously into either the side or the hind leg of nude mice. ^{31}P spectra were measured initially after 6–10 weeks, when tumors had reached a diameter of about 17–25 mm.

^{31}P NMR at 7 T

A standard in vivo probe head was used with a Bruker AM 300 SWB (15 cm vertical bore). The two-turn spiral surface coil (17 mm external diameter) was double-tuned for ^{1}H/^{31}P and gave a 180° pulse for ^{31}P of 24 µs at the surface of the measured object. Spectra (SW = 10 kHz, TD = 4K, AQ = 0.20 s) were acquired with pulse lengths of 5, 10, and 20 µs and a repetition time T_r of 2 s. Under these

[1] Chirurgische Universitätsklinik, Abt. Urologie und Poliklinik, W-6900 Heidelberg, FRG.
[2] Zentrale Spektroskopie, DKFZ, 6900 Heidelberg, FRG

conditions 80% of the total signal came from depths up to 6, 8, and 10 mm, respectively. Inverse-gated ^{1}H decoupling (4 watts, BB mod.) was applied and in favorable cases gave improved resolution in the PME region. Routinely, 600 scans (20 min) were taken. Lorentz-Gauss resolution enhancement and polynomial baseline correction were applied to all spectra.

In Vivo NMR Without Anesthetic (Fig. 1)

Mice were not anesthetized for NMR but were placed in a homemade restriction cage (Fig. 1). This allowed stable and reproducible positioning of tumors over the surface coil. Mice could be routinely subjected to 1- to 2-h measurement periods repeated daily.

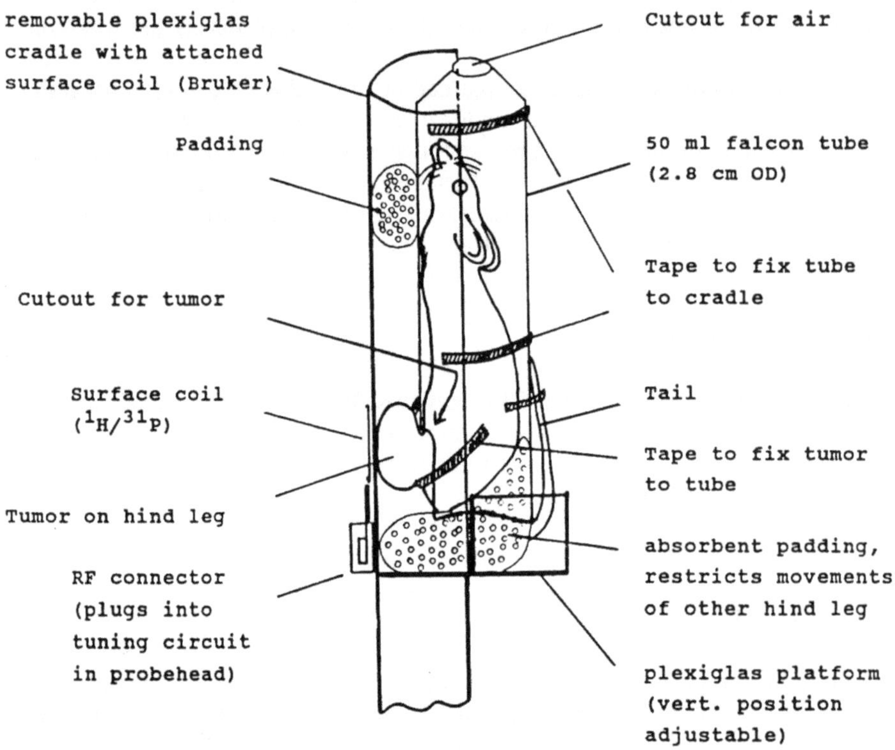

Fig. 1

Results

Even tumors less than 17 mm in diameter can be reasonably homogeneous with little necrosis as indicated by a narrow P_i resonance (pH = 7.0–7.1) and high nucleotide level in spectra obtained with different pulse widths (Fig. 2). The low PCr/NTP ratio indicates that there is little contamination from underlying muscle. Various homogeneous tumors having neutral pH show *no significant differences in PCr or nucleotide levels.*

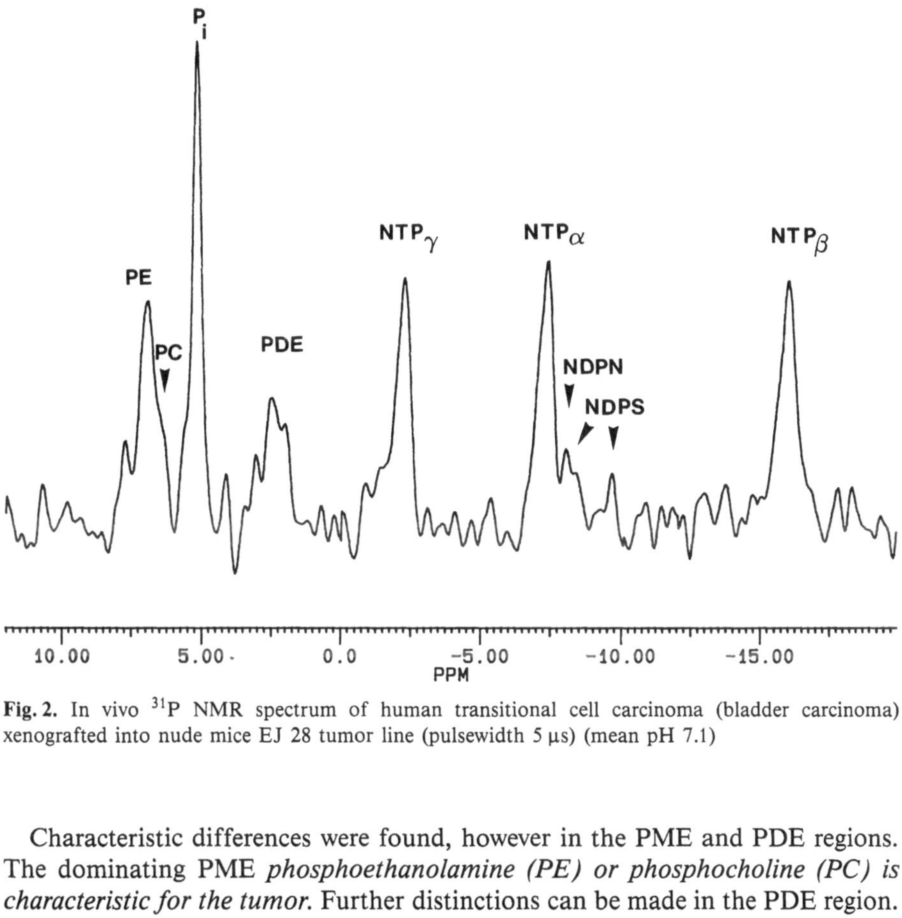

Fig. 2. In vivo ^{31}P NMR spectrum of human transitional cell carcinoma (bladder carcinoma) xenografted into nude mice EJ 28 tumor line (pulsewidth 5 μs) (mean pH 7.1)

Characteristic differences were found, however in the PME and PDE regions. The dominating PME *phosphoethanolamine (PE) or phosphocholine (PC) is characteristic for the tumor.* Further distinctions can be made in the PDE region. Figure 3 shows spectra from a renal cell carcinoma metastasis established as a xenograft in several nude mice. The tumor was reasonably homogeneous in form (about 10 weeks after implantation), resulting in a well-resolved spectrum of an apparently well-vascularized tumor of neutral pH (3A). A single interferon treatment (50000 units in 0.1 ml saline administered subcutaneously) had little effect on the metabolic state of this tumor (3B, C).

Some of the tumors examined were heterogeneous (necrotic) and gave broader spectra with a lower mean and larger spread in pH and significantly lower nucleotide levels. The level of PE appeared to drop at lower pH. GPC also appeared to decrease as the tumor became necrotic. In parallel studies of tumor cell cultures we found that phospholipid metabolite levels are very sensitive to the pH of the medium. In Fig. 4 a second mouse with a visibly heterogeneous (lumpy) tumor

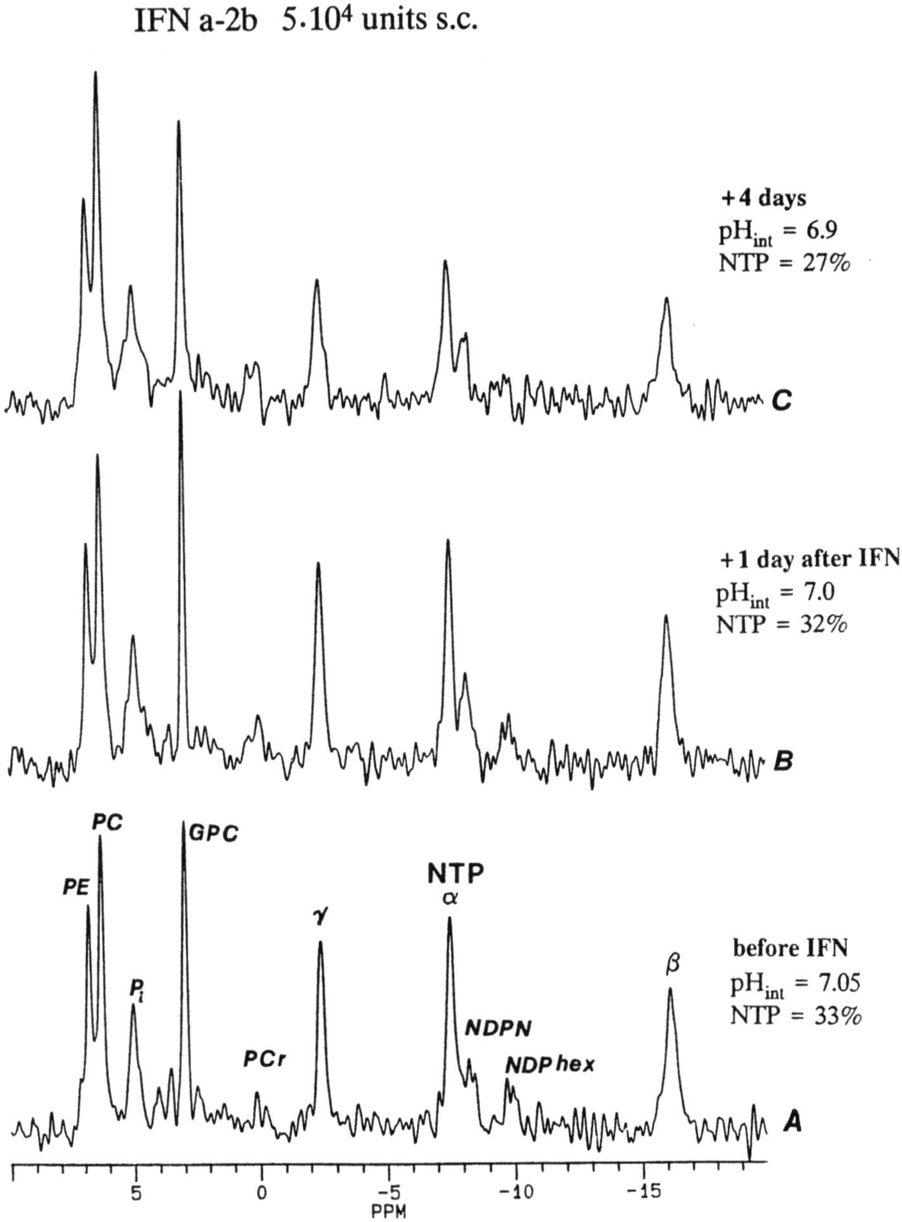

Fig. 3. In vivo ^{31}P NMR (7 T, 40 min) brain metastasis from human renal cell carcinoma xenograft in nude mouse (homogeneous tumor) IFN a-2b $5 \cdot 10^4$ units s.c.

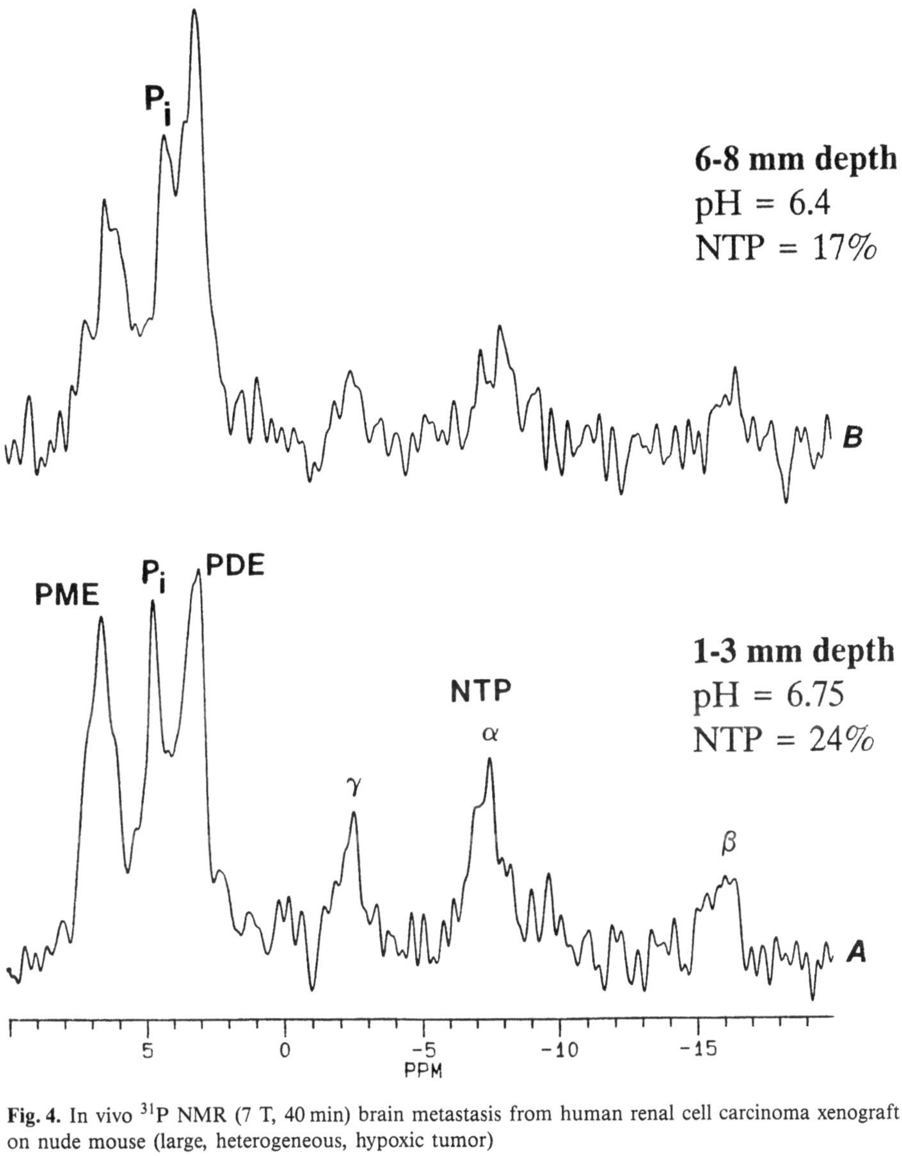

Fig. 4. In vivo ^{31}P NMR (7 T, 40 min) brain metastasis from human renal cell carcinoma xenograft on nude mouse (large, heterogeneous, hypoxic tumor)

mass was examined. The poorer quality of the spectra reflect this heterogeneity and a significant acidosis (hypoxia, necrosis). Fig. 5 shows the results of treating this tumor with interferon α-2b (Intron A, Essex Pharma). As a result a dramatic decay of NTP and phosphoesters as well as liberation of P_i could be demonstrated.

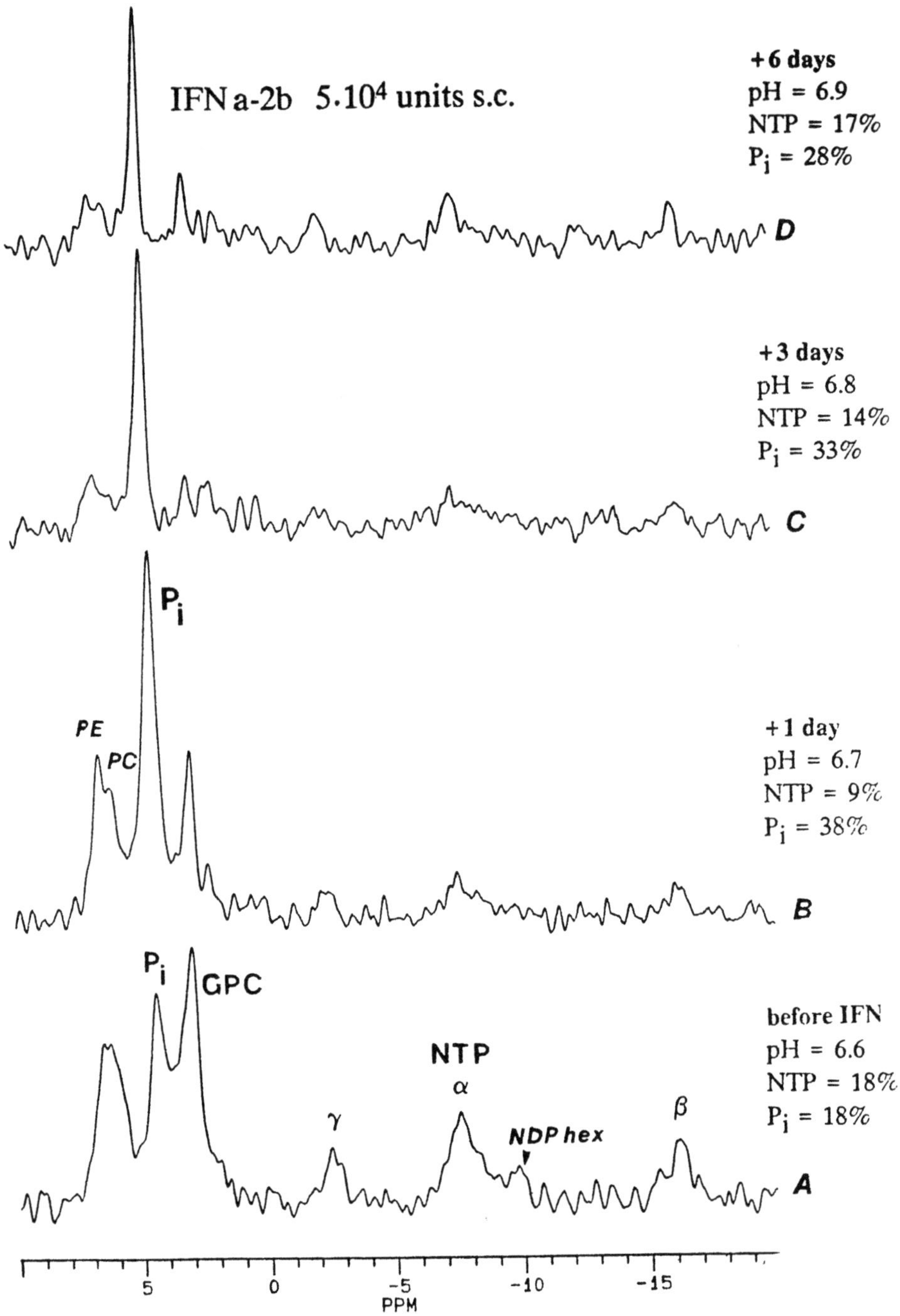

Fig. 5. In vivo ^{31}P NMR (7 T, 40 min) brain metastasis from human renal cell carcinoma xenograft on nude mouse (hypoxic tumor) IFN a-2b $5 \cdot 10^4$ units s.c.

Conclusion

Our preliminary results show that the immediate effects of therapy of renal cell carcinoma on tumor metabolism can be monitored by means of ^{31}P NMR. The amounts of PC, PE, and GPC change in response to therapy, such as, for example, immunotherapy.

References

Daly PF, Cohen JS (1989) Magnetic resonance spectroscopy of tumors and potential in-vivo clinical applications: a review. Cancer Res 49:770–779

Hull WE, Kuesel AC, Graschew G, Lorenz W, Thielmann HW (1990) High-field ^{31}P NMR studies of several human tumor cell lines. Comparisons in basement membrane gel culture and in solid tumors (abstracts). Magn Reson Med 9:845

Steen RG (1989) Response of solid tumors to chemotherapy monitored by in-vivo ^{31}P nuclear magnetic resonance spectroscopy: a review. Cancer Res 49:4075–4085

Characterization of a Differentiation Antigen Defined by Monoclonal Antibody Due ABC 3*

K. DECKEN[1], P. SIETH[2], S. SCHLICHTHERLE[1], T. EBERT[1], and B. J. SCHMITZ-DRÄGER[1]

Abstract

Monoclonal antibody Due ABC 3 recognizes a differentiation antigen in urologic epithelia. This antigen is expressed in proximal tubular epithelium as well as in renal cell carcinomas and in urothelial carcinomas. The epitope recognized by this antibody was shown to be part of the carbohydrate structure of a glycolipid, a structure related to Lewis X blood group antigen (CD 15). Occurrence of this antigen in lipid extracts from kidney tissue and transitional cell carcinoma cell lines was assayed by immuno-TLC.

Introduction

The monoclonal antibody (Mab) Due ABC 3 recognizes a differentiation antigen of urologic epithelia. This antigen is expressed by proximal tubular epithelia of the kidney (59/59) and the majority of renal cell carcinomas (70/120) and transitional cell carcinomas (25/28). In normal urothelium the few positive cases (7/26) show predominant staining of umbrella cells. Cross-reactivity is seen in tissue-infiltrating leukocytes of the granulocytic lineage, some gynecologic tumors, and gastrointestinal epithelia (Schmitz-Dräger et al. 1988; Decken et al. 1991). In urothelial tumors expression of the differentiation antigen occurs independently of tumor grade. Thus, the Mab supports an immunocytologic diagnosis of urothelial tumors from urine samples (Nakamura et al. 1989; Schmitz-Dräger et al. 1991). Since the degree of expression of the antigen correlates to tumor grade in renal cell cancer it qualifies as a prognostic marker in kidney tumors (Schmitz-Dräger 1989). The aim of this study was to analyze the biochemical nature of the antigen recognized by Mab Due ABC 3.

Materials and Methods

Cell Culture. Bladder tumor cell lines SW1710, SD, TCC-Sup and 5637 were cultured as monolayers in plastic flasks or on coverslips as well. Incubation was performed in Dulbecco's minimal essential medium (DMEM, Biochrom, Berlin,

* This work was supported by the Bundesminister für Forschung und Technologie (grant 01GA8701/7) and the Minister für Wissenschaft und Forschung des Landes Nordrhein-Westfalen.

[1] Urologische Klinik; [2]Pathologisches Institut, Abt. für Neuropathologie, Moorenstraße 5, W-4000 Düsseldorf 1, FRG.

FRG) supplemented with 15% fetal bovine serum (FBS, Biochrom), 100 IU/ml penicillin, and 100 µg/ml streptomycin at 37 °C in a humidified atmosphere with 5% CO_2. SW 1710 cells were provided with an additional 0.4 U/ml of bovine insulin (Hoechst). Passages were made from confluent cultures using 0.05% trypsin plus 0.02% EDTA.

Enzyme Treatment. For characterization of the antigen SW 1710 cells cultured on coverslips were treated with different agents (Table 1): neuraminidase from *Clostridium perfringens* (Sigma, St. Louis, Mo/10 mU/coverslip in 0.1 *M* acetate buffer pH 5.2), periodate (0.01 *M* in 0.1 *M* acetate buffer pH 5.2), acetate buffer control (0.1 *M* pH 5.2), acetate buffer (0.1 *M* pH 4.0), Dulbecco's PBS without calcium and magnesium (pH 7.2), sodium hydroxide (0.05 *M* pH 11.0), methanol/chloroform (2+1) and formaldehyde (3.7%). After treatment at room temperature coverslips were washed in PBS, fixed in acetone/formaldehyde solution (5%/1% in PBS) followed by hydrogen peroxide (0.5%) in cold methanol. Cells were incubated with undiluted Mab Due ABC 3 culture supernatant and bound Mab was visualized by immunoperoxidase reaction with a peroxidase-conjugated rabbit anti-mouse serum (Jackson Immunoresearch Laboratories, West Grove, Pa) diluted at 1:200 in PBS and DAB as chromogenic substrate.

Table 1. Biochemical protperties of Due ABC 3 Antigen

Treatment		Antigen stability
Heat		Stable up to 70 °C
Acid		Stable up to pH 4
Alkali		Stable up to pH 11
Periodate		Sensitive
Neuraminidase	EC 3.2.1.18	
from *Clostridium perfringens*		Sensitive
from *Vibrio cholerae*		Stable
Proteases		
trypsin	EC 3.4.21.4	Stable
proteinase K	EC 3.4.21.14	Stable
papain	EC 3.4.22.2	Stable
dispase	EC 3.4.22.4	Stable
collagenase	EC 3.4.24.3	Stable
proteinase E	EC 3.4.24.4	Stable
Chloroform/methanol		Sensitive
Formalin		Stable

Adsorption Assay. The sensitivity of Due ABC 3 antigen to heat and protease treatment was assayed with suspended SW 1710 cells (10^6/ml DMEM). Aliquots of 1 ml were incubated at 37 °C, 56 °C, 70 °C, 80 °C, 90 °C, and 100 °C for 5 min and chilled by addition of 2 ml of ice-could DMEM. To test for protease sensitivity 1-ml aliquots were incubated for 15 min at 37 °C with trypsin (0.05%), papain (0.2%), dispase (2.4 U/ml), proteinase K, proteinase E, and collagenase

(1 mg/ml). Digestion was stopped by addition of 1 ml FBS. After heat or protease treatment cells were washed and resuspended in 200 μl DMEM, then 25 μl Mab (culture supernatant) were added and incubated for 45 min at room temperature and an additional 45 min at 4 °C. After sedimentation of the cells the supernatant was incubated on coverslip cultures and stained by immunoperoxidase reaction.

Thin Layer Chromatography (TLC). SW 1710, 5637, SD, and TCC-Sup cells as well as benign kidney tissue were extracted overnight with chloroform/methanol (2+1) and centrifuged at 3000×*g* after addition of potassium chloride (1/2 vol 0.5 *M* KCl). The organic phase was collected and dried under nitrogen. Dry total lipid extracts were solved in chloroform and separated on aluminum silica plates (Merck, Darmstadt, FRG) with chloroform (5 vol), methanol (4 vol), and calcium chloride (1 vol 0.2%). After separation TLC plates were dried and blocked with bovine serum albumine (BSA, 2% in PBS = PBSA). Undiluted culture supernatant from hybridomas Due ABC 3 and Leu M1 (ATCC, Rockville, Mt) was added and bound Mab was detected with biotinylated anti-mouse serum (1:50 in PBSA) and peroxidase-conjugated avidin (1:100 in PBSA, Vector, Burlingame, Calif) stained with α-chloronaphthol.

Results

The antigen recognized by Mab Due ABC 3 is stable to heat up to 70 °C, while antigenicity of the cells is lost at temperatures beyond 70 °C. The antigen is stable to a wide range of pH values (pH 4 to pH 11) and to all proteases tested so far (Table 1). In contrast to these observations, periodate oxidation completely destroys the structure of the antigen, thus providing evidence that the antigen may be of a carbohydrate nature. Reduction of antigenicity after chloroform/methanol extraction argues for a lipid as responsive antigen. Neuraminidase treatment of the antigen yields contrary results: the antigen is sensitive to neuraminidase from *Clostridium* but not from *Vibrio*. These data suggest some kind of

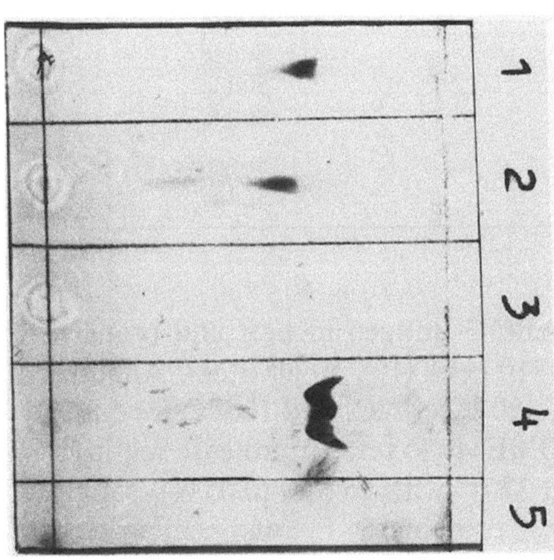

Fig. 1. Thin layer chromatogram stained with Mab Due ABC 3. Thin layer chromatographic separation of total lipid extracts from transitional cell carcinoma cell lines SW 1710 (lane 1), 5637 (lane 2), SD (lane 3), and TCC-Sup (lane 5), and from normal kidney tissue (lane 4) stained with Mab Due ABC 3

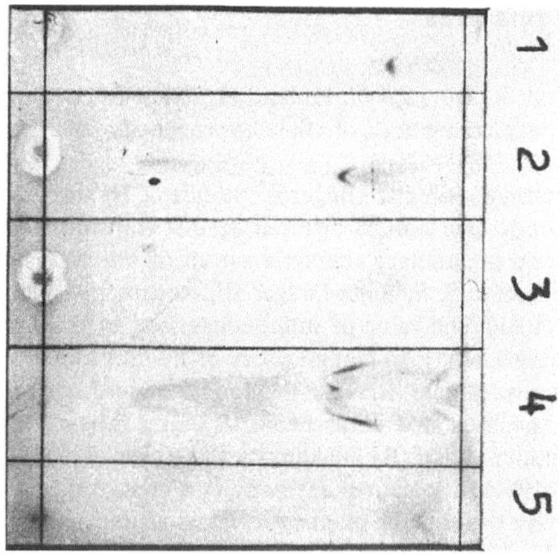

Fig. 2. Thin layer chromatogram stained with Mab Leu M1. Thin layer chromatographic separation of total lipid extracts from transitional cell carcinoma cell lines SW1710 (lane 1), 5637 (lane 2), SD (lane 3), and TCC-Sup (lane 5), and from normal kidney tissue (lane 4) stained with Mab Leu M1

glycolipid, possibly a ganglioside, giving the antigenic structure to Mab Due ABC 3.

Immunostaining of TLC plates with separations of lipid extracts from TCC cell lines or kidney tissue by Mab Due ABC 3 yielded, in a lipid band (Fig. 1) that was stained more weakly by Mab Leu M1, a Mab reacting with CD 15 or Lewis X (Le^x) hapten (Fig. 2). The Due ABC 3 band did not occur in lipid extracts from cells that were immunocytochemically negative for Due ABC 3, but did occur in extracts from positive cells as well as from benign kidney.

Discussion

Cell fractionation and TLC analysis showed a significance preference of Mab Due ABC 3 to bind to a carbohydrate structure on a glycolipid. The histologic and biochemical analyses point to Le^x or a related structure as the antigen responsible, while the contradictory results from neuraminidase treatment of cell extracts leave it unresolved whether Due ABC 3 recognizes Le^x itself, a nonsialylated derivative of Le^x, or the sialoyl-Le^x ganglioside, which is reported to be the main ganglioside of human kidney (Rauvala 1976).

The Le^x hapten is known to occur both on glycolipids and on glycoproteins, the latter usually with relative molecular masses of 185 K or 200 K. This suggests that other Mabs which exhibit an immunohistological binding pattern similar to that of Mab Due ABC 3 might bind to a related structure. Therefore the possibility cannot be ruled out that, for example, Mab 486P 3/12, which was reported to recognize a CEA-like glycoprotein of 200 K molecular mass (Arndt et al. 1987), might be directed against a Le^x-related hapten on this glycoprotein. Since the results of the biochemical analysis provide no evidence of a protein nature of the ABC 3 antigen, it is tempting to speculate that Mab 486P 3/12 and Due ABC, 3 recognize different epitopes on the same hapten. Further testing of this hypothesis might provide a better understanding of membrane glycosylation.

References

Arndt R, Dürkopf H, Huland H, Donn F, Loening T, Kalthoff H (1987) Monoclonal antibodies for characterization of the heterogeneity of normal and malignant transitional cells. J Urol 137:758–763

Decken K, Schmitz-Dräger BJ, Rohde D, Nakamura S, Ebert T, Ackermann R (1991) Monoclonal antibody Due ABC 3 directed against transitional cell carcinoma. I. Production, specificity analysis and preliminary characterization of the antigen. J Urol (in press)

Nakamura S, Schmitz-Dräger BJ, Rottmann-Ickler C, Decken K, Pfitzer P, Bojar H, Ackermann R (1989) The value of immunocytology in the diagnosis of bladder cancer. J Urol 141:319A

Rauvala H (1976) Gangliosides of human kidney. J Biol Chem 251:7517–7520

Schmitz-Dräger BJ (1989) Monoklonale Antikörper gegen urologische Tumoren – Produktion: Spezifität und klinische Anwendung. Thesis, Medical Faculty, University of Düsseldorf

Schmitz-Dräger BJ, Nakamura S, Decken K, Pfitzer P, Rottmann-Ickler C, Ebert T, Ackermann R (1991) Monoclonal antibody Due ABC 3 directed against transitional cell carcinoma. II. Prospective trial on the diagnostic value of immunocytology using monoclonal antibody Due ABC 3. J Urol (in press)

Schmitz-Dräger BJ, Rohde D, Peschkes C, Ebert T, Ackermann R (1988) Monoklonale Antikörper gegen Harnblasenkarzinome – ein Beitrag zur Verbesserung der Diagnostik? Akt Urol 19:117–123

Lymphocyte Subpopulations and Tumor Necrosis Factor During Interferon-α2b and Interleukin-2 Therapy in Patients with Metastasized Renal Cell Cancer

A. MANSECK[1], B. MANSOURI TALEGHANI[2], and M. WIRTH[1]

Abstract

Treatment of patients with metastasized renal cell cancer with interferon-α2b (IFN-α2b) and interleukin-2 (IL-2) initially led to a drop in the total lymphocyte count and in all lymphocyte subpopulations with the exception of CD-19-positive cells. Upon termination of therapy, there was an excessive increase in all lymphocyte subpopulations. No correlation between the kinetics of the lymphocyte subpopulations and the clinical outcome of the patient was demonstrated. Significant stimulation of tumor necrosis factor-α (TNF-α) as a result of the treatment was not detected. This may indicate that stimulation of TNF-α by IL-2 is not an important effector mechanism.

Introduction

There is still no standard treatment for metastasized renal cell carcinoma. Hormone therapy has proved to be of no therapeutic value [4] and no effective chemotherapeutic drugs are available. Immunomodulation with IFN-α2b and IL-2 has been described in the literature as a new and promising treatment for metastasized renal cell carcinoma [1, 2, 5, 9, 12–15, 17–23]. Since only some renal tumors respond to this form of treatment, it would be of great interest to determine what group of patients profit from immunomodulation. In order to ascertain which patients respond well to a combined treatment of IL-2 and IFN-α2b and to better understand the way in which this treatment modality works, tests to investigate the immunostimulation caused by these substances are necessary. One possible way to solve these questions may be to study the effect of IFN-α2b and IL-2 on various lymphocyte subpopulations in the peripheral venous blood of patients with renal cell carcinoma. The question of whether IL-2 leads to increasing levels of TNF-α in the sera of these patients was also investigated.

Materials and Methods

Ten patients with metastasized renal cell carcinoma underwent treatment with recombinant IFN-α2b (Essex Pharma) and recombinant IL-2 (EuroCetus). Patient

[1] Urologische Klinik und Poliklinik; [2]Medizinische Klinik, Hämatologie, der Universität, Josef-Schneider-Str. 2, W-8700 Würzburg, FRG.

age was between 44 and 65 years (average 53 years). All patients had pulmonary metastases. In three cases the primary tumor had not been removed or there had been local recurrence of the tumor. In the bone scan metastases were evident in 3 patients. All patients had a Karnofsky index greater than 80% prior to the commencement of treatment. No patient had received antitumor therapy in the 12 weeks immediately prior to immunomodulation treatment. Patients with cerebral metastases, serious heart disease, or acute intercurrent diseases were not included in the study. The patients were each treated for 5 days with IFN-α2b 10×10^6 IU/m^2 administered subcutaneously. After a break of 2 days, IL-2 3×10^6 CU/m^2 and day were administered by continuous intravenous infusion (1 CU = 1 Cetus Unit = 6 IU).

Cell Surface Markers

The lymphocyte subpopulations were determined using a flowcytometer (EPICS-V, Coulter) by means of the following monoclonal antibodies: CD 2, CD 4, CD 8, CD 10, CD 19, CD 24, CD 71, and HLA-DR (CD nomenclature according to the 4th International Working Committee for Human Leukocyte Differentiation Antigens). The monoclonal antibodies were supplied by Ortho, T-cell Sciences, and Dakopatt. Tumor necrosis factor-α was determined with the Quantikine human TNF-α immunoassay (RD System/USA). Blood samples were taken from the patients prior to the commencement of treatment, on days 2 and 4 of IFN-α treatment and days 2 and 4 of IL-2 treatment, and after termination of IL-2 therapy (Table 1).

Table 1. Treatment schedule of IFN-α 2b and IL-2

Interferon α-2b ←→							Interleukin-2 ←→				
1	2	3	4	5	6	7	8	9	10	11	12

Results

None of the ten patients showed an objective response to the treatment. Three patients were in a stable phase. Figure 1 shows the absolute lymphocyte count during treatment. During treatment with IFN-α2b, no significant change in the lymphocyte subpopulations was observed. On day 2 of the IL-2 therapy, there was a decline in all the lymphocyte subpopulations determined, with the exception of the CD 19-positive B-cells. On day 4 of the interleukin-2 therapy no further changes in the lymphocyte subpopulations were detected. An excessive increase in the lymphocyte subpopulations took place after termination of the treatment, which then exceeded their absolute count prior to the treatment. In Figs. 2 and 3, the lymphocyte subpopulations during immunotherapy are presented as examples. In Fig. 4,

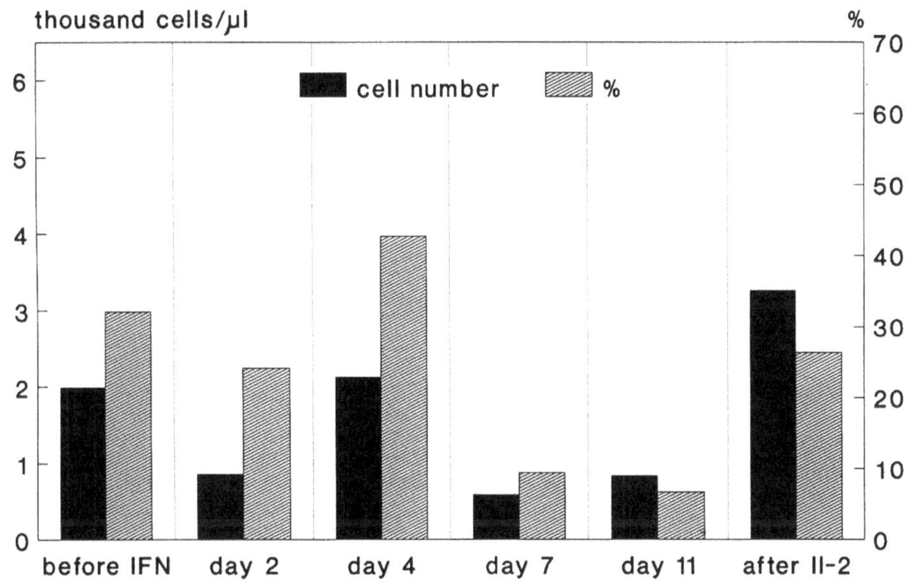

Fig. 1. Total number and ratio of lymphocytes before, during and after IFN-α2b and IL-2 therapy

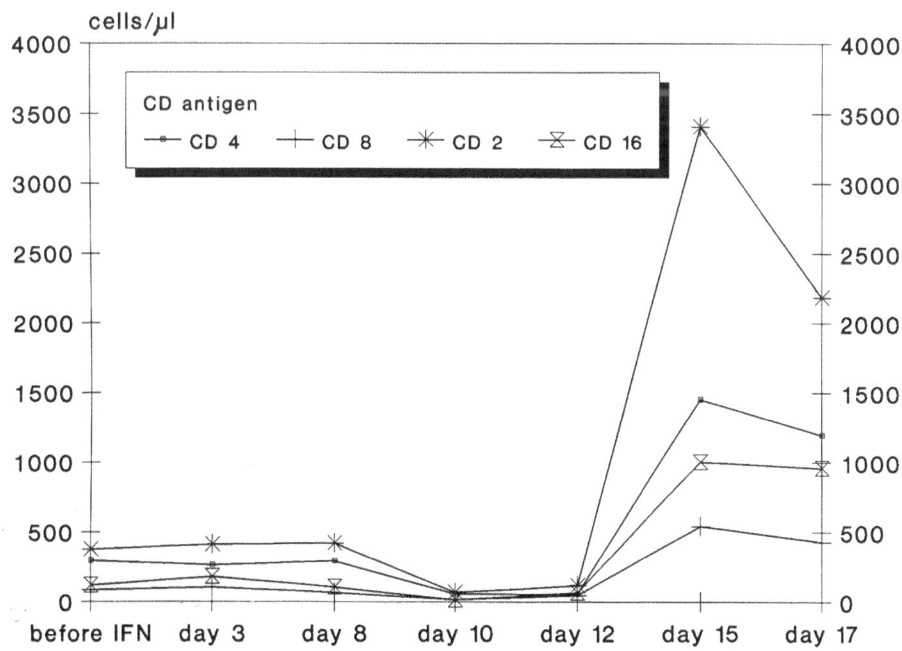

Fig. 2. Total number of lymphocyte subpopulations before, during, and after IFN-α2b and IL-2 therapy

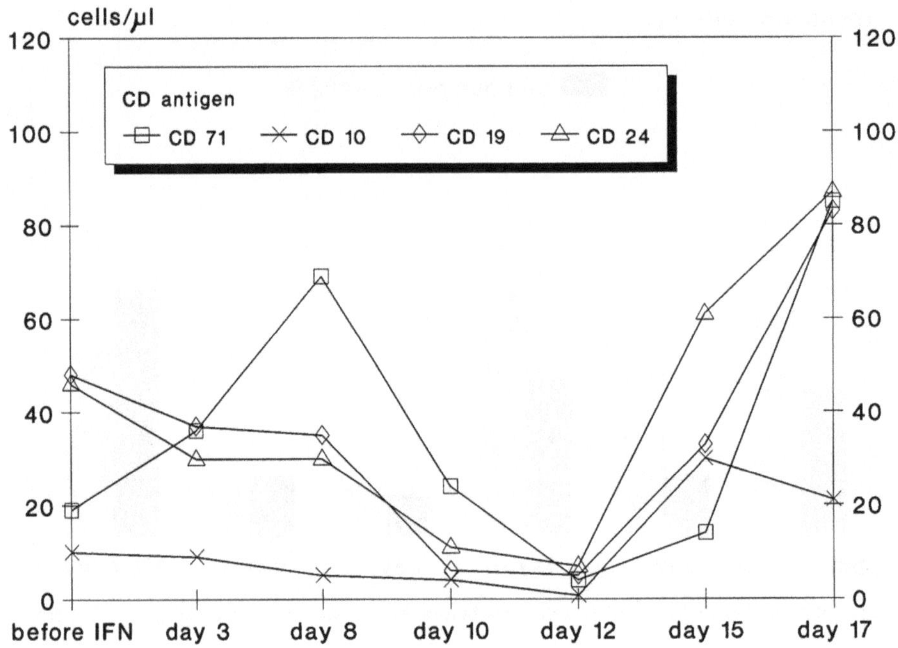

Fig. 3. Total number of lymphocyte subpopulations before, during, and after IFN-α2b and IL-2 therapy

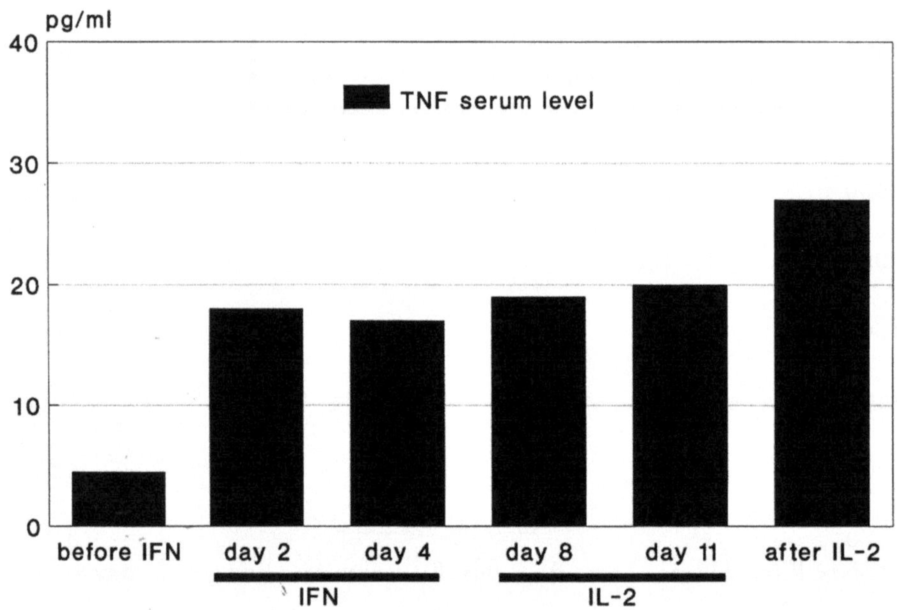

Fig. 4. TNF-α serum levels before, during, and after IFN-α2b and IL-2 therapy

the TNF-α serum level of all patients during the course of therapy is presented. All the TNF-α values determined were slightly above the lower detection limit of the test kit used. No significant changes before, during, or after treatment were observed.

Discussion

A significant increase in TNF-α serum levels after continuous IL-2 infusion could not be proved in our study. The administration of IL-2 as a bolus injection resulted in other studies in an increase of TNF-α serum levels [11, 16]. After bolus injection of IL-2 in patients with renal cell cancer tumor remission was observed by Rosenberg et al. in 31% [21]. However, this bolus injection led to severe side effects. Less side effects were observed by continuous infusion of IL-2 as reported by West et al. [23]. These authors also showed that continuous infusion of IL-2 as well as a bolus injection leads to tumor remission in patients with renal cell carcinoma. A significant increase in TNF-α serum levels, which could not be proved with continuous infusion of IL-2 in our study, may not, therefore, be essential for the success of IL-2 therapy. During treatment with interleukin-2, a rapid drop in the total lymphocyte count was observed. Upon termination of interleukin-2 infusion, there was a rapid increase in the lymphocyte count, to a level exceeding that recorded prior to the commencement of treatment. These kinetics were more marked among the T-cell subpopulations than among the B-cell subpopulations. The markers characteristic of lymphocyte activation (CD 71, HLA-DR) behaved similarly. In our study, however, it was not possible to establish a correlation with the proportion of various lymphocyte subpopulations during treatment and those patients revealing stable disease. It would not, therefore, be possible to make any premature statements concerning the success of the IFN-α2b and IL-2 therapy on the basis of a determination of lymphocyte subpopulations and, in particular, of the number of activated T-cells.

References

1. Ackermann R (1988) Immunologische Aspekte in der Behandlung des Nierenkarzinoms. In: Staehler G (ed) Das Nierenkarzinom. Springer, Berlin Heidelberg New York Tokyo, S 104–114
2. Atzpodien J (1990) Home therapy with recombinant interleukin-2 and interferon-α2b in advanced human malignancies. Lancet 335:1509–1512
3. Blay JY et al (1990) Correlation between clinical response to interleukin-2 therapy and sustained production of tumor necrosis factor. Cancer Res 50:2371–2374
4. Bono AV (1986) Steroid hormones and hormonal treatment in renal cell carcinoma. In: DeKernion JB, Pavone Macaluso M (eds) Tumors of the kidney, vol 13. Williams & Wilkins, Baltimore, pp 205–227
5. Budd TJ et al (1989) Phase I clinical trial of interleukin-2 and α-interferon: toxicity and immunologic effects. Cancer Res 49:6432–6436
6. DeKernion JB (1986) Treatment of advanced renal cell carcinoma. Traditional methods and innovative approaches. J Urol 130:2–7
7. Dinarelle CA, Mier JW (1986) Interleukins. Ann Rev Med 37:173–178
8. Domzig W et al (1983) Interleukin-2 dependence of human natural killer (NK) cell activity. J Immunol 130:1970–1973

9. Fowler JE (1986) Failure of immunotherapy for metastatic renal cell carcinoma. J Urol 135:22–25
10. Grimm EA et al (1982) Lymphokine-activated killer cell phenomenon. J Exp Med 155:1823–1841
11. Gumlo BT et al (1988) Circulating cytokines in patients with metastatic cancer treated with recombinant interleukin-2 and lymphokine activated killer cells. Cancer Res 48:5864–5867
12. Hefeneider SH et al (1983) In vivo interleukin-2 administration augments the generation of alloreactive cytolytic T lymphocytes and resident killer cells. J Immunol 130:222–227
13. Kriegmair M, Hofstetter A (1989) Interferontherapie in der Urologie. Urologe [A] 28:116–121
14. Krown SE (1987) Interferon treatment of renal cell carcinoma. Cancer 59 [Suppl]:647–651
15. Marumo K et al (1989) Immunologic study of human recombinant interleukin-2 (low-dose) in patients with advanced renal cell carcinoma. Urology 33:219–225
16. Mier JW et al (1988) Induction of circulating tumor necrosis factor (TNF-α) as the mechanism of the febrile response to IL-2 in our patients. J Clin Immunol 82:426–436
17. Miltenburg AMM et al (1988) Lymphokine-activated killer cells lyse human renal cancer cell lines and cultured normal kidney cells. Immunology 63:729–731
18. Neidhard JA et al (1984) Interferon-α therapy of renal cancer. Cancer Res 44:4140–4143
19. Otto U et al (1988) Die Behandlung des metastasierten Nierenkarzinoms mit rekombinantem α-2- oder γ-Interferon. Onkologie 11:185–194
20. Reem GH, Yeh NH (1984) Interleukin-2 regulates expression of its receptors and synthesis of γ interferon by human T lymphocytes. Science 225:429–430
21. Rosenberg SA et al (1989) Combination therapy with interleukin-2 and α-interferon for the treatment of patients with advanced cancer. J Clin Oncol 7:1863–1874
22. Urba WJ et al (1990) Immunomodulatory properties and toxicity of interleukin-2 in patients with cancer. Cancer Res 50:185–192
23. West WH et al (1987) Constant infusion of recombinant interleukin-2 in adoptive immunotherapy of advanced cancer. N Engl J Med 316:898–905

Effects of Buthionine Sulfoximine Mediated Glutathione Depletion in Chemoresistant Human Renal Cell Carcinomas

G. MICKISCH[1,2], H. BIER[3], R. TSCHADA[1], and P. ALKEN[1]

Abstract

Defined resistance factors play a substantial role in the characterization of chemoresistance. Glutathione metabolism is apparently involved in the expression of high chemoresistance in human renal cell carcinoma. In 35 renal cell carcinomas, primary monolayer cultures were generated, the glutathione content enzymatically determined, and depletion of glutathione instigated by buthionine sulfoximine, a specific inhibitor of glutathione biosynthesis, was studied. Furthermore, the degree of chemoresistance against doxorubicin and carboplatin was determined in an MTT microculture assay and the possibility of modulation of resistance by buthionine sulfoximine was examined.

The glutathione content amounted to 81 ± 26 nM/mg protein. A high degree of chemoresistance waa associated with increased levels, a low degree with reduced levels. With appropriate culture conditions, the glutathione content could be reduced to approximately 30% of the control value. Thus, a distinct potentiation of carboplatin cytotoxicity could be detected and doxorubicin resistance was still measurably subdued.

Introduction

The tripeptide glutathione (GSH) and its associated enzymes involved in the GSH-redox-cycle exert substantial cell protection against damage caused by metal ions, irradiation, oxidation, and cytotoxic compounds (Arrick and Nathan 1984). Early studies demonstrated that houseflies can become resistant to the insecticide DDT (dichlorodiphenyltrichloroethane) via GSH-dependent dehydrochlorination (Lipke and Kearns 1959). Recent publications indicate a possible role of the GSH metabolism in producing chemoresistance towards cytotoxic compounds like anthracyclines, alkylating agents, and platinum complexes (Russo et al. 1986a).

Human renal cell carcinomas (RCCs) display a characteristically high degree of chemoresistance. Several isoenzymes of glutathione S transferase (GGT), a key enzyme of GSH-related cellular activities, have been traced in human RCCs (Shea

[1] Urologische Klinik, Klinikum Mannheim der Universität Heidelberg, Theodor-Kutzer-Ufer, W-6800 Mannheim 1, FRG.
[2] Laboratory of Molecular Biology, National Cancer Institute, National Institutes of Health, Bethesda, MD 20892, USA.
[3] Hals-Nasen-Ohrenklinik, Klinikum Mannheim der Universität Heidelberg, Theodor-Kutzer-Ufer, W-6800 Mannheim 1, FRG.

et al. 1988; Harrison et al. 1989), and we have previously linked raised GSH metabolism to the in vitro degree of chemoresistance against doxorubicin (Mickisch et al. 1990b) and carboplatin (Mickisch et al. 1990d).

A modulation of the GSH content may change the response of tumor cells to chemo- or radiotherapy (Meister 1988). Augmentation of oxothiazolidine-4-carbonylate (Williamson et al. 1982) or by glutathione esters (Anderson et al. 1985) may induce increased cell protection; a reduction of diethylmaleate, vitamin K_3) selenocysteine, sodium selenite, acetominophene, deprivation of L-cysteine or buthionine sulfoximine (BSO) may lead to sensitization (reviewed in Stewart and Evans 1989). Substances which block GSH biosynthesis, in particular, were shown to yield potent and specific GSH depletion (Griffith and Meister 1979). BSO is mainly used at present, because it does not inhibit GSH synthetase as earlier compounds did due to the introduction of a large, terminal S-alkyl group (Meister 1988). BSO acts on an earlier stage of the GSH formation by interfering with the γ-glutamyl cysteine synthetase (Fig. 1). This chemical modification resulted in markedly reduced neurotoxicity.

The present study examines whether BSO reduces the GSH content of primary human RCCs and also focuses on the question whether this effect may lead to modulation of chemoresistance against doxorubicin (ADM) and carboplatin (CP).

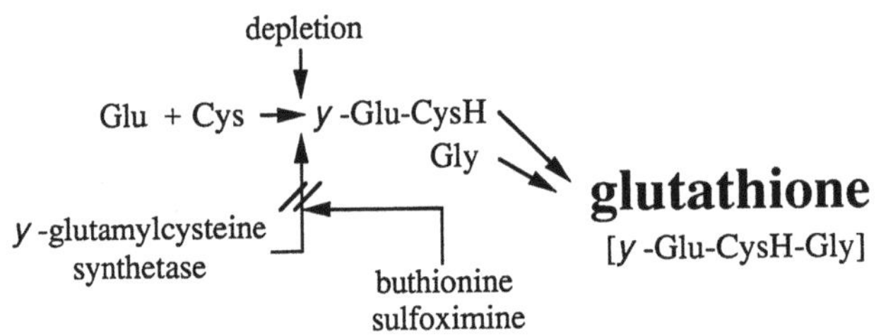

Fig. 1. Interaction of buthionine sulfoximine with GSH biosynthesis. (Modified after Griffith and Meister 1979)

Materials and Methods

Cell Ccultures

Representative samples from separate parts of 35 human RCCs were surgically obtained and processed under sterile conditions within 1 h after operation. The tumor segments were carefully freed from fat, connective tissue, and necrotic areas. Hematoxylin-eosin-stained smears were used as a matter of routine in order to rule out major admixture of nontumorous material. Single-cell suspensions were mechanically prepared, filtered through multilayer textile gauze (pore size 50–100 μm; SSGF) and purified by Ficoll centrifugation (density 1.07, 400×g, 10 min, 4 °C; Seromed) after addition of 5 mg% DNase (Boehringer Mannheim). Cell viability and content of tumor cells were examined by the trypan dye exclusion test (final concentration 0.16%; Flow) and by HE-stained smears, respectively. Using exclusively specimens from well-defined and small RCCs (max. diameter 5 cm), the primary cell suspensions contained approx. 80% viable cells; more than 90% were classified cytologically as tumor cells. Cell suspensions were plated in monolayer flasks (Flow) containing culture medium (RPM 1640-, supplemented with 20% synthetic NU serum; Flow) at a density of 5×10^6 cells per flask.

Test Conditions

Cell cultures were maintained until an exponential growth phase was reached (cell counts). Cells were exposed to different concentrations of BSO (50–400 μ*M*; Sigma) for varying periods of time. Initial experiments showed that the use of primary cell cultures without attaining a growth phase yielded substantially inferior results. All experiments were run in triplicate; subsequently, the GSH content was analyzed.

Determination of the Glutathione Content

Tumor specimens were first mechanically disintegrated (Potter Ellwejn) and then homogenized by ultrasound (Ultraturrax). The protein content was determined from aliquots of the solution using Folin-phenol reagent. The extinction was measured at 578 nm (Spectronic 1001) with bovine serum albumin as a protein standard. The homogeneous tissue solution was centrifuged at $5000 \times g$ for 20 min and the supernatant retained. After precipitation of the proteins by perchloric acid (Merck) and adjusting to pH 7.4 (EDTA buffer), the total GSH content was examined enzymatically using Tietze's method (Tietze 1969). Measurements included the time-dependent formation of 2-nitro-5-thiobenzoic acid read at 420 nm, and the GSH content was calculated from a standard curve (Boehringer Mannheim). Experiments were run in triplicate; hemolyzed vials were rejected. Values were expressed as n*M*/mg protein or as a percentage of control levels to establish the effect of BSO-induced depletion.

MTT Microculture Assay

To determine the degree of chemoresistance, 2×10^4 tumor cells per well were distributed by multichannel pipettes into 96-well, flat-bottomed microculture plates (Flow), and the MTT test was carried out as reported earlier (Mickisch et al. 1990a). Exposure time to ADM and CP was 16 h; subsequently, MTT solution (Sigma) was added at 20 μl/100 μl cell suspension, and incubation continued for further 4 h. MTT formazan crystals were dissolved in DMSO (Merck) and extinction was measured at 540 nm in a microculture plate reader (Titertek Multiskan MKII). Four replicate wells determined each point. The values were expressed as percentages of the untreated trial groups.

To investigate whether BSO induces a modulation of chemoresistance, we assessed in parallel cell cultures which were pretreated with BSO as described and were then exposed to a constant concentration of ADM (3 μg/ml) or CP (7.5 μg/ml) followed by the MTT test. The results were expressed as percentages of levels in control groups which contained the same amount of chemotherapeutic agent but were not preincubated with BSO.

All reagents were of p. a. grade and were, if not otherwise stated, purchased from Boehringer Mannheim.

Methods of statistical analysis included Student's *t* test, applying the Bonferroni-Holm correction for curves (Holm 1979).

Results

BSO exhibited a time- and concentration-dependent reduction of the GSH content in cultivated human RCCs (Fig. 2).

Using the MTT staining procedure, human RCCs were separated into highly and less resistant carcinomas with reference to the number of surviving tumor cells in the presence of a variety of anticancer agents (Fig. 3). Despite apparent

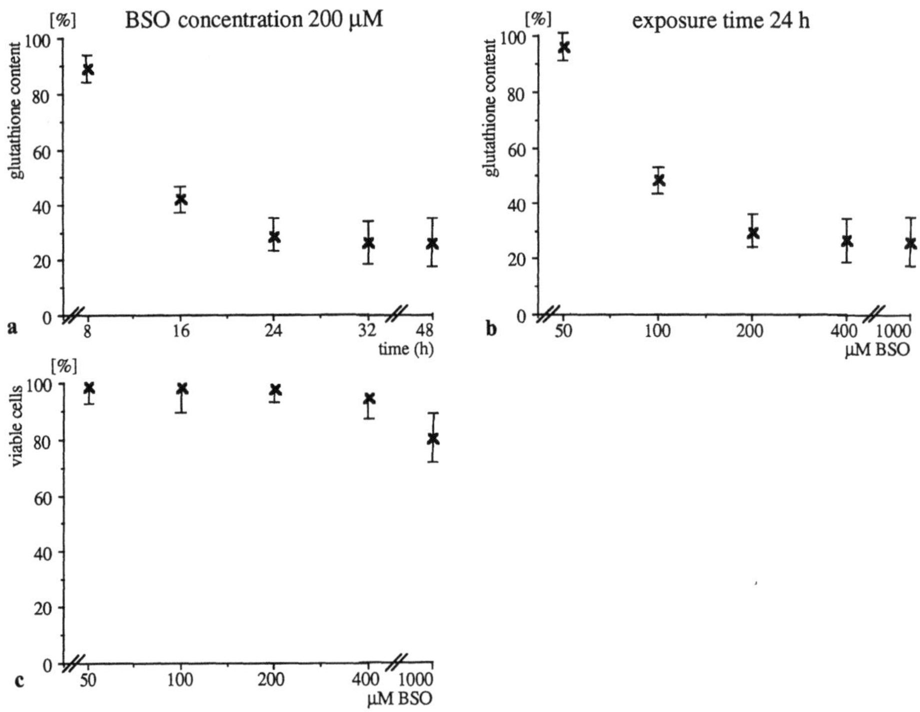

Fig. 2 a – c. Effects of buthionine sulfoximine on cultured human renal cell carcinomas. **a** Time dependence, **b** concentration-related activity, **c** cytotoxicity (BSO alone)

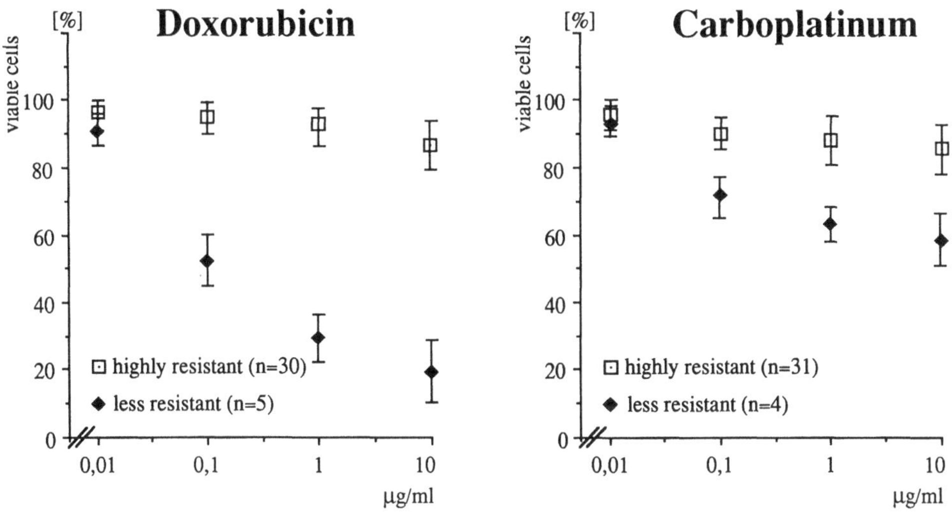

Fig. 3. Determination of the degree of chemoresistance in an MTT microculture assay

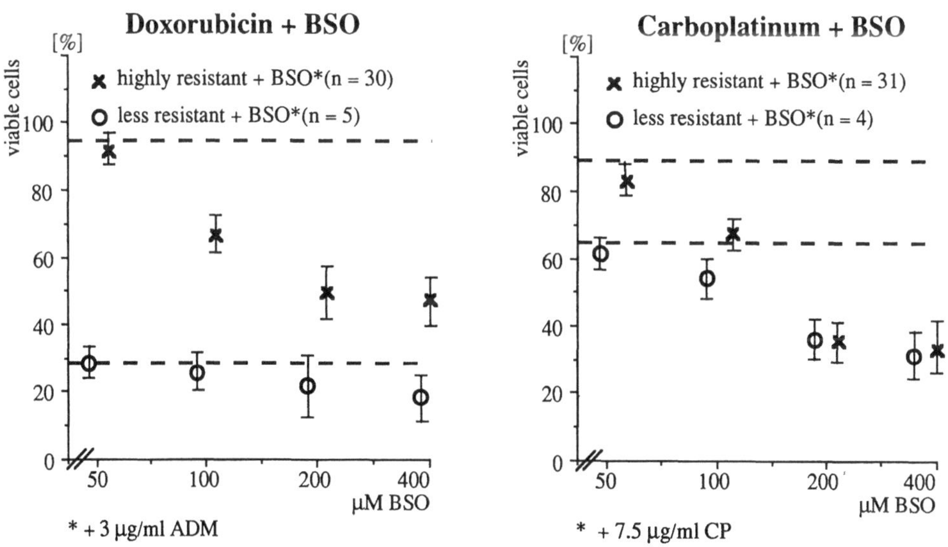

Fig. 4. Buthionine sulfoximine-induced reversal of chemoresistance. Values expressed as percentage of control groups containing only 3 mg/µl ADM or 7.5 mg/µl CP. *Upper dotted lines* indicate the effect of the chemotherapeutic agent alone on highly resistant tumors, *lower dotted lines* the effect on less resistant tumors. Chemoresistance data derived from Fig. 3

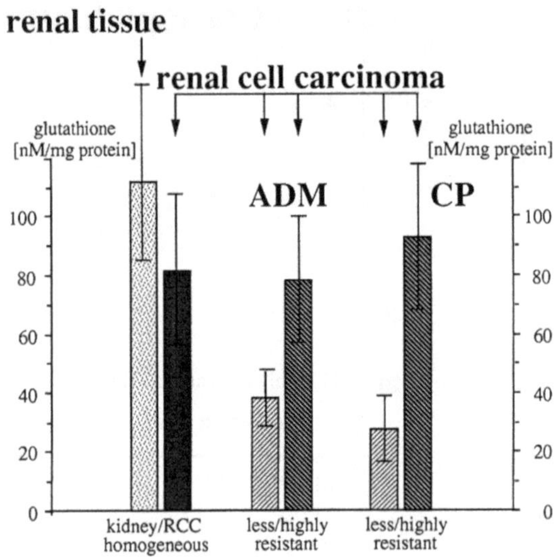

Fig. 5. Distribution of GSH content in accordance with histology and degree of chemoresistance. Chemoresistance data derived from Fig. 3

differences in the quantity of live cells, the level of significance was not reached in the case of CP due to the low number of chemoresponders.

A wide range of BSO concentrations failed to cause increased cell killing of human RCCs in cell culture exposed for 24 h (Fig. 2). However, pretreatment with BSO for 24 h and subsequent incubation with a constant amount of chemotherapeutic agent for 16 h resulted in a BSO-dependent modulation of cell viability. Highly ADM-resistant tumors responded to BSO concentrations of 100 μM and greater with a significant reduction in the number of surviving cells ($p<0.05$; Fig. 4); less ADM-resistant tumors did not. Both highly and less CPP-resistant tumors were influenced by pretreatment with BSO (Fig. 4). In highly resistant carcinomas this effect became significant for 100 μM/24 h or greater ($p<0.02$).

The GSH content of normal renal tissue distantly excised from tumor-bearing kidneys amounted to 112 ± 29 nM/mg protein, whereas RCCs had 81 ± 26 nM/mg protein. On distributing the individual values obtained in accordance with the degree of chemoresistance as detailed in Fig. 3, high ADM or CP resistance revealed concentrations of 80 ± 21 or 92 ± 34 nM/mg protein respectively; low resistance was associated with 41 ± 10 or 29 ± 11 nM/mg protein respectively (Fig. 5).

Discussion

Obviously, a concentration of 200 μM BSO for 24 h gives optimal results in human RCCs (Fig. 2). Similar findings were reported for established cell lines derived from ovarian (Hamilton et al. 1985), colon (Jordan et al. 1987), or breast carcinoma (Kramer et al. 1988).

BSO incubation of primary human RCCs leads to a reduction of the GSH content to approx. 30% of the value obtained in untreated controls (Fig. 2), whereas in established cell lines a decrease of more than 90% could be demonstrated (Kramer et al. 1988). In vivo administration of BSO reduces the GSH content of mouse kidneys to about 20% (Griffith and Meister 1979). Our data supports two possible explanations. Since BSO acts as an inhibitor of GSH synthesis (Meister 1988), any BSO-related effects need cell growth. Freshly prepared primary cell suspensions contain cells in different phases of these cell cycle. Our initial experiments have shown that the cultures yield not only a larger variation of values, but also a reduction of the GSH content of less than 50%. In contrast, plating these cultures in monolayer flasks and attaining an exponential growth phase (see Materials and Methods) section resulted in an substantial improvement (Fig. 2). Furthermore, primary cell cultures consist of heterogeneous cell populations, unlike cloned cell lines. In particular, in RCCs, significant differences in the GSH content of different cell clones from the same tumor could be ascertained in flow cytometric analysis (Shrieve et al. 1988).

A relative response to ADM could be detected in only a few cases ($n = 5$), while for CP no efficacy was exhibited as regards the different degrees of in vitro chemoresistance (Fig. 3). This may correspond to the characteristically high degree of chemoresistance evaluated in clinical trials (Torti 1983).

BSO alone in a wide concentration range has no cytotoxic effects in tumor cell lines. This finding was confirmed in human RCCs (Fig. 2). In vivo administration of BSO exclusively exerts no cytotoxic side effects in mice (Griffith and Meister 1979; Page et al. 1987), although one study reported tissue damage in liver and kidneys of beagle dogs receiving extremely high concentrations (Smith et al. 1987).

More than 60 studies published so far have compiled evidence that BSO significantly reduces the GSH content of cell lines of tumors from human and other sources (Stewart and Evans 1989). In addition, sensitization against radiation of hypoxic cells (Shrieve and Harris 1986) and against chemotherapy (Russo et al. 1986b) has been described. The majority of these reports investigated alkylating agents, anthracyclines, and platinum complexes since their antineoplastic effects depend partially on oxidative DNA damage and may therefore be modulated by the GSH-triggered intracellular reduction potential (Arrick and Nathan 1984). There were variations in the extent of how effectively resistance was reversed from study to study and between the chemotherapeutic agents employed. This is generally believed to result from a tumor-dependent GSH metabolism (Stewart and Evans 1989). In fact, even within one study group varying results were reported when different tumors were examined (Andrews et al. 1986). In multiple myeloma, however, which displays a high GSH content, BSO-mediated GSH depletion did not potentiateicity (Bellamy et al. 1989).

On assessing tumors of urological interest, BSO-induced sensitization of murine bladder carcinoma to cyclophosphamide metabolites has been demonstrated (Tomashewsky et al. 1985). In vivo studies revealed that survival times of tumor-bearing mice were significantly enhanced by combining BSO with chemotherapy and that toxicity was not a limitation (Ozols et al. 1987). In general, BSO did not increase toxicity in normal tissues such as bone marrow (Russo et al. 1986a; Ono and Shrieve 1987), which is assumed to be due to an abundant GSH content in the latter.

The GSH content of primary human RCCs in tissue culture can be markedly reduced by BSO (Fig. 2); this effect leads to circumvention of chemoresistance (Fig. 4). CP resistance was most profoundly reversed, but high ADM resistance was still measurably subdued (Fig. 4).

When we related GSH content to the in vitro degree of chemoresistance (Fig. 5), these results were confirmed. Hence, it appears that GSH metabolism plays an important role in the expression of chemoresistance in human RCCs, thus adding to the evidence for another biochemical pathway instigating multidrug resistance apart from the classical P-170 glycoprotein-mediated multidrug resistance of human RCCs (Mickisch et al. 1990c).

References

Anderson ME, Powrie F, Purie RN, Meister A (1985) Glutathione monoethyl ester: preparation, uptake by tissues, and conversion to glutathione. Arch Biochem Biophys 239:538–548

Andrews PA, Murphy MP, Howell SB (1986) Differential sensitization of human ovarian carcinoma and mouse L1210 cells to cisplatin and melphalan by glutathione depletion. Mol Pharmacol 30:643–650

Arrick BA, Nathan CF (1984) Glutathione metabolism as a determinant of therapeutic efficacy. Cancer Res 44:4224–4232

Bellamy WT, Dalton WS, Meltzer P, Dorr RT (1989) Role of glutathione and its associated enzymes in multidrug-resistant human myeloma cells. Biochem Pharmacol 38:787–793

Griffith OW, Meister A (1979) Potent and specific inhibition of glutathione synthesis by buthionine sulfoximine (S-*n*-butyl homocysteine sulfoximine). J Biol Chem 254:7558–7560

Hamilton TC, Winker MA, Louie KG, Batist G, Behrens BC, Tsuruo T, Grotzinger KR, McKoy WK, Young RC, Ozols RF (1985) Augmentation of adriamycin, melphalan, and cisplatin cytotoxicity in drug-resistant and sensitive human ovarian carcinoma cell lines by sulfoximine mediated glutathione depletion. Biochem Pharmacol 34:2583–2586

Harrison DJ, Kharbanda R, Bishop D, McLelland LI, Hayes JD (1989) Glutathione-S-transferase isoenzymes in human renal carcinoma demonstrated by immuno-histochemistry. Carcinogenesis 10:1257–1260

Holm S (1979) A simple sequentially rejective multiple test procedure. Scand J Statist 6:65–70

Hromas RA, Andrews PA, Murphy MP, Burns CP (1987) Glutathione depletion reverses cisplatin resistance in murine L1210 leukemia cells. Cancer Let 13:9–13

Jordan J, d'Arcy Doherty M, Cohen GM (1987) Effects of glutathione depletion on the cytotoxicity of agents toward a human colonic tumour cell line. Br J Cancer 55:627–631

Kramer RA, Zakher J, Kim G (1988) Role of the glutathione cycle in acquired and de novo multidrug resistance. Science 241:694–696

Lipke H, Kearns CW (1959) DDT dehydrochlorinase. 1. Isolation, chemical properties, and spectrophotometric assay. J Biol Chem 234:2123–2128

Meister A (1988) Glutathione metabolism and its selective modification. J Biol Chem 263:17205–17208

Mickisch G, Fayta S, Keilhauer G, Schlick E, Tschada R, Alken P (1990a) Chemosensitivity testing of primary human renal cell carcinoma by a tetrazolium-based microculture assay (MTT). Urol Res 18:131–136

Mickisch G, Bier H, Bergler W, Bak M, Tschada R, Alken P (1990b) P-170 glycoprotein, glutathione and associated enzymes in relation to chemoresistance of primary renal cell carcinomas. Urol Intern 45:170–176

Mickisch GH, Koessig J, Keilhauer G, Schlick E, Tschada RK, Alken PM (1990c) Effects of calcium antagonists in multidrug resistant primary human renal cell carcinomas. Cancer Res 50:3670–3674

Mickisch GH, Roehrig K, Koessig J, Forster S, Tschada RK, Alken PM (1990d) Mechanism and modulation of multidrug resistance in primary human renal cell carcinoma. J Urol 144:755–759

Ono K, Shrieve DC (1987) Effect of glutathione depletion by L-buthionine sulf-oximine on the cytotoxicity of cyclophosphamide in single and fractionated doses to EMT6/SF mouse tumors and bone marrow. J Natl Canc Inst 79:811–815

Ozols RF, Louie KG, Plowman J, Behrens BC, Fine RL, Dykes D, Hamilton TC (1987) Enhanced melphalan cytotoxicity in human ovarian cancer in vitro and in tumor-bearing nude mice by buthionine sulfoximine depletion of glutathione. Biochem Pharmacol 36:147–153

Page JG, Carlton BD, Smith AC, Kastello MD, Grieshaber CK (1987) Preclinical toxicology and pharmacokinetic studies of buthionine sulfoximine (BSO, NSC-326231) in CD2F1 mice. Proc AACR 28:440

Russo A, Tochner Z, Phillips T, Carmichael J, DeGraff W, Friedman N, Fisher J, Mitchell JB (1986a) In vivo modulation of glutathione by buthionine sulfoximine: effect on marrow response to melphalan. Int J Radiat Oncol Biol Phys 12:1187–1189

Russo A, Carmichael J, Friedman N, DeGraff W, Tochner Z, Glatstein E, Mitchell JB (1986b) The roles of intracellular glutathione in antineoplastic chemotherapy. Int J Radiat Oncol Biol Phys 12:1347–1354

Shea TC, Kelly SL, Henner WD (1987) Identification of an anionic form of glutathione transferase present in many human tumors and human tumor cell lines. Cancer Res 48:527–533

Shrieve DC, Harris JW (1986) Effects of glutathione depletion by buthionine sulfoximine on the sensitivity of EMTe/SF cells to chemotherapy agents or X radiation. Int J Radiat Oncol Biol Phys 12:1171–1174

Shrieve DC, Bump EA, Rice GC (1988) Heterogenity of cellular glutathione from a murine fibrosarcoma or a human renal cell carcinoma detected by flow cytometric analysis. J Biol Chem 263:14107–14114

Smith AC, Page JG, Carlton BD, Kastello MD, Grieshaber CK (1987) Preclinical toxicology and pharmacokinetic studies of buthionine sulfoximine (BSO, NSC-326231) in beagle dogs. Proc AACR 28:440

Stewart DJ, Evans WK (1989) Non-chemotherapeutic agents that potentiate chemotherapy efficacy. Cancer Treat Rev 16:1–40

Tietze F (1969) Enzymic method for quantitative determination of nanogram amounts of total and oxidized glutathione: applications to mammalian blood and other tissues. Anal Biochem 27:502–522

Tomashewsky P, Astor M, White R (1985) Relationship between thiol depletion and chemosensitization in a transplantable murine bladder tumor. J Natl Cancer Inst 74:1233–1238

Torti FM (1983) Treatment of metastatic renal cell carcinoma. In: Torti FM (ed) Urologic cancer: chemotherapeutic principles and management. Springer, Berlin Heidelberg New York Tokyo, pp 85, 123–143

Williamson JM, Bottcher B, Meister A (1982) Intracellular cysteine delivery system that protects against toxicity by glutathione synthesis. Proc Natl Acad Sci USA 79:6246–6249

Renin-Producing Renal Cell Carcinoma – Clinical and Experimental Investigation of a Special Form of Renal Hypertension

J. STEFFENS[1], R. BOCK[2], H. U. BRAEDEL[1], E. ISENBERG[1], C. P. BÜHRLE[3], and M. ZIEGLER[1]

Hypertension as a consequence of unilateral or bilateral renovascular or renoparenchymal disease occurs in 5%–7% of the total hypertensive population (Berglund et al. 1976). Renal hypertension is thus the most common cause of secondary hypertension. A rare cause of renal hypertension is a renal tumour with autonomous renin production. This form of renal hypertension is thus the consequence of "primary reninism" (Conn et al. 1972). Three different types of renin-producing tumours are known: tumours of the juxtaglomerular cells (Robertson et al. 1967), nephroblastomas (Ganguly et al. 1973) and renal cell carcinomas (Hollifield et al. 1977).

We studied 129 of our own patients with renal cell carcinoma, seeking a possible causal pathogenetic relationship between tumour and hypertension. For this purpose the plasma renin activity (PRA) was determined in the peripheral venous blood and selectively in renal vein blood and the renin content measured in homogenates of tumour tissue and of tumour-free ipsilateral renal cortex. To detect secondary hyperaldosteronism, aldosterone was determined in peripheral venous blood. Immunohistochemical methods were used to identify the source of renin production within the tumour. An attempt was also made to demonstrate autonomous renin production in cell culture.

Material and Methods

In a group of 129 consecutive patients presenting with renal cell carcinoma there were 41 (31.8%) with hypertension. In all 129 patients the *plasma renin activity* (PRA) was determined in peripheral venous blood and selectively in renal venous blood using a commercial renin RIA (Baxter Travenol Diagnostics, Cambridge, MA, USA). In 57 patients a conventional aldosterone RIA (Abbott Diagnostics, Wiesbaden, FRG) was used to measure the *aldosterone* concentration in the peripheral venous blood in addition to determination of the PRA.

For calculation of the *tissue renin content* 1 g tumour tissue and 1 g adjacent tumour-free renal cortex were excised from the removed tumour kidney, placed in a test tube, treated with phosphate buffer (pH 7.4) and homogenised. The homogenates were centrifuged for 10 min at 4000 rpm. The renin contents of the two tis-

[1] Urologische Klinik und Poliklinik; [2] Anatomisches Institut der Universität des Saarlandes, W-6650 Homburg/Saar, FRG.
[3] Physiologisches Institut der Universität, Im Neuenheimer Feld 326, W-6900 Heidelberg 1, FRG.

sue samples were determined in the supernatant using a commercial renin RIA (Pasteur, Paris, France).

The *protein content* in the homogenates of tumour and renal cortex were determined by the biuret method and for each tissue specimen the renin content was expressed as a fraction of the protein content (μg renin/g protein).

For the *immunohistochemical* examination 1-g portions of tumour tissue and adjacent cortex tissue were fixed in Bouin's fluid and processed by the peroxidase-antiperoxidase (PAP) method. We used a polyclonal renin antibody produced in our own laboratory which binds active and inactive renin. The dilution of the primary antiserum was 1 : 2000. Renal cortex was incubated as positive control. Sections of renin-positive tumour tissue were stained with haematoxylin to identify tumour epithelial cells and counterstained with Schiff's reagent to evaluate the capillaries.

Determination of renin in *cell culture*: in each of 7 cases, tumour tissue obtained under sterile conditions was cut into pieces measuring 2×2 mm, placed in a culture box at 37 °C in an atmosphere of 5% CO_2 and 95% air and left to grow for 6 months. Each culture vessel contained 10 ml culture medium which was changed every other day. Dulbecco's modified Eagle's medium (DMEM) (Gibco Biocult, Karlsruhe, FRG) was the basic culture medium used. We added 1 ml/100 ml penicillin-streptomycin (10000 IU/ml), 1 ml/100 ml non-essential amino acids and 10% fetal calf serum to the commercially available synthetic medium. The renin activity in the culture medium was determined using the renin RIA (see above). If there was a measurable renin concentration the cultured cells were examined immunohistochemically using the renin antibody prepared in our own laboratory (see above).

Results

Clinical Findings

In 5 out of 41 hypertensive patients with renal cell carcinoma tumour nephrectomy led to normotension. In a sixth patient the blood pressure fell from 190/90 mmHg to 165/90 mmHg. These six patients (14.6%) no longer required antihypertensive treatment. In the remaining 35 patients the blood pressures were still raised after tumour nephrectomy and further antihypertensive medication was necessary.

PRA, Plasma Aldosterone and Tissue Renin

Peripheral PRA was within the normal range in all tumour patients. In 6/41 (14.6%) patients' selective determination of PRA in renal vein blood showed a difference between the two kidneys. The tumour kidney to contralateral kidney ratio for PRA in these patients was between 4 and 7 while in the remaining 123 cases the ratio was less than 1.5 (Fig. 1). A ratio of more than 1.5 was only found in the 6 patients whose blood pressure decreased or returned to normal after nephrectomy.

Two of the 57 patients in whom the peripheral aldosterone concentrations were measured had renal vein renin ratios above 1.5. Only these two patients were found to have secondary hyperaldosteronism with hypernatraemia and hypokalaemia.

Significantly higher renin concentrations in the renal tumour tissue than in tissue from the adjacent tumour-free cortex of the ipsilateral kidney were only found in the six patients with raised PRA in the blood from the renal vein of the tumour kidney (Fig. 2). The renin content/g protein in the tumour homogenate was on av-

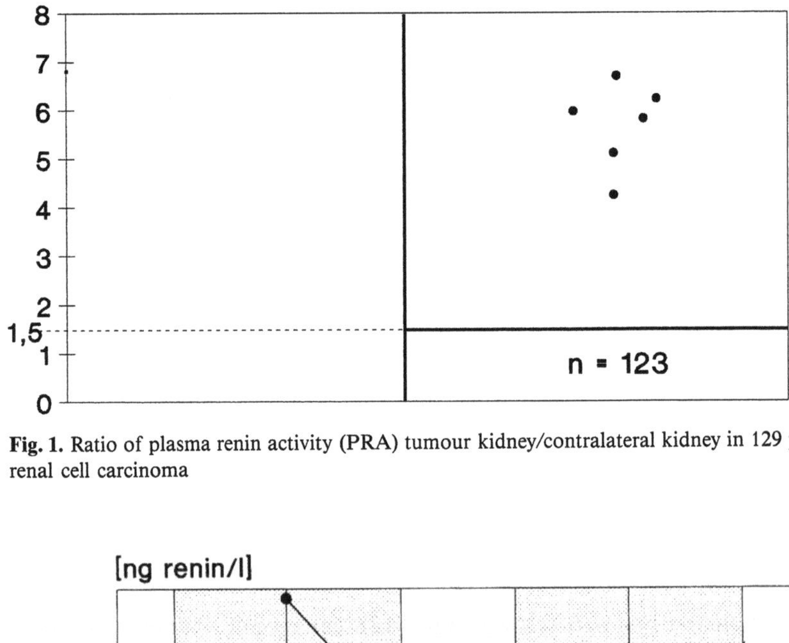

Fig. 1. Ratio of plasma renin activity (PRA) tumour kidney/contralateral kidney in 129 patients with renal cell carcinoma

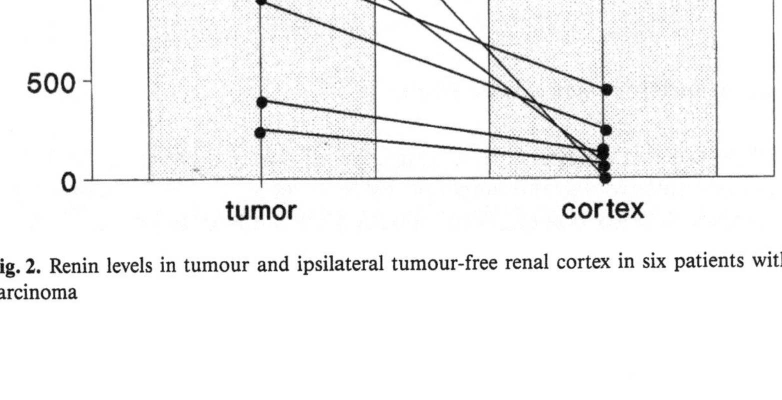

Fig. 2. Renin levels in tumour and ipsilateral tumour-free renal cortex in six patients with renal cell carcinoma

erage 1.7 µg renin/g protein, while that in the renal cortex homogenate averaged 0.1 µg renin/g protein ($p < 0.05$).

Angiographic Findings

The tumour kidneys of the six hypertensive patients with elevated levels of renin activity in the plasma of the ipsilateral renal vein and raised renin concentrations in the tumour tissue presented no characteristic angiographic findings. The tumour diameters varied between 3 and 10 cm. Four tumours were located centrally and two peripherally. All the tumours were hypervascular, but there was no evidence of compression of renal arteries or of arteriovenous fistula.

Morphological Findings

In the immunohistochemical assays renin was only demonstrated in the tumours of the six patients who also had elevated renin levels in the corresponding renal vein plasma and tumour tissue homogenates. The antigen was found in the walls of the tumour capillaries in cells which were irregularly distributed and sometimes arranged in clusters (Fig. 3a). The cells often possessed cytoplasmic processes and were thus distinguishable from the epithelioid cells of the juxtaglomerular apparatus which were labelled in the adjacent tumour-free tissue of the renal cortex.

Demonstration of Renin in Cell Culture

In three patients with hypertension and elevated renin concentrations in plasma and tissue we were able to demonstrate autonomous renin production of the tumour tissue grown in culture. The explants, which were composed of variously compact tissue pieces, survived in culture for 6 months. During this period, renin activity was demonstrated continuously in the incubation medium in three successive cell generations of the same tumour tissue. Immunohistochemical examination showed renin-positive cells which corresponded morphologically to the renin-positive endothelium cells demonstrated immunohistochemically in tumour tissue (Fig. 3b).

Discussion

A rare cause of renal hypertension is a renin-producing renal tumour. The autonomous renin production by such tumours was described by Conn et al. (1972) as primary reninism. Although most reports of renin-producing tumours only describe individual cases (Conn et al. 1972; Ganguly et al. 1973; Hollifield et al. 1977; Robertson et al. 1967), their clinical and pathogenetic significance by far exceeds their frequency.

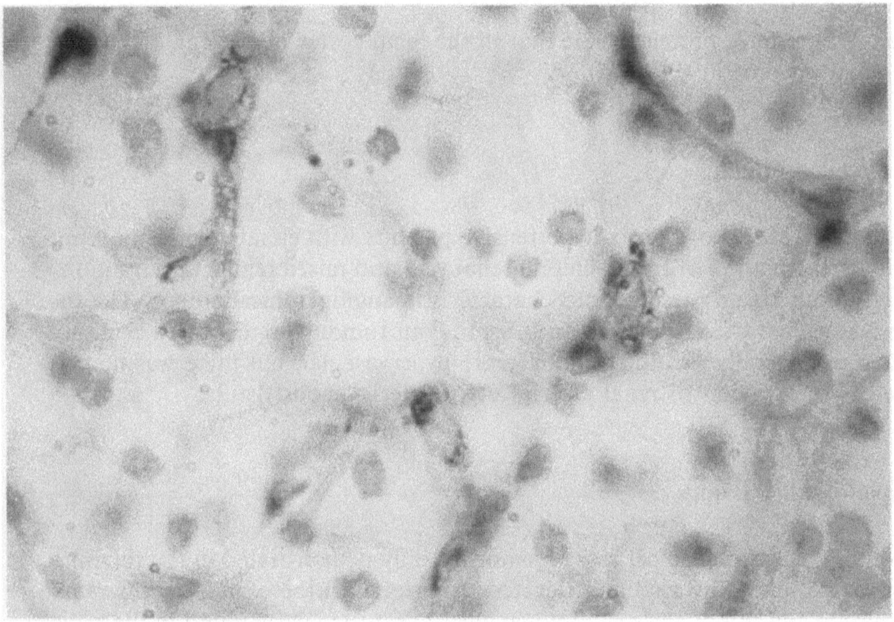

a

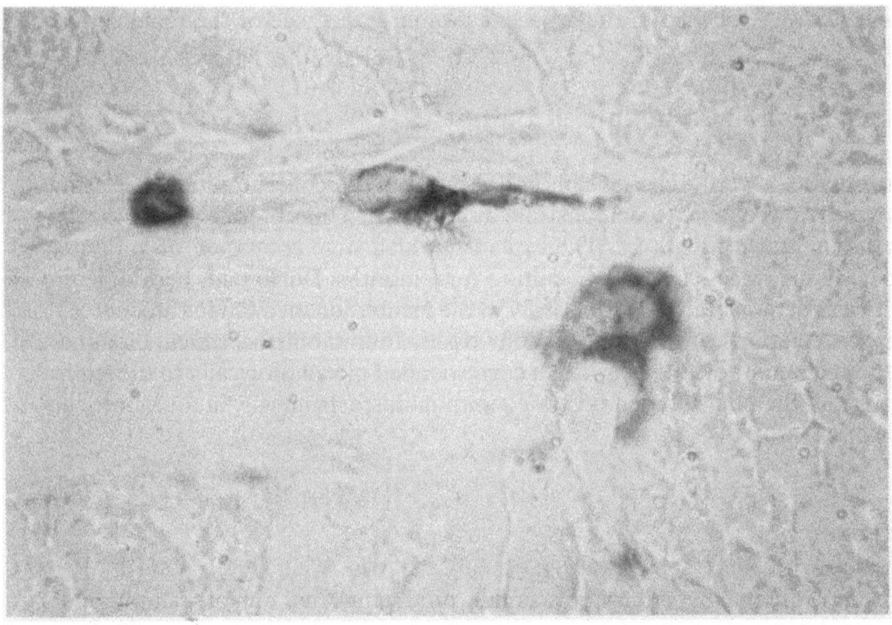

b

Fig. 3a. Renin-positive endothelial cells arranged in clusters. Tumour cells counterstained with haematoxylin. Original magnification ×100. **b** Immunohistochemical demonstration of renin-positive endothelial cells in a renal cell carcinoma grown in cell culture. Original magnification ×100

The fact that in six patients the blood pressure returned to normal after tumour nephrectomy suggested that there was a relationship between tumour and hypertension. The high ratio found on selective determination of renin in the renal veins was indicative of renin-induced hypertension. While in renal hypertension of other origin a ratio of more than 1.5 is a sign of renal hypertension (Ziegler et al. 1983), in the six tumour patients the ratio was between 4 and 7.

Since the peripheral PRA was within the normal range in all tumour patients, measurement of the active renin in the peripheral blood is not suitable either as a tumour marker in renal cell carcinoma or for elucidation of renal hypertension.

Secondary hyperaldosteronism as an indirect indication of primary reninism was found in only two patients, who also had elevated renal vein renin ratios. It follows from this that activation of the renin-angiotensin-aldosterone system must play a central role in the pathogenesis of tumour-related renal hypertension.

The introduction of immunohistochemical techniques has made it possible to demonstrate renin morphologically in the cells using special antibodies (Taugner et al. 1979). By using Schiff's reagent for examination of the capillaries we were able to assess the location of the renin-positive cells in our own tumour material. The morphology and location suggest that they are endothelial cells. It is known that these cells have the capacity for renin production. Lilly et al. (1985) and Kifor and Dzau (1987) were able to demonstrate renin expression by aortic endothelial cells in cell culture. In our own population the renin-positive endothelial cells were found only in the six renal cell carcinomas with hypertension which were associated with elevated renin levels in plasma and tissue. None of the other tumours examined displayed any renin-positive cells. We do not yet know the role played by the renin-angiotensin system in renal tumours. The close relationship between renin-positive endothelial cells and blood vessels in the renal cell carcinoma suggests that angiotensin II might represent a growth factor for blood vessels which increases the vascularisation of the tumour.

The results of our investigations show that 14.6% of renal cell carcinomas can, as paraneoplastic syndrome, cause hypertension through increased secretion of active renin produced in the endothelial cells. This increased renin secretion can only be detected by selective collection of blood from the renal veins and not by determination of the PRA in peripheral blood. Determination of renin in tumour homogenate and extracts from ipsilateral tumour-free renal cortex and cell culture investigations show that increased levels of renin found in the tumour are responsible for the renal hypertension.

The differential diagnostic considerations for raised blood pressure should therefore include a renal tumour as cause of the hypertension, and an ultrasonographic examination of the kidneys should be performed at every check-up examination. While the most common type of tumour in elderly patients is renal cell carcinoma and in children Wilms' tumour, in young patients the possibility of a small benign tumour of the juxtaglomerular apparatus (Robertson et al. 1967) must also be considered. Such tumours can be located by selective determination of PRA and selective angiography. In the case of small tumours the hypertension can be treated causally by organ-sparing tumour resection. In the case of larger neoplasms tumour nephrectomy is at the same time treatment of the hypertension.

References

Berglund G, Andersson O, Wilhelmsen L (1976) Prevalence of primary and secondary hypertension: studies in a random population sample. Br Med J 2:554–559

Conn JW, Cohen EL, Lucas CP, McDonald WJ, Mayor GH, Blough WM, Eveland WC, Bookstein JJ, Lapides J (1972) Primary reninism, hypertension, hyperreninemia and secondary hyperaldosteronism due to renin-producing juxtaglomerular cell tumors. Arch Int Med 130:682–696

Ganguly A, Gribble J, Tune B, Kemson RL, Luetscher JA (1973) Renin-secreting Wilms tumour with severe hypertension. Ann Intern Med 79:835–837

Hollifield JW, Page DL, Smith C, Michelakis AM, Staab E, Rhamy R (1977) Renin-secreting clear cell carcinoma of the kidney. Arch Int Med 135:859–864

Kifor J, Dzau VJ (1987) Endothelial renin-angiotensin pathway: evidence for intracellular synthesis and secretion of angiotensins. Circ Res 60:422–428

Lilly LS, Pratt RE, Alexander RW, Larson DM, Ellison KE, Gimbrone MA Jr, Dzau VJ (1985) Renin expression by vascular endothelial cells in culture. Circ Res 57:312–318

Robertson PW, Klidjian A, Harding LK, Walters G, Lee MR, Robb-Smith AHT (1967) Hypertension due to a renin-secreting renal tumour. Am J Med 43:963–976

Taugner Ch, Poulsen K, Hackenthal E, Taugner R (1979) Immunohistochemical localization of renin in mouse kidney. Histochemistry 62:19–27

Ziegler M, Mast GJ, Braedel HU (1983) Gefäßerkrankungen der Niere. In: Hohenfellner R, Zingg EJ (eds) Urologie in Klinik und Praxis. Thieme, Stuttgart, pp 1294–1310

II. Andrology and Testicular Cancer

Experimental Approach for Assessment of Tumor Biology in Clinical Stage I Nonseminomatous Germ Cell Tumors (NSGCT)

E. P. ALLHOFF[1], S. LIEDKE[1], C. WITTEKIND[2], C. STIEF[1], H.-J. SCHMOLL[3], W. DE RIESE[1], and B. SCHNEIDER[4]

Introduction

Until the late 1970s, the standard therapy for stage 1 nonseminomatous germ cell tumors (NSGCT) consisted of orchiectomy and subsequent retroperitoneal lymphadenectomy, the latter implying staging as well as having a therapeutic function. However, the disadvantage of retroperitoneal lymphadenectomy is the morbidity not only of the operative procedure but also the loss of ejaculation associated with the removal of the sympathetic fibers. For this reason, in 1981 Peckham et al. (1982) introduced the paradigm of the "wait and see" strategy, which schedules patients after orchiectomy for close follow-up only. The encouraging relapse rate of 17% published at that time led to the adoption of the protocol at the Department of Urology of Hannover Medical School. After a decade, analysis of our cases revealed a progression rate of 34.6%, which prompted us to evaluate vascular invasion as predictive factor in stage 1 NSGCT, for better identification of those patients who would not benefit from surveillance only.

Patients, Material, and Method

So far, 107 patients have been managed according to the "wait and see" protocol in our department, and have been followed closely with a median follow-up of 44 months (range 4–100 months). While 70 patients exhibited no evidence of disease, 37 relapses in 37 patients were noted to date, giving a relapse rate of 34.6% (Liedke et al. 1990).

Due to the referral to our department of the majority of patients after orchiectomy exclusively for the "wait and see" strategy, archival tissue of the primary tumor could be obtained for further evaluation only in 50 cases (35 patients with no evidence of disease, 15 patients with metastases).

From the paraffin blocks 4- to 6-µm serial sections were taken and stained with hematoxylin-eosin as well as immunohistochemically for the expression of blood group isoantigens. The latter method was adopted from a procedure developed earlier for tumor biology studies in bladder cancer (Allhoff et al. 1986). The monoclonal primary antibodies necessary for this purpose were purchased from

[1] Urologische Klinik; [2] Pathologisches Institut; [3] Zentrum für Innere Medizin, Abt. Hämatologie und Onkologie; [4] Zentrum Biometrie, Medizinische Hochschule, Konstanty-Gutschow-Str. 8, W-3000 Hannover 61, FRG.

DAKO and used as follows: anti A, code no. A 581, 1:60, 60 min/anti B; code no. A 582, 1:40, 60 min/anti H; code no. A 583, 1:80, 30 min. These were applied with the chromogen DAB using the avidin-biotin method (Camon, Vector-Stain ABC Kit, PK 4002).

Substitution of the primary antibody by buffer solution as well as the employment of each primary antibody absorbed with the homologous antigen served as negative control. As positive control a tissue section known to be positive for the respective antigen was always included in the staining procedure. The staining of erythrocytes and endothelium allowed precise identification of vascular invasion.

Interpretation of the features displayed after both conventional and immunohistochemical staining was performed by our reference pathologist (C.W.)

Results

The population investigated appears at first sight selected, but statistical evaluation reveals that the incidence of relapse in the 50 patients studied did not differ significantly from that of the entire group ($p = 0.35$).

Vascular invasion was identified in the primary tumors of 4 (11.4%) of the 35 patients with no evidence of disease at follow-up, whereas it had occurred in the tumors of 4 (26.6%) of the 15 patients with spread disease.

Staining of the endothelial lining using the method outlined above was clearly superior to the conventional HE technique in precisely identifying vascular invasion. Figure 1 demonstrates convincingly the improvement in differentiating of

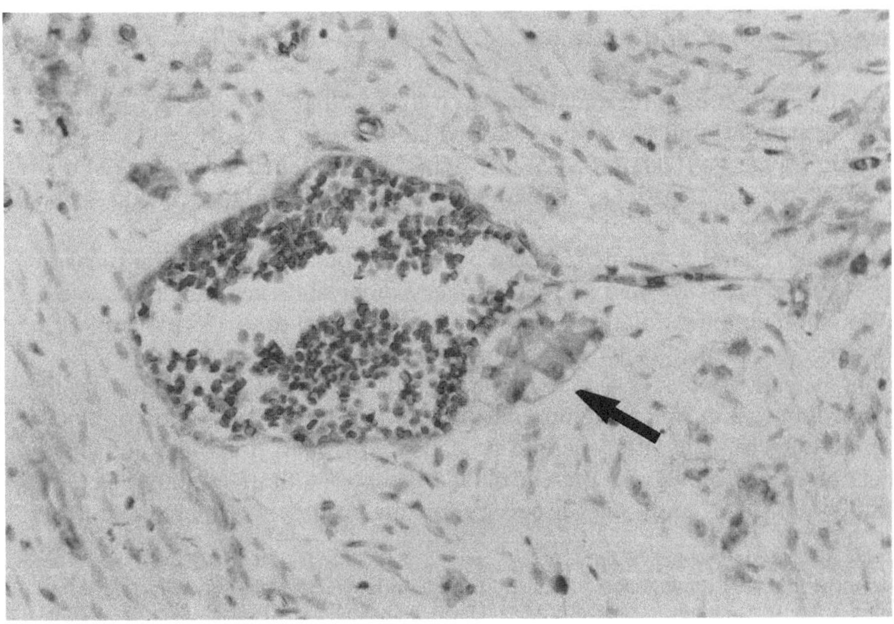

Fig. 1. Tumor cell clone, not penetrating, but bulging out the endothelial lining

the various histological structures at the microscopic level. The phenomenon of vascular invasion was more strongly correlated to disseminated disease than to lack of disease recurrence. According to χ^2 distribution statistical significance was attained at the 0.1 level (one-sided test, $p = 0.09$) (Pearson 1900).

Discussion

The negative impact of retroperitoneal lymphadenectomy resulting in loss of ejaculation as well as the introduction of such imaging modalities as CT and ultrasonography made the strategy of "wait and see" acceptable in the early 1980s. However, the encouraging 17% relapse rate was soon replaced by a relapse-free rate of only 68% at 4 years (Freedman et al. 1987).

Our clinical data, with a relapse rate of 34.6%, are almost identical to results noted by our English colleagues and are also based on a larger group of patients and a more conclusive, because longer, follow-up. It becomes obvious that the biological behavior of NSGCTs has been considerably underestimated in early reports, and that at least adequate predictors must be available if continuation of a "wait and see" policy is to be justified.

Freedman et al. described four features which independently predicted relapse: invasion of testicular veins, invasion of testicular lymphatics, absence of yolk sac elements, and presence of undifferentiated tumor (Freedman et al. 1987). Just recently, Pont et al. concluded that low- and high-risk patients with stage 1 NSGCT can be identified by evaluation of blood vessel invasion and pointed out that embryonal carcinoma and vascular invasion might be related prognostic factors (Pont et al. 1990). In a retrospective study Moriyama et al. found the presence or absence of vascular invasion to be strongly correlated to concomitant lymph node involvement or subsequent appearance of other metastatic disease. In 29 tumors with vascular invasion 25 patients were seen with tumor spread, whereas spread was noted in only 3 out of 16 patients whose primaries lacked vascular involvement (Moriyama et al. 1985).

Our investigation confirms the observation made by the authors cited (Freedman et al. 1987; Moriyama et al. 1985; Pont et al. 1990) that vascular invasion can be regarded as a reliable, statistically significant predictor for the metastatic potential of NSGCT. As also shown in our study, the criterion of vascular invasion cannot be considered an absolute parameter but rather an epiphenomenon which allows distinction between majorities. Furthermore, the problems in identifying vascular involvment with certainty become obvious when one considers the processing of soft testicular tissue specimens, with the possibility of misinterpreting gaps as "vessels" and accidentally intraluminally placed tumor cells as "penetrated neoplasm". The technique developed by our group and outlined above thus improves recognition of the histopathological structures and reduces the number of false-positive findings.

The major argument against retroperitoneal lymphadenectomy so far has been the loss of ejaculation associated with the standard surgical procedure. However, a nerve-sparing modified form of retroperitoneal lymphadenectomy, pioneered at Indiana University, has recently been reported to preserve ejaculation in 100% of cases along with no evidence of disease. Thus, there is no reason to bypass retroperitoneal lymphadenectomy in favor of surveillance on the basis of surgical morbidity (Donohue et al. 1990). However, reliable risk factors might allow identification of those patients whose tumors lack metastatic potential, so that even the operation can be foregone without compromising adequate tumor therapy.

The factors described here are hampered by the retrospective nature of the study and the lack of evidence of their independence. A prospective study therefore is needed which should include the variables currently suggested to be of predictive value, especially the feature of hyperpentaploidy, which was recently reported by our group to be highly significant (Allhoff et al. 1990).

References

Allhoff EP, Liedke S, Wittekind C, de Riese W, Lenis G, Tanke H, Jonas U (1990) DNA-content in NSGCT/CS I: a new prognosticator for biologic behaviour. J Cancer Res Clin Oncol 116 [Suppl]:592

Allhoff EP, Franzen W, Stroms A, Engelking R (1986) Monoclonal antibodies in evaluating the biological potential in urothelial cancer. In: Greten H, Klapdor R (eds) Clinical relevance of new monoclonal antibodies. Thieme, Stuttgart New York, pp 219–230

Donohue JP, Thornhill JA, Foster RS, Rowland RG, Bihrle R (1990) The evolution of surgical templates and nerve sparing technique in retroperitoneal lymphadenectomy (RPLND) for low stage testis cancer. J Urol 143:395A

Freedman LS, Jones WG, Peckham MJ, Newlands ES, Parkinson MC, Oliver RTD, Read G, Williams CJ (1987) Histopathology in the prediction of relapse of patients with stage I testicular teratoma treated by orchidectomy alone. Lancet 8:294–297

Liedke S, Allhoff EP, Jonas U (1990) "Wait and see" in nonseminomatous germ cell tumors clinical stage I: a critical assessment after eight years. J Urol 143:147A

Moriyama N, Daly JJ, Keating MA, Lin CW, Prout GR (1985) Vascular invasion as a prognosticator of metastatic disease in nonseminomatous germ cell tumors of the testis. Cancer 56:2492–2498

Pearson K (1990) On the criterion that a given system of deviations from the probable in the case of a correlated system of variables is such that it can be reasonably supposed to have arisen from random sampling. Phil Mag V 50:157

Peckham MJ, Husband JE, Barrett A, Hendry WF (1982) Orchidectomy alone in testicular stage I non-seminomatous germ-cell tumours. Lancet ii:678–680

Pont J, Höltl W, Kosak D, Machacek E, Kienzer H, Julcher H, Honetz N (1990) Risk-adapted treatment choice in stage I nonseminomatous testicular germ cell cancer by regarding vascular invasion in the primary tumor: a prospective trial. J Clin Oncol 8:16–20

Turbidimetrical Determination of Inflammatory Parameters in Seminal Plasma

M. ZELLNER, P. FORNARA, A. DICHTL, K. EDER, and A. G. HOFSTETTER[1]

Introduction

Proof of microbial inflammation being given in approximately 50% of patients with chronic prostatitis, only the so-called vegetative urogenital syndrome or anogenital syndromes must be considered in the remaining 50%.

Radial immunodiffusion as a method to investigate increased concentrations of acute phase proteins (albumin, complement 3c, immunoglobulins A and G) in ejaculum has been described (Hofstetter 1974) as being of diagnostic value in addition to routine methods such as urine bacteriology, urethral smear, expressed urine, and ejaculum culture. However, this technique cannot be used in clinical routine because of its cost in time and financial resources. As an alternative to radial immunodiffusion, the feasibility of turbidimetry as a simple, rapid, and less expensive test system was examined.

Materials and Methods

Principle of Radial Immunodiffusion

The precipitation of antigen-antibody complexes in a gel occurs in the equivalence range (concentration of antigen : antibody = 1 : 1) only. Specimens of unknown antigen concentration are placed in the center of a gel plate containing a defined concentration of antibody. Due to the radial diffusion of the antigen, a precipitation ring occurs at the range of equivalent concentrations after 2–3 days. The diameters of the precipitation zones are measured. Using a calibration curve, the antigen concentration can be determined.

Principle of Turbidimetry

Solutes of antigen-antibody complexes are able to absorb light. The test kit contains a defined concentration of specific antibodies. The quantitative measurement of antigens in solution occurs by a surplus of antibodies, i.e., in the rising part of the curve of Heidelberger and Kendall (Fig. 1).

The quantitative determination of antigen is founded on the kinetic measurement of the cloudiness of the solution caused by the formation and precipitation

[1] Urologische Klinik und Poliklinik der Universität Klinikum Großhadern, Marchioninistraße 15, W-8000 München 70, FRG.

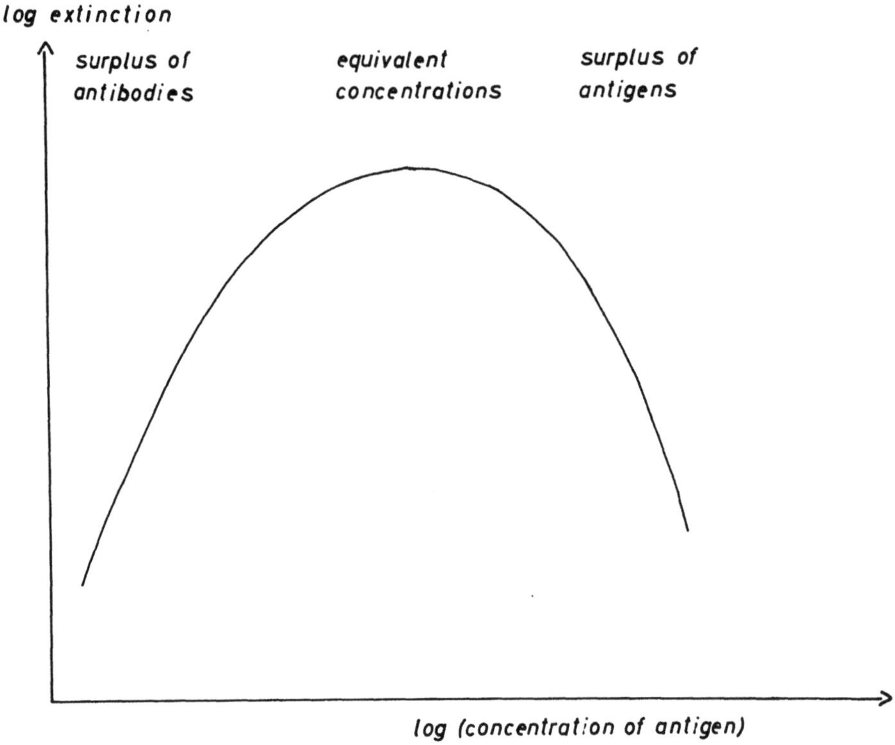

Fig. 1. Curve of Heidelberger and Kendall

of antigen-antibody complexes. By simultaneous measurement of the maximum reaction speed measured during the rising part of the curve of Heidelberger and Kendall and the time required, it is possible to ascertain an antigen concentration with certainty.

To verify the clinical value of turbidimetry, measurement of albumin, immunoglobulins A and G, complement 3c, and C-reactive protein in the ejaculum of 45 patients was performed by radial immunodiffusion and turbidimetry. The samples used were ejaculum from patients with serious clinical conditions and from healthy subjects.

After liquefaction of the ejaculum (after an average of 30 min) at a temperature of 37 °C, centrifugation was done at 4000 rpm for about 15 min. Then the liquid fraction was examined.

Results

To illustrate the results, the values found by turbidimetry were set on the *y* axis while the values from radial immunodiffusion were set on the *x* axis of a graph. If both methods were equivalent, the values must lie on the bisector of an angle (i.e., the reference curve).

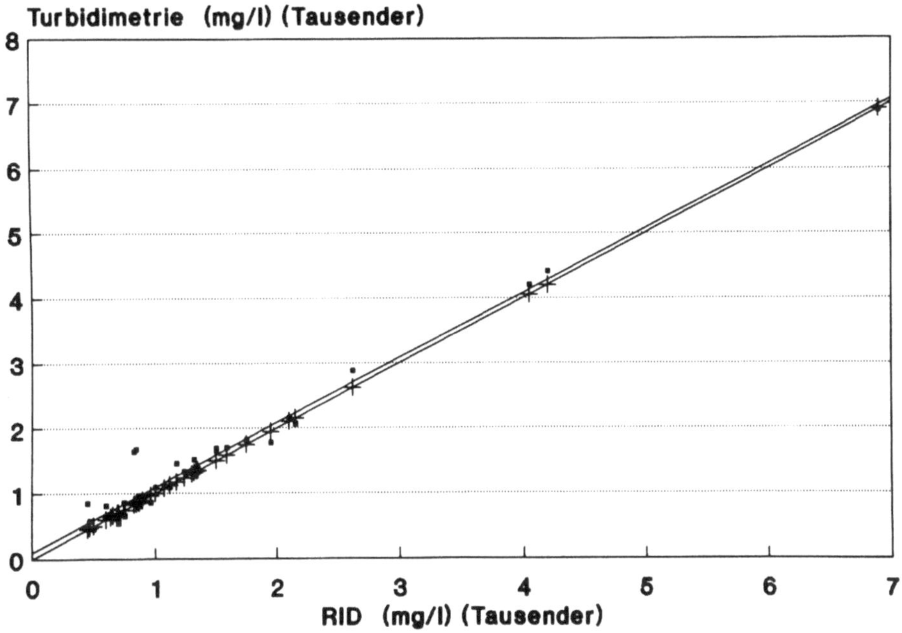

Fig. 2. Albumin: results of turbidimetry and radial immunodiffusion (scales in thousands). +, reference curve; ■, results

Albumin

The range of values of albumin was 447–6900 mg/l. This is in accordance with the extent of variation in an inhomogeneous group of patients. The average discrepancy to turbidimetrical values was ±14.1%.

The graphic evaluation (Fig. 2) shows good correlation between the measurement values obtained by the different methods. Turbidimetry tended to produce rather higher values than radial immunodiffusion, but the results were at comparable levels.

Immunoglobulin G

The values for immunoglobulin G varied between 4.6 and 283.6 mg/dl. The mean discrepancy between the two methods was ±11.35%. The graphic evaluation (Fig. 3) also shows excellent correlation between the methods. Values measured by radial immunodiffusion values were little higher but always by the same amount.

Immunoglobulin A

The values for immunoglobulin A varied between 0.0 and 102.6 mg/dl. The graphic evaluation (Fig. 4) shows clearly the proportionality of results within a

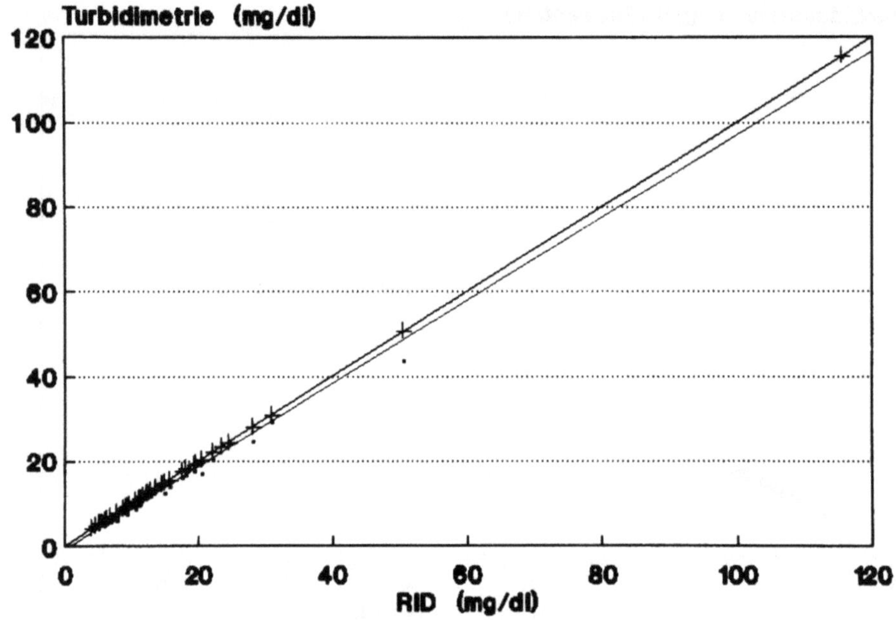

Fig. 3. Immunoglobulin G: results of turbidimetry and radial immunodiffusion. +, reference curve; ■, results

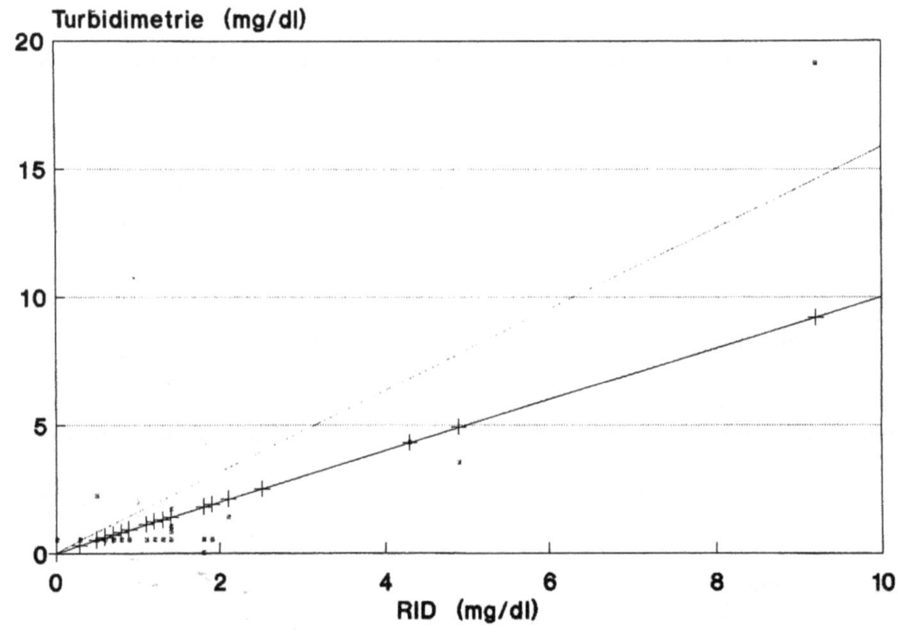

Fig. 4. Immunoglobulin A: results of turbidimetry and radial immunodiffusion. +, reference curve; ■, results

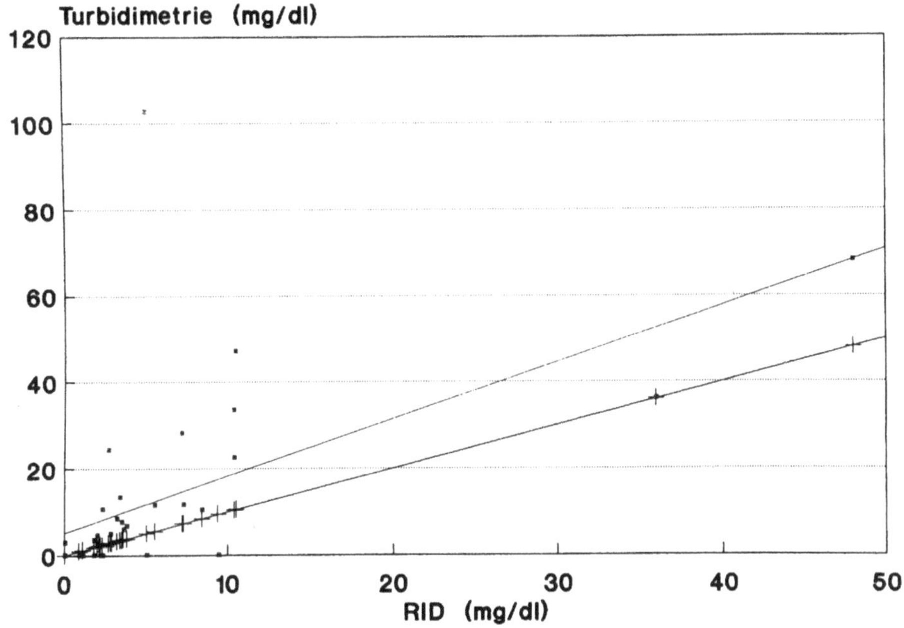

Fig. 5. Complement 3c: results of turbidimetry and radial immunodiffusion. +, reference curve; ■, results

range of 10 mg/dl. Turbidimetry, however, gave almost constantly markedly higher values. In some cases major differences were obtained.

Since an increased immunoglobulin A level is most distinctly seen in inflammatory processes, a greater precision of values measured by turbidimetry was expected compared to immunodiffusion.

Complement 3c

The values determined for complement 3c were between 0.0 and 19.1 mg/dl. In the range of values up to 5 mg/dl we found a good correlation between the methods for complement 3c too (Fig. 5). In occasional cases, however, we saw extreme differences between turbidimetry and immunodiffusion. An analysis of microbiological findings will have to show whether the turbidimetry results were correct or too high.

C-Reactive Protein

The findings for C-reactive protein (Fig. 6) were similar. C-reactive protein was not detectable by radial immunodiffusion at all, while the values measured by turbidimetry were in the range of 0.0–2.2 mg/dl.

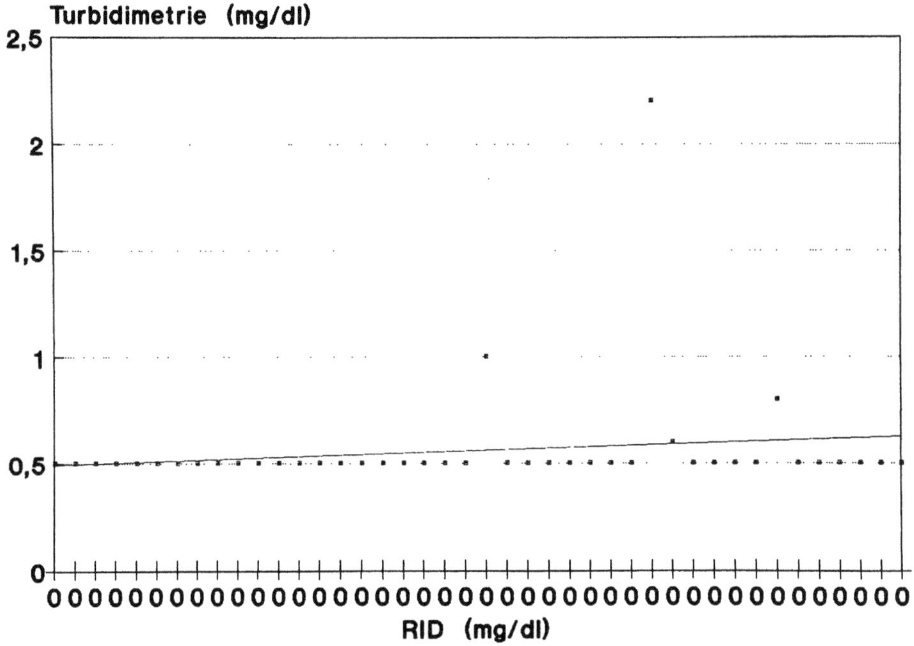

Fig. 6. CRP: results of turbidimetry and radial immunodiffusion. +, reference curve; ■, results

Discussion

Up to now turbidimetry has been used especially for the determination of plasma proteins. However, it seems to be quite suitable for quantitative measurement of acute-phase proteins in seminal plasma. In addition to the advantages of lower costs and easier, automated practicability, the decisive advantage of turbidimetry is that the results are available immediately after the specimen is obtained.

Our results certainly suggest the possibility of utilizing turbidimetry routinely in the diagnostic investigation of male adnexitis. In addition to the variables analyzed so far, we feel encouraged to add further measurements of acid-α_1-glycoprotein, α_1-antitrypsin, haptoglobin, and transferrin.

Reference

Hofstetter AG et al. (1974) Immunelektrophoretische Untersuchungen im Serum und Ejakulat bei der chronisch rezidivierenden Adnexitis des Mannes. Verh Ber Dtsch Ges Urol 25:342–344

The Arteries of the Spermatic Cord and Testis: A Dynamic Angiographic Study and Its Clinical Relevance

M. SCHARDT, M. MEYER-SCHWICKERATH, and H. RÜBBEN[1]

Introduction

Since Silber and Kelly (1976) successfully performed autotransplantation of the cryptorchid testis in 1975, the use of microsurgical procedures involving the spermatic cord and testis has steadily increased and vascular microsurgery has become a part of operative urology (Belker 1980; Kadawaki and Yakami 1979; Osterwitz and Fahlenkamp 1987). All the more important, therefore is a profound knowledge of the anatomy and vascular supply of the testis and spermatic cord for the assessment and understanding of intraoperative hazards, complications, and postoperative results.

Few publications so far have dealt with the vascular anatomy of the spermatic cord and testis (Ben-Menachem et al. 1974; Kahn and Frates 1968; Koischwitz 1973; Kormano and Nordmark 1977; Nordmark et al. 1977).

In 1981 we reported for the first time on postmortem sequential angiography of the spermatic cord and testis using a contrast medium of particularly low viscosity (Kormano and Nordmark 1977). Our angiographic studies help to explain the different results reached by various authors involved with research on the vascular system of the spermatic cord and testis.

Materials and Methods

Forty testicles were obtained by orchiectomy or at autopsy. Using a surgical microscope, a blunt cannula was inserted into either the testicular artery or the arteria ductus deferentis. A hydrous contrast medium with a median viscosity of 350 centipoise and a median particle size of 0.5–0.7 μm was injected. A very fine granulated industrial X-ray film (Strukterix NDT.AGFA) was exposed to 50–60 kV and 200–400 mAs utilizing a fine-focus X-ray tube. Turning and tilting the organ placed directly onto the film, X-ray exposures were obtained in different paths of rays and projections, allowing precise analysis of the arterial system of the spermatic cord (Fig. 2). Sequential exposures were performed injecting contrast medium in steps of 0.1–0.25 ml, covering all phases of vascular filling (Fig. 1). Finally, the specimens were fixed in 4% formaldehyde solution. Histological slides of 5×4 cm were prepared from some of the testicles.

[1] Urologische Klinik der Universität/Gesamthochschule, Hufelandstr. 55, W-4300 Essen 1, FRG.

Results

Three arteries coming from different regions supply the spermatic cord and testis. The testicular artery originates directly from the abdominal aorta. The deferential artery branches off the internal iliac artery. The cremasteric artery derives from the external iliac artery.

Angiography of the Testicular Artery (Figs. 1–3)

Four to six centimeters before reaching the testis, the variably coiled testicular artery passes one or two major branches to the upper and lower pole of the epididymis. The arteria testis propria splits into two to four branches perforating the tunica albuginea at the mediastinum testis. The branches then run to the ventral margin of the testis between the tunica albuginea and the testicular parenchy-

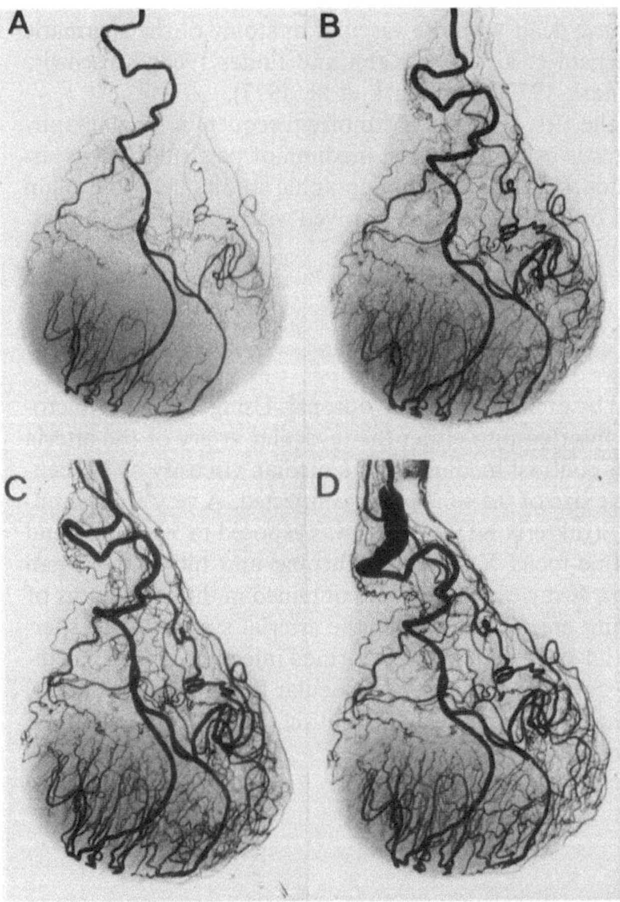

Fig. 1. Sequential exposures following injection of contrast medium in steps of 0.1–0.25 ml

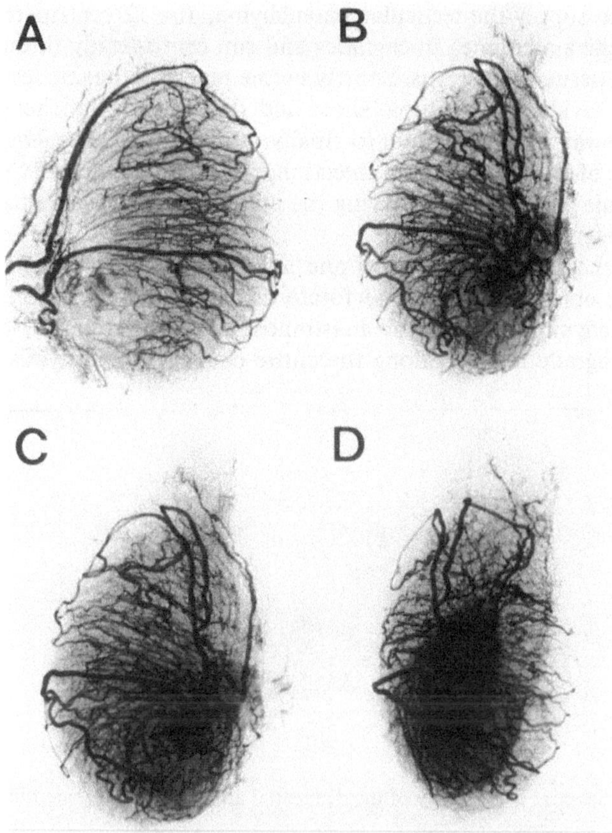

Fig. 2. By turning and tilting the organ, exposures were obtained in different planes of projection

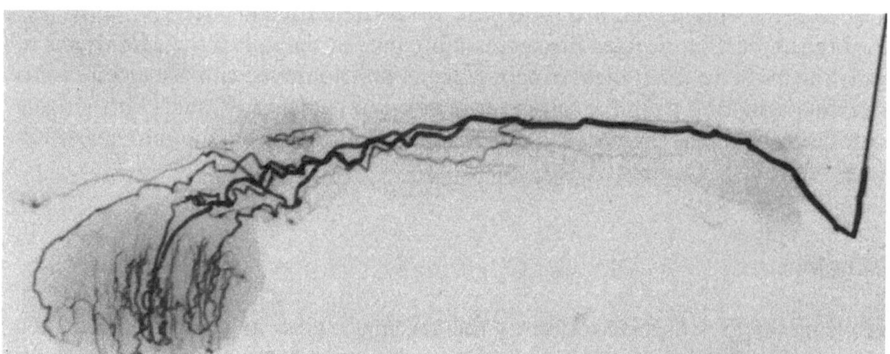

Fig. 3. The testicular artery splits into three branches perforating the tunica albuginea at the mediastinum testis. The tunica vaginalis was removed and the epididymis separated from the testis

ma. To supply the testicular parenchyma, 10–12 centripetal arteries branch off the tunica albuginea in cascades and run centripetally through the interstitial fibrous tissue of the testis. Shortly before reaching the rete testis, the centripetal arteries divide into multiple short and thin-walled branches turning as recurrent rami away from the hilum to finally ramify in the parenchym. Even in the early phase of contrast medium injection, the epididymal artery, originating from the testicular artery and supplying the epididymis, reveals a broad anastomosis with the deferential artery.

At the region of the upper and lower pole of the epididymies, minor branches of the epididymal artery perforate the tunica albuginea or supply the testicular parenchyma. Multiple tiny anastomoses with the cremasteric arteries are filled in a retrograde manner along the entire course of epididymis.

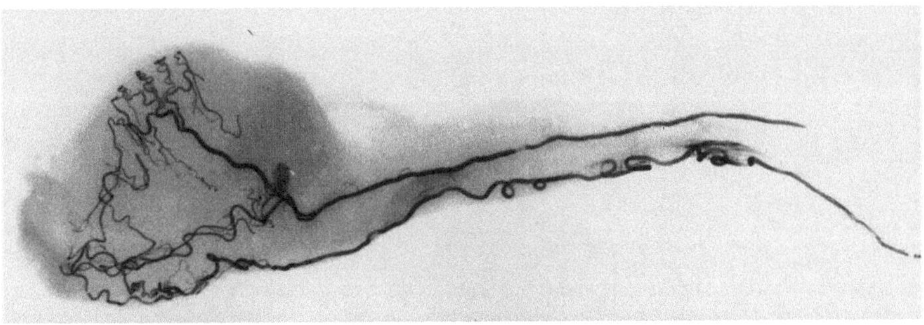

Fig. 4. Selective angiography of the deferential artery with retrograde filling of the testicular artery

Angiography of the Deferential Artery (Fig. 4)

The deferential artery runs together with the deferential duct to the lower pole of the epididymis, where it divides. One branch supplies the lower pole and anastomizes with the epididymal artery arising from the testicular artery.

Another branch perforates the tunica albuginea at the tail of the epididymis to supply the testis. In the testicular parenchyma, anastomoses with the arteria testis propriae originating from the testicular artery can be demonstrated. Further tiny anastomoses with the cremasteric artery are filled in a retrograde manner at the epididymal tail.

Discussion

Knowledge of the vascularization of the spermatic cord and testis should be a fundamental of male reproductive medicine (Konrad et al. 1988). Despite a large number of surgical procedures involving the spermatic cord and testis to improve testicular and seminal maturation, few reports of systematic research into vascular anatomy exist (Kormano and Nordmark 1977). In the few angiographic studies of the testis and spermatic cord, only selective demonstration of the testicular artery was described, performed either by intravital catheterization and injection of a common water-soluble contrast medium or by postmortem corrosion following injection of acrylic solution.

We are the first to selectively demonstrate the deferential artery in sequential angiography (Fig. 4). It runs along the spermatic cord to the epididymal tail, where it anastomoses with the cremasteric arteries and the epididymal artery arising from the testicular artery. Its branches perforate the tunica albuginea to supply the testicular parenchyma. With further injection of contrast medium into the vascular system, the complete vascularization of the testis, epididymis, and spermatic cord can be visualized. These constant results explain the relatively low rate of atrophy (18%) following the Fowler-Stephensen procedure for abdominal testis. To mobilize the abdominal testis the testicular artery is separated with only the deferential artery being spared, together with a vascularized peritoneal flap (long loop vas), to supply the testis (Osterwitz and Fahlenkamp 1987). In contrast to the studies of Konrad et al. (1988), our angiography demonstrates an adequate blood supply to the epididymis by the deferential artery through a system of epididymal anastomoses.

Our experimental results reflect the clinical experience of a low complication rate in surgery of the spermatic cord and testicular biopsy, due to the extensive network of anastomoses between the three arterial systems of the spermatic cord and testis.

References

Belker AM (1980) Urologic microsurgery – current perspectives: orchidopexy and testicular homotransplantation. Urology 15:103

Ben-Menachem Y, De Berardinis MC, Salimas R (1974) Localization of intra-abdominal testes by selective testicular arteriography: a case report. J Urol 112:493

Kadawaki H, Yakami T (1979) Basic study of microsurgical orchidopexy for high undescended testis; assessment of clinical applicability. J Pediatr Surg 14:544–550

Kahn PC, Frates RE (1968) The value of angiography of the small branches of the abdominal aorta. Am J Roentgenol 102:407

Koischwitz D (1973) Röntgenologischer Nachweis eines Hodentumors bei Kryptorchismus. Fortschr Röntgenstr 119:639

Konrad G, Wurzer B, Gebhardt T, Strittmatter T (1988) Die Blutversorgung des Hodens und ihre Bedeutung für die Klinik. 9. Symposium für Experimentelle Urologie 17.–18.6.1988 Abstract Nr. 13

Kormano M, Nordmark L (1977) Angiography of the testicular artery. III. Testis and epididymis analysed with a magnification technique. Acta Radiol Diagn 18:925

Meyer-Schwickerath M, Müller K-M (1981) Angiographische und morphologische Befunde bei Hodentumoren. Urologe [A] 20:58–62

Nordmark L, Bjersing L, Domellöf L, Hjämas K, Nyberg G (1977) Angiography of the testicular artery. II. Cryptorchism and testicular agenesis. Acta Radiol Diagn 18:167

Osterwitz H, Fahlenkamp D (1987) Klinische Hodentransplantationen. Übersichten zu Indikationsstellung, Operationstechniken und Ergebnissen bei der Auto-, Allo- und Esotransplantation. Z Urol Nephrol 80:525

Silber SJ, Kelly J (1976) Successful autotransplantation of an intraabdominal testis to the scrotum by microvascular technique. J Urol 115:452–4

Vitale R, Kahdemi M, Seebode JJ (1974) Selective gonadal angiography for testicular localization in patients with cryptorchism. Surg Forum 25:538

Comparison of Duplex Sonography and Color-Coded-Flow Duplex Sonography for Evaluation of Erectile Dysfunction

K. LANG[1], W. SCHANTZEN[2], B. M. CRAMER[2], and J. W. THÜROFF[1]

Introduction

Duplex sonography has been established as a standard study for evaluation of erectile dysfunction (Lue et al. 1985; Müller 1988; v. Wallenberg-Pachaly et al. 1989; Porst et al. 1988). Color-coded-flow duplex sonography, which is a technological refinement of duplex ultrasonography, has not yet been evaluated with regard to its possibilities, advantages, and disadvantages.

Material and Methods

In 25 patients complaining of erectile dysfunction we compared findings by duplex sonography and color-coded-flow duplex sonography. The age of the patients was between 17 and 76 years (mean 58 years). The standard work-up of patients included history, physical examination, hormonal assessment, pharmacosonography, and, additionally, cavernosography in some cases.

For duplex sonography we used an Acuson 128 computed duplex ultrasound system. For pharmacosonography we injected 10 μg prostaglandin E_1 into the cavernous bodies. Pharmacosonography was performed first using duplex sonography and repeated on another day using color-coded-flow duplex sonography.

Arterial diameters and systolic peak flow velocities of proximal and distal sections of deep penile arteries on either side were measured before and after injection of prostaglandin E_1.

Results

Eleven patients had arteriogenic impotence, five neurogenic impotence, one patient had a venous leak, and eight patients had normal organic erectile function. Sonography revealed flow velocity patterns compatible with arteriogenic and nonarteriogenic impotence (Fig. 1).

The findings in patients with arteriogenic and those with nonarteriogenic impotence were analyzed separately. Analyses included the amount of time necessary to complete the studies and the accuracy of flow velocity measurements.

[1] Urologische Klinik; [2] Radiologische Klinik, Klinikum Barmen, Heusnerstr. 40, W-5600 Wuppertal, FRG.

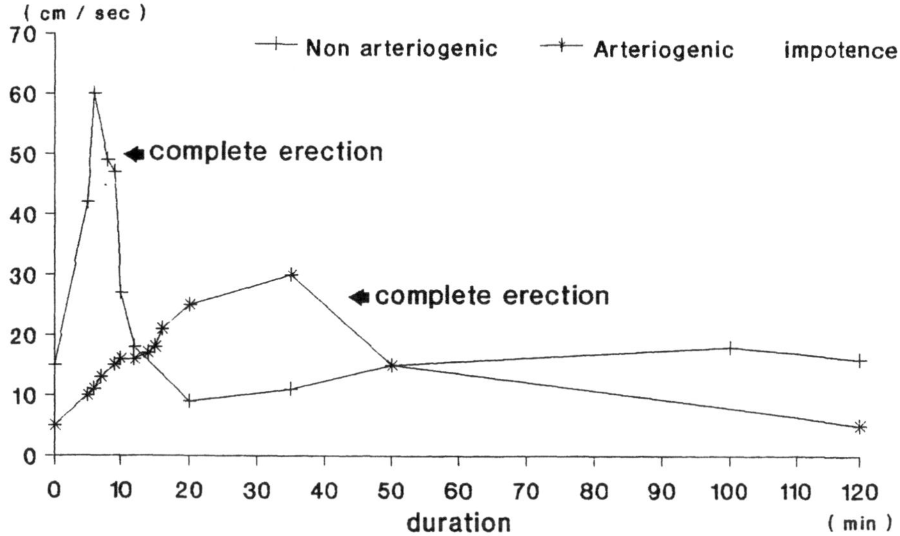

Fig. 1. Systolic flow velocity after intracavernous injection of 10 µg prostaglandin E_1 in typical cases of arteriogenic and nonarteriogenic erectile dysfunction

The duration of duplex sonography versus color-coded-flow duplex sonography was analysed for two periods:

1. From the beginning of study until injection of prostaglandin E_1 (Table 1) and
2. from injection until the end of the study (Table 2).

Table 1. Time from beginning of study until injection of prostglandin E_1

	Duplex sonography	Color-coded-flow duplex sonography	Significance
Arteriogenic erectile dysfunction	12 min 00 s	9 min 40 s	n.s.
Nonarteriogenic erectile dysfunction	14 min 00 s	11 min 30 s	$p<0.05$

Table 2. Time from injection of prostaglandin E_1 to end of study

	Duplex sonography	Color-coded-flow duplex sonography	Significance
Arteriogenic erectile dysfunction	19 min 40 s	17 min 50 s	n.s.
Nonarteriogenic erectile dysfunction[a]	10 min 50 s	8 min 10 s	$p<0.05$

[a] In this group five examinations could not be completed due to flow reduction at full erection: four duplex sonography, one color-coded-flow duplex sonography.

The amount of time necessary to complete studies in patients with nonarteriogenic erectile dysfunction was significantly longer with duplex sonography than with color-coded-flow duplex sonography. In addition, it was possible to identify intercavernous shunts and distal ramifications of the deep penile arteries by color-coded-flow duplex sonography but not by conventional duplex sonography.

Analysis of the accuracy of measurement of flow velocity relates to theoretical considerations and the ease and speed of actual measurements but lacks objective control, e.g., by direct flow measurement. The velocity of flow is determined by measuring the Doppler shift in frequency between transmitted ultrasound and the ultrasound reflected back from a moving target (bloodstream). The velocity as measured by Dopplersonography represents only a partial vector of the total real velocity. The total velocity must be calculated by correcting for the angle between the axis of flow and the axis of the Doppler ultrasound beam (Fig. 2) according to the formula:

$$V = \frac{\Delta f}{\cos \alpha}$$

We found color coding of flow useful for rapid and easy detection of arteries, especially in young patients with thin-walled vessels. Color coding of flow was most important for rapid and precise angle correction in measurements after prostaglandin E_1 injection in patients with nonarteriogenic erectile dysfunction, where the usable time for measurements before full erection is limited.

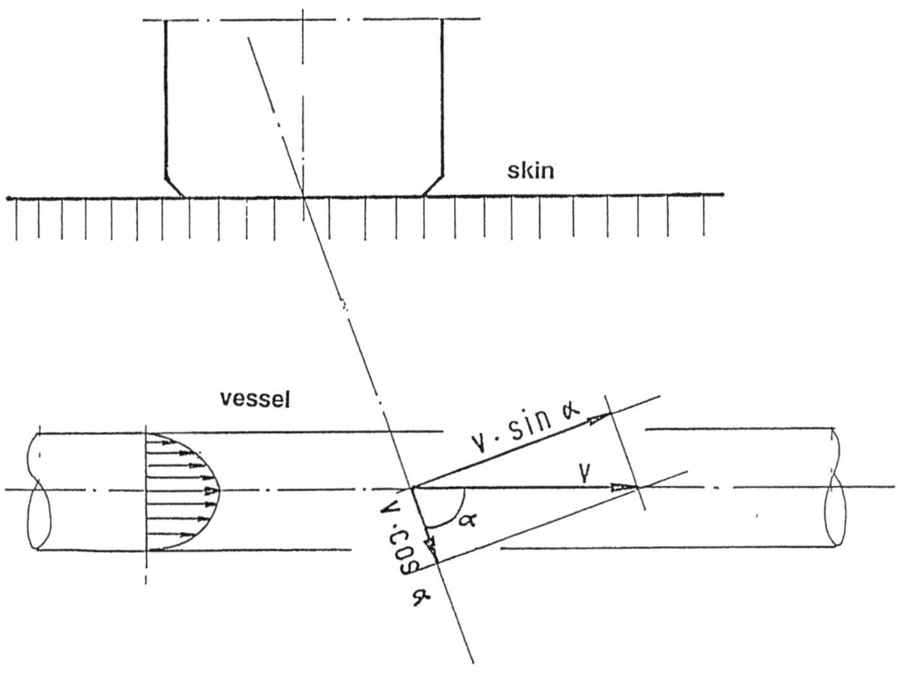

Fig. 2. The relation between the actual flow velocity and the measured flow velocity depends on the angle α between the axis of flow and the axis of the ultrasound beam

Conclusions

In our study, color-coded-flow duplex sonography allowed easier and more rapid imaging of thin-walled arteries. This effect was especially useful in examination of young patients with nonarteriogenic impotence. In this group of patients the time period usable for duplex sonography after injection of the vasoactive substance is limited by the reduction in arterial flow with increasing rigidity (Table 3). However, this was unimportant in patients with arteriogenic impotence because

1. Thickened arterial walls were much easier to identify on conventional duplex sonography and
2. a prolonged arterial inflow resulted in an extended tumescence phase until full rigidity was reached.

Table 3. Duration of tumescence until erection after injection of prostaglandin E_1[a]

Arteriogenic erectile dysfunction	23 min (17 – 30 min)
Nonarteriogenic erectile dysfunction	11 min (8 – 30 min)

[a] Six patients did not reach full erection after 30 min: five arteriogenic, one non-arteriogenic erectile dysfunction (venous leak).

Summary

For evaluation of erectile dysfunction color-coded-flow duplex sonography appears superior to conventional duplex sonography because it allows easier and more rapid identification of vessels. This is especially important in patients with non-arteriogenic impotence, with thin-walled vessels and anatomic variations, in whom completion of duplex sonography before decrease of arterial flow due to increasing rigidity can be a problem. Rapid identification of the axis and direction of flow by color coding of flow and corresponding angle correction appears to increase the accuracy of flow velocity measurement. At the present time we feel that the high cost of equipment is the main disadvantage of color-coded-flow duplex sonography.

References

Lue TF, Hricak H, Marich KW, Tanagho EA (1985) Evaluation of vasculogenic impotence with high resolution ultrasonography and pulsed Doppler spectrum analysis. Radiology 155:777

Müller SC, Lue TF (1988) Evaluation of vasculogenic impotence. Urol Clin North Am 15:65

Nürnberger N, Hirsch P (1990) Velocity profile of penile arteries in erectile dysfunction assessed by color doppler imaging (abstract). Eur Urol 18 [Suppl 1]:15

Porst H, Ahlen H, Köster O, Scholaut KH (1988) Vergleich von Papaverin-induzierter Dopplersonographie und Angiographie in der Diagnostik der erektilen Dysfunktion. Urologe [A] 27:8–13

Wallenberg-Pachaly H, Voges G, Schild H, Müller SC (1989) Vergleich von Beckenangiographie, gepulster Dopplersonographie und PBI in der Abklärung der erektilen Impotenz. Akt Urol 20:24–28

Registration of Cavernous Electrical Activity and its Interpretation *

CH. G. STIEF, M. DJAMILIAN, W. DE RIESE, E. P. ALLHOFF, A. KRAMER, and U. JONAS[1]

Introduction

Due to the lack of tests for the cavernous autonomic nervous system, the somatosensory penile innervation has usually been examined to elucidate the neurogenic factor in impotence. The latency of the bulbocavernous-reflex (BCR-L) has been measured (Siroky et al. 1979), but recent publications have cast some doubts on the relevance of this procedure to autonomic neuropathy (Lavoisier et al. 1989). Gerstenberg and Wagner were the first to approach this major drawback in the diagnosis of erectile dysfunction when they suggested the registration of cavernous smooth muscle activity (1989). In this paper we describe the registration of cavernous electrical activity with different data processing methods than those published by Gerstenberg and Wagner.

Patients and Methods

One hundred and eighty-two consecutive patients with erectile dysfunction were evaluated multidisciplinarily in our impotence clinic (Stief et al. 1988). A further 39 patients from our urological ward with normal erectile function underwent single potential analysis of cavernous electrical activity (SPACE). Another 32 patients with erectile dysfunction were referred from other departments (especially the diabetes clinic) or centers especially for SPACE.

With the patient in a sitting position, a coaxial needle electrode (Dantec 9013 L; length 4 cm, surface of the tip 0.07 mm^2) was inserted laterally into the cavernous body until the tip of the electrode was located in the center of the cavernous body. Usually, the needle electrode was inserted into the left cavernous body. To assess whether cavernous electrical activity was synchronous in different areas of the penis, two needles were inserted into each cavernous body or proximally and distally into one cavernous body in more than 50 patients. The potentials were processed by an electrophysiological unit (Wiest Space Recorder, Munich, FRG): paper speed was 5 mm/s. The cut-off frequencies were 2–2000 Hz for the first 71 patients, then set at 0.5–500 Hz. The upper cut-off frequency of the Wiest thermowriter was 100 Hz. Amplification was mostly at 50 μV/unit. Because all normal patients showed abnormal potentials up to 15 min after introduction

* This work was supported by a grant from the Deutsche Forschungsgemeinschaft (Sti 96/2-1).

[1] Urologische Klinik, Medizinische Hochschule, Konstanty-Gutschow-Str. 8, W-3000 Hannover 61, FRG.

of the needle electrode, SPACE evaluation was started 20 min after needle electrode introduction. After 25 min registration of cavernous electrical activity during flaccidity, audiovisual sexual stimulation was applied for another 25 min, the examiner leaving the room. At the end of audiovisual stimulation, the examiner evaluated the erectile response by inspection, palpation, and interrogation. Recording was then continued for another 10 min.

Results

Electrical activity of the cavernous smooth muscles could not be registered in one impotent and two normal patients. When we changed the lower cut-off frequency to 0.5 Hz in the second normal patient with no recorded activity (overall patient no. 71), potentials were easily recorded. Starting with this patient, we therefore chose 0.5 Hz as the lower cut-off frequency. Lowering of the cut-off frequency from 2 to 0.5 Hz resulted in an increase in amplitude of about 80%–250%.

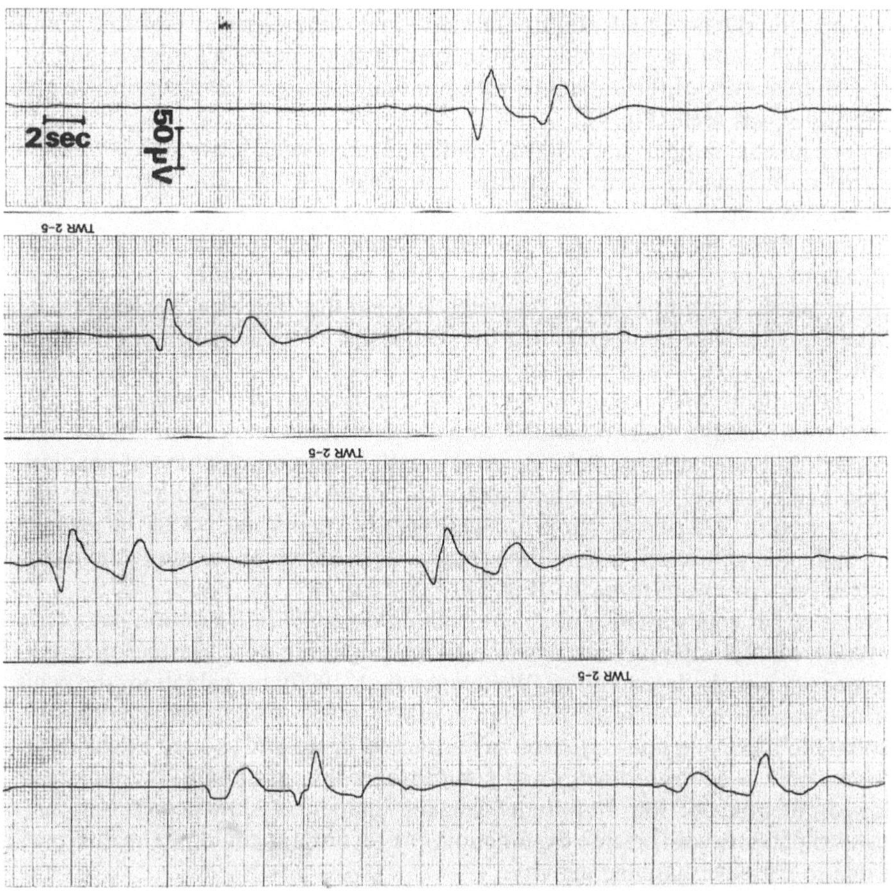

Fig. 1. Continuous recording of cavernous electrical activity in a normal patient shows similar potentials with a low frequency; cut-off frequencies are 2–2000 Hz

In 34/38 *normal* patients with recorded activity, the potentials were similar. The potentials started with a positive depolarisation or with a brief negative followed by a positive depolarisation. At cut-off frequencies of 2–2000 Hz, the length of the potentials was 3–12 s (mean 9.5, SD 0.3); the amplitude was 60–250 μV (mean 153, SD 31); polyphasity was 5–11 (mean 8.5, SD 0.3). At cut-off frequencies of 0.5–500 Hz, the length was 8–18 s (mean 12.8, SD 2.8); the amplitude 250–750 μV (mean 444, SD 109), and the polyphasity 8–22 (mean 13.8, SD 3.3). The shape of the potentials was very uniform for the same individual, although the frequency varied considerably depending on the degree of relaxation of the patient. Frequency was 0.6–2.6 potentials/min (Fig. 1). Simultaneous recording of cavernous electrical activity in both cavernous bodies showed synchronization of the potentials (Fig. 2). More superficial or deeper positioning of the electrode did not significantly alter the potentials.

To evaluate a possible influence of stress on the cavernous electrical activity, SPACE was performed about 1 h before surgery in two normal patients. In both patients, a wavelike electrical activity with small potentials in these waves but no specific bigger potentials was recorded (Fig. 3).

Comparing the potentials during flaccidity and tumescence or erection, a uniform change could be observed: with increasing tumescence and rigidity, an increase in frequency of the potentials with simultaneous decrease in amplitude and polyphasity was seen (Fig. 4).

In one normal patient, both normal and abnormal potentials were recorded. In another normal patient, only a wavelike baseline activity without specific potentials was recorded.

In the patients with presumed *upper motor neuron lesions* (complete traumatic spinal cord injury above T 11), potentials with a duration from 28 s to over 2 min were recorded. The amplitude of the potentials and the time between the passages of the baseline were comparable to the recordings of potentials in normal patients.

In the patients with presumed *peripheral autonomic nerve lesions* (e.g., after cystoprostatectomy), short potentials with a significantly reduced amplitude were recorded. In these patients, short potentials with a fast convex phase of depolarisation and a slower repolarisation phase of concave shape ("whip") were frequently seen. In 3/5 of the cystoprostatectomised patients and 1/3 of the patients who had undergone extirpation of the rectum, normal potentials and pathological electrical activity were recorded (Fig. 5).

In 11/14 patients with insulin-dependent *diabetes mellitus* (duration more than 20 years), multidisciplinary examination showed signs highly suggestive of cavernous smooth muscle degeneration (Wetterauer et al. 1990): on palpation, the penis in these patients felt much smaller than in other patients. All patients had a poor response to intracavernous injection of vasoactive drugs and showed extensive venous leakage in cavernosometry and cavernosography. In SPACE, these patients showed potentials of low amplitude, irregular shape and slow depolarisation.

In two patients with erectile dysfunction, the recordings could not be interpreted due to wavelike baseline activity.

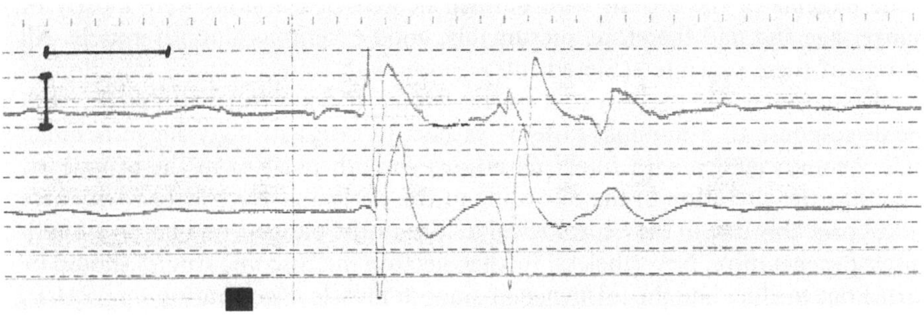

Fig. 2. Simultaneous continuous recording of cavernous electrical activity in both cavernous bodies shows synchronisation of cavernous electrical activity in both cavernous bodies in the normal man; cut-off frequencies are 0.5–500 Hz, the *horizontal bar* is 5 s, the *vertical bar* 100 µV

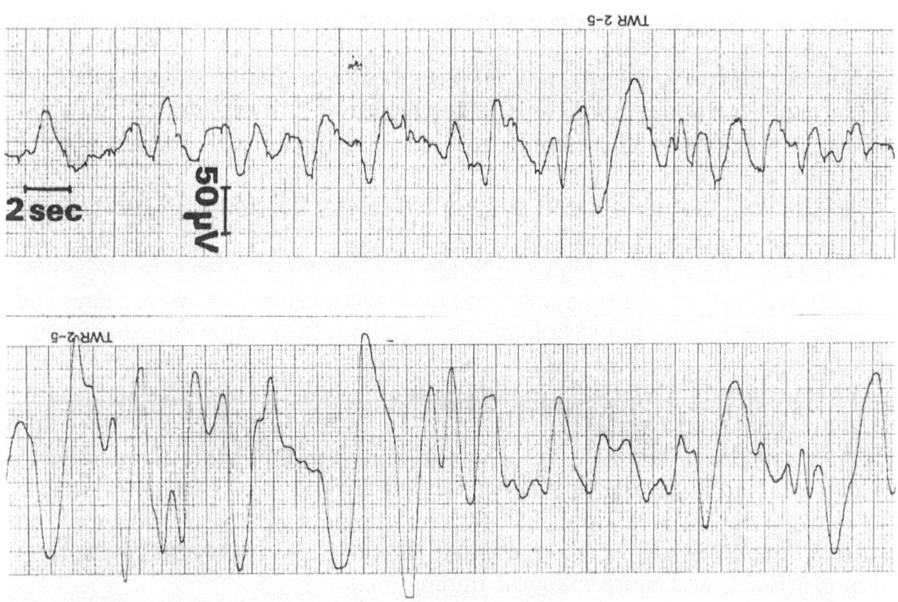

Fig. 3. Recording of a 29-year-old patient with varicocele 1 h prior to surgery. Cut-off frequencies are 2–2000 Hz

Discussion

The reproducible recordings and the similarity of the potentials in normal patients as well as the different recordings during full erection to audiovisual stimulation on one hand and after intracavernous injection of vasoactive drugs on the other strongly suggest that the recordings are not artefacts. The potentials recorded in normal patients are similar to smooth muscle potentials recorded in other smooth muscle organs in other species (Wagner 1976).

The patients in the groups with defined neurological lesions were mostly of younger age and had therefore, presumably, good cavernous smooth muscle. All but one of these patients achieved full erection with intracavernous injection of 0.5 ml papaverine (15 mg/ml) and phentolamine (0.5 mg/ml) or less. This full erectile response to a minimal dose of vasoactive drugs strongly suggests intact penile hemodynamics with intact cavernous smooth muscles in these patients. Therefore, the alteration in the recording of the cavernous electrical activity here is most probably due to the neurological lesions of the patients and not to smooth muscle degeneration. Nevertheless, further electron microscopic studies should be carried out to elucidate the influence of smooth muscle degeneration on SPACE.

The coexistence of normal potentials and pathological electrical activity in 7/12 patients having undergone radical cystoprostatectomy or after abdominoperineal extirpation of the rectum may be a sign of partial destruction of the autonomic cavernous supply. In the patients with insulin-dependent diabetes of onset more than 20 years ago and signs of extensive cavernous smooth muscle degeneration in the clinical work-up, significant changes of cavernous electrical activity were found. The low amplitude and the slow depolarisation of the potentials are suggestive of cavernous smooth muscle degeneration. This assumption correlates well with the electron microscopic findings in patients with venous leakage (Persson et al. 1989).

Our findings in normal patients suggest that during flaccidity, the contractions of the cavernous smooth muscle cells are synchronized by the sympathetic tone. This results in a potential of high amplitude and long duration that can be simultaneously recorded in different areas of both cavernous bodies. With increasing tumescence and rigidity to physiological stimulation, the sympathetic tone is dramatically reduced, resulting in non-synchronisation of the contractions of the smooth muscle cells. This results in potentials of decreased amplitude and length, but in an increase in frequency.

SPACE may be a minimally invasive and reproducible diagnostic method to evaluate autonomic cavernous innervation; the diagnosis of cavernous smooth muscle degeneration seems possible. Further comparative studies with electron microscopic controls are needed to evaluate the correlation between our interpretation of SPACE and morphological findings.

References

Gerstenberg TC, Nordling J, Hald H, Wagner G (1989) Standardized evaluation of erectile dysfunction in 95 consecutive patients. J Urol 141:857

Lavoisier P, Proulx J, Courtois F, Carful F (1989) Bulbocavernous reflex. J Urol 141:311

Persson C, Diederichs W, Lue TF, Yen TS, Fishman I, McLin PH, Tanagho ET (1989) Correlation of altered ultrastructure with clinical arterial evaluation. J Urol 142:1462

Siroky MB, Sax DS, Krane RJ (1979) Sacral signal tracing. J Urol 122:661

Stief CG, Bähren W, Gall H, Scherb W (1988) Functional evaluation of penile hemodynamics. J Urol 139:734

Wagner G (1976) Contractility of myometrial transplants. In: Coutinhu EM, Fuchs F (eds) Physiology and genetics of reproduction, part B. Plenum, New York

Wetterauer U, Stief CG, Kulvelis F, Staubesand J, Sommerkamp H (1990) The electron microscopic ultrastructure of cavernous tissue in erectile dysfunction. J Urol 143:509A

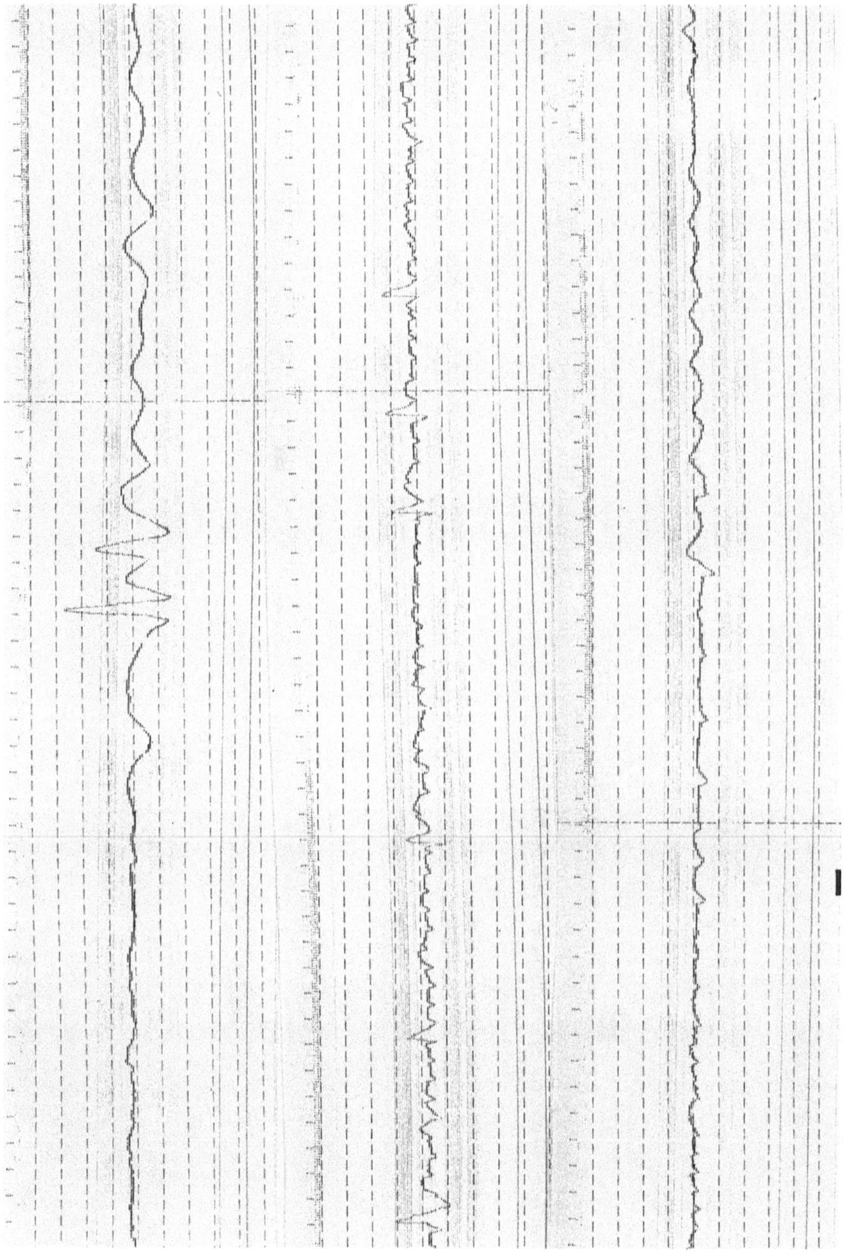

Fig. 4. The *upper tracing* shows the recording during flaccidity in a normal patient (one large potential); the *middle line* shows the electrical activity during tumescence to audiovisual sexual stimulation. The *lower tracing* shows the electrical activity during full erection. Cut-off frequencies are 0.5 – 500 Hz, the *horizontal bar* is 5 s, the *vertical bar* 100 µV

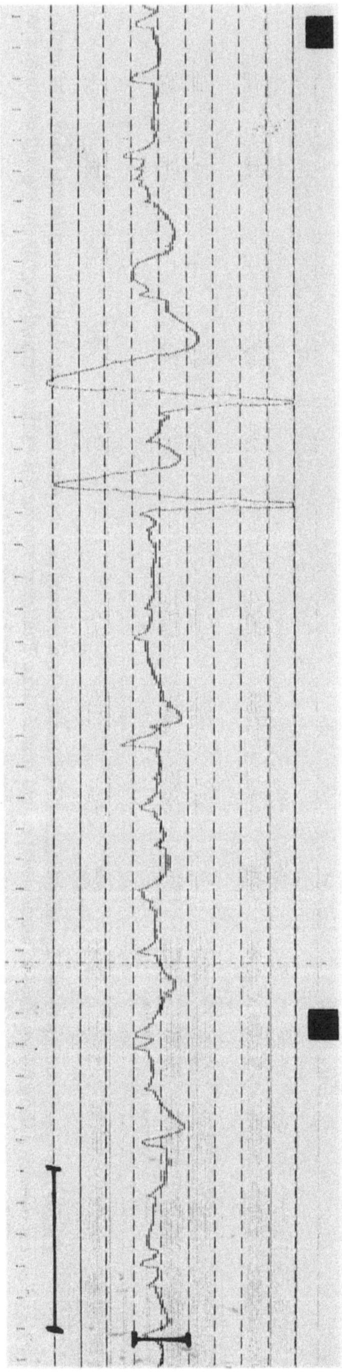

Fig. 5. One year after radical prostatectomy, SPACE shows abnormal as well as normal potentials in a 65-year-old impotent man. The *horizontal bar* is 5 s, the *vertical bar* 100 µV; cut-off frequencies are 0.5 – 500 Hz

III. BPH, Prostate Cancer

Imprint and Scrape Cytology: Advantages and Possible Uses in Urology

H. AL-ABADI, R. FRIEDRICHS, V. BORGMANN, I. ROTTER, and R. NAGEL [1]

Introduction

Imprint and scrape cytology are variations of a form of applied cytology that is only rarely used here in Germany. While as a techniques they are fundamentally different from exfoliative and aspiration cytology (i.e., fine needle biopsy), in some ways they are also related to these two methods. They are employed for diagnostic purposes in scientific research and in the training and continuing training of cytologists and urologists interested in cytology (Al-Abadi and Nagel 1988a, b; Müller and Böhm 1974; Shidham et al. 1984; Skopa et al. 1990).

Material and Methods

In the period between 1983 and 1989 imprint and scrape cytology were performed intraoperatively in addition to rapid frozen section diagnosis in 953 cases.

Several cytological preparations were made from each tissue sample, either by lightly pressing the freshly cut surface of the tissue onto a slide or by scraping it. The preparations were fixed with Merckofix fixation spray and stained using a variation of Panaicolaou's method developed by ourselves for rapid diagnosis. They were ready for evaluation after 3–4 min (see Figs. 1–5).

Results

The cytological findings were compared with the rapid frozen section diagnoses (Table 1) and the definitive histopathological diagnoses of the tissues embedded in paraffin. The results agreed in 99.8% of cases. The rate of false-positive results was 0.2% and there were no false-negative findings. Kidney tumors were found in 31% cases, tumors of the testis in 23%, bladder tumors in 23%, tumors of the renal pelvis and ureter in 17%, and other categories of tumor or tissue or suspected malignancy in 6%.

[1] Urologische Klinik und Poliklinik der Freien Universität, Klinikum Rudolf Virchow, Standort Charlottenburg, Spandauer Damm 130, W-1000 Berlin 19, FRG.

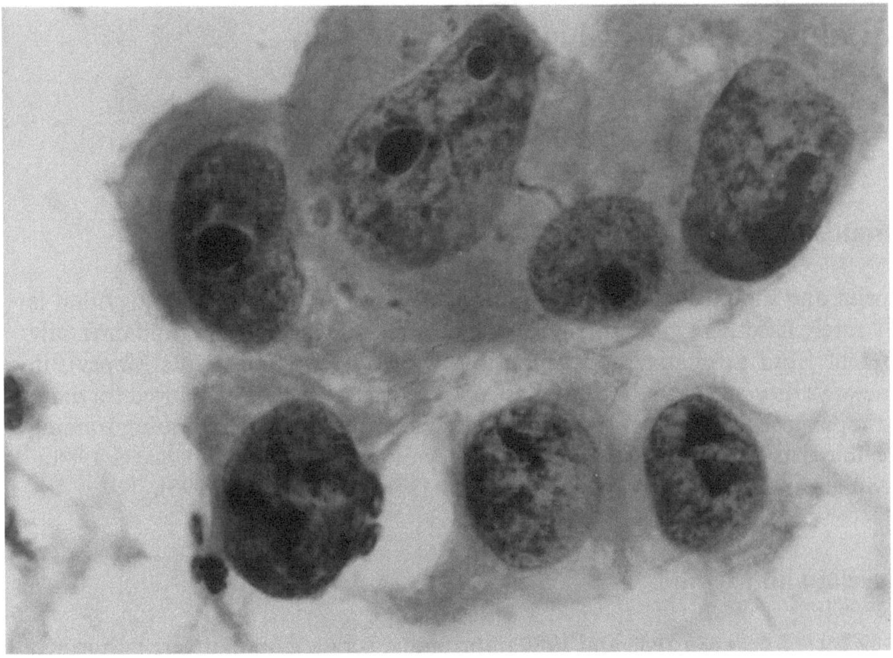

Fig. 1. Imprint smear of a kidney tumor. Hyperchromatic, polymorphic epithelial nuclei with prominent polymorphic nucleoli. Grade III carcinoma of the renal cells, ×1000

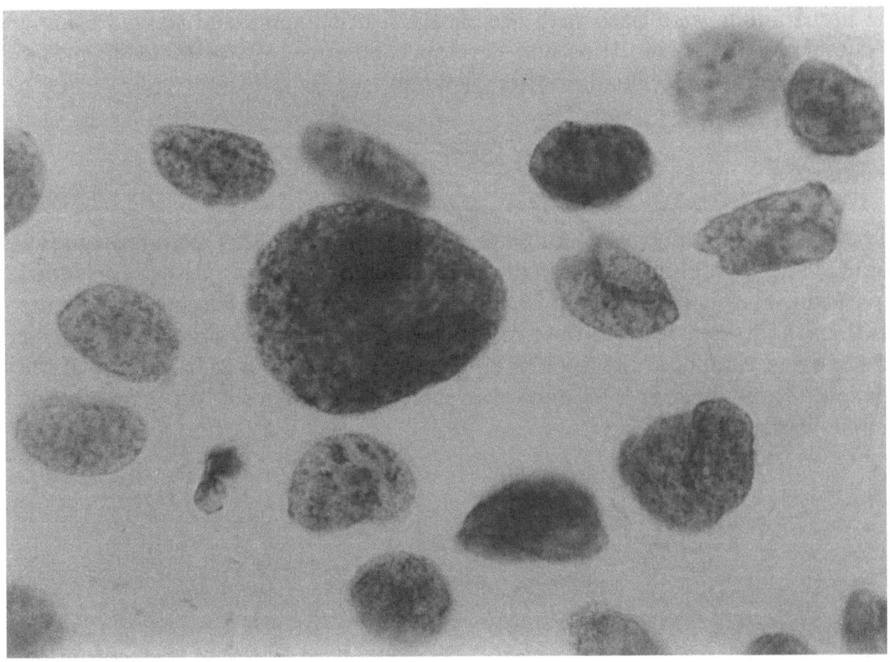

Fig. 2. Imprint smear with Feulgen's reaction. Strongly stained, tumor nuclei occurring singly. No artefacts. (DNA measurement) ×1000

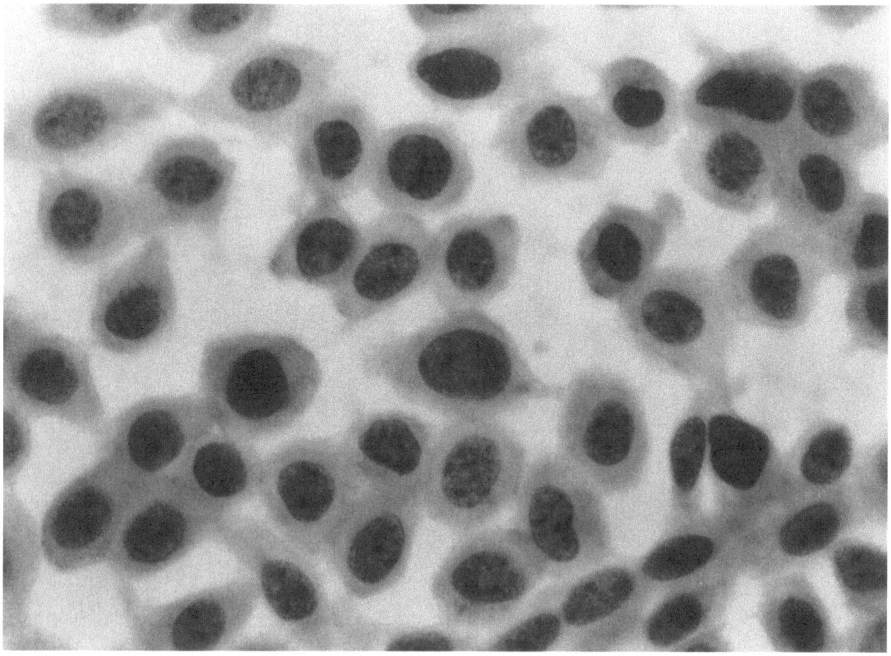

Fig. 3. Imprint cytology of tumors of the renal pelvis. Moderate nuclear polymorphism and hyperchromatism. Grade II urothelial carcinoma, ×400

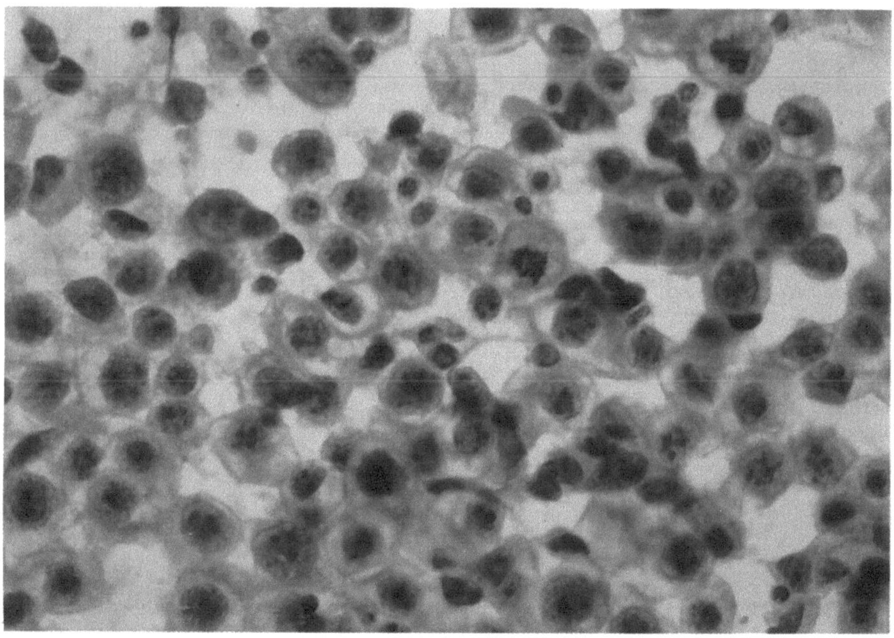

Fig. 4. Imprint cytology of tumors of the testis. Typical seminoma with polymorphic, hyperchromatic germinal cell epithelium with tumor cell mitoses, prominent nucleoli and typical inflammatory infiltrate. Papanicolaou stain, ×400

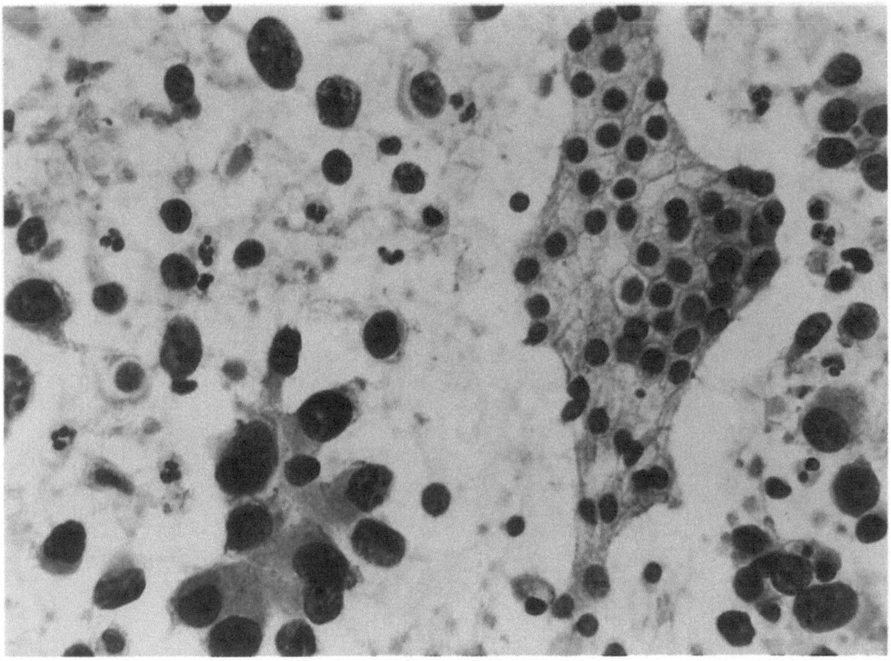

Fig. 5. Imprint cytology in transurethral resection of the prostate. Normal clusters of cells from prostate epithelium with typical reticular structure and abundant hyperchromatic and distinctly polymorphic epithelial nuclei from a grade II urothelial carcinoma infiltrating the prostate, ×400

Table 1. Imprint and scrape cytology vs rapid frozen section ($n = 953$)

Cytological diagnosis	Correct diagnosis		False-positive diagnosis		False-negative diagnosis		Suspected		Total
	n	%	*n*	%	*n*	%	*n*	%	
Imprint and scrape cytology									
Benign	181	98.9	1	0.5	–	–	1	0.5	183
Malignant	767	99.6	1	0.1	–	–	2	0.2	770
Rapid frozen section									
Benign	169	92.3	4	2.18	2	1.09	8	4.37	183
Malignant	732	95.0	9	1.16	11	1.40	18	2.30	770

Conclusions

Our investigations have shown that imprint and scrape cytology are excellent methods and should be employed more as a routine measure, since in experienced hands they are a much faster alternative to histological rapid frozen section diagnosis. They are also suitable for use in scientific research, especially since they can be used in combination with single-cell DNA cytophotometry and for immunocytochemical evaluation (Al-Abadi and Nagel 1988a, b).

References

Al-Abadi H, Nagel R (1988a) Prognostische Bedeutung von Ploidie und proliferativer Aktivität beim lokal fortgeschrittenen Prostatakarzinom. Akt Urol 19:182–186

Al-Abadi H, Nagel R (1988b) Prognostic relevance of ploidy and proliferative activity of renal cell carcinoma. Eur Urol 15:271–276

Müller H-A, Böhm W (1974) Vergleichende imprint-zytologische und histologische Untersuchungen an menschlichen Speicheldrüsentumoren. Verh Dtsch Ges Pathol 58:504

Shidham VB, David NV, Grover S, Kher AV (1984) Role of scrape zytology in rapid intraoperative diagnosis. Value and limitations. Acta Cytol 28:477–482

Scopa Ch-D, Melachrinou M, Apessou D, Bonikus D (1990) Tissue imprints in surgical pathology. A rapid intraoperative diagnostic aid. Diagn Cytopathol 6:5–8

^{31}P-NMR Spectroscopy and ^{1}H Imaging of the Prostate – Differences between Benign Hyperplasia and Cancers

F. HERING and S. MÜLLER[1]

Introduction

Conventional magnetic resonance imaging (MRI) of the prostate used strictly noninvasively by means of volume coils or surface coils operating at the periphery of the body fails in predicting tumor stage correctly, especially in distinguishing tumor infiltration of the capsule or infiltration of the seminal vesicles.

Stimulated by Narayan and Hricak (1987), who recently reported differences in the metabolite concentrations of benign prostate hyperplasia (BPH) and prostate carcinomas using a transrectal probe for ^{31}P spectroscopy, we developed a transrectal probe designed for spectroscopy and imaging. The advantage of a transrectal probe is a high filling factor and consequently MR spectra of high sensivity.

Material and Methods

In this study we used a similar experimental set-up for investigation of the human prostate. However, in contrast to previous reports, a further step of experimental simplification was attained by acquiring both ^{31}P spectra and ^{1}H images with a single transrectal transmit-receive surface coil.

All experiments were performed using a Siemens Magnetom 63/84 operating at 1.5 Tesla. ^{31}P spectra and ^{1}H images were obtained using a 2-cm surface coil protected by a smoothly rounded cover of hard plastic. The probe is digitally positioned under the prostate. The tuning and matching circuit of the probe is placed in a Faraday box close to the coil and can be manipulated from outside the magnet. A second tuning capacitor can be added by a switch and permits tuning the probe to ^{1}H or ^{31}P (Fig. 1).

Several different strategies for ^{1}H imaging with the transmit-receive surface coil were explored to avoid image artefacts due to flip-angle variations close to the surface coil. The best results were obtained with FISP sequences and slice orientations parallel to the surface coil plane.

^{31}P spectra of the peripheral zone of the prostate were acquired in 10–20 min using a 180° pulse at the coil center. Shimming was done with the same coil tuned to ^{1}H.

In addition, extracts of prostate carcinoma tissue obtained by transurethral resection were measured in vitro in a Bruker MSL 400 System at 162 MHz and compared with the in vivo results.

[1] Urologische Klinik und MR-Zentrum, Universitätsklinik Basel, Spitalstrasse 21, 4031 Basel, Switzerland.

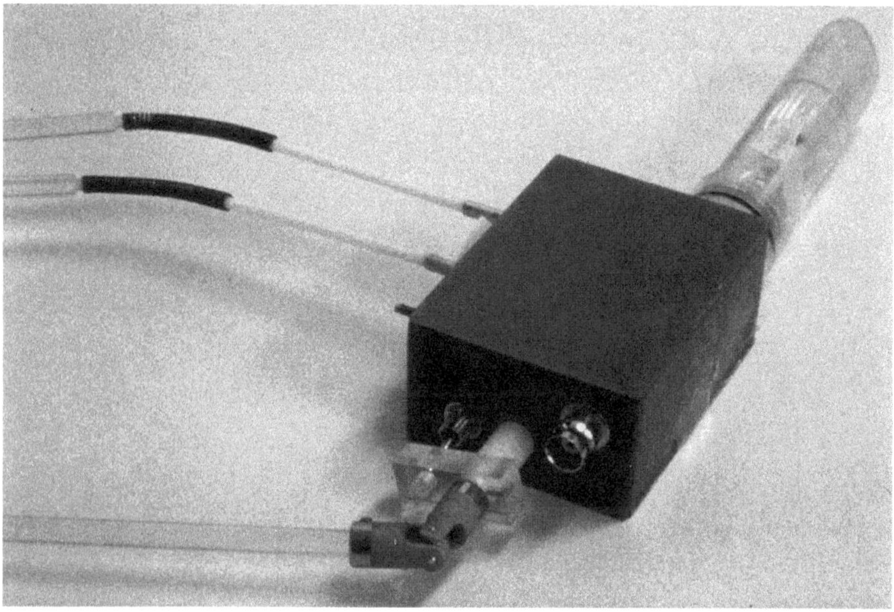

Fig. 1. Transrectal transmit-receive surface coil for obtaining both ^{31}P spectra and ^{1}H images

To date, 20 patients (10 with BPH and 10 with prostate carcinomas) have been investigated.

Results

As an example, we show the ^{31}P spectra of one patient with BPH, one patient with prostate carcinoma stage T4 N2, and the in vitro spectrogram of the tissue of the last patient obtained by TUR (Fig. 2).

There are no differences in the ATP and ADP spectra, but generally lower phosphomonoester/ATP ratios in patients with prostate carcinoma. The same observation was made by Thomas, a coworker of the San Francisco based group who in 1987 reported similar ^{31}P spectra using a transrectal probe (Thomas et al. 1989).

The ^{31}P spectra of a patient radically prostatectomized for pT3 pNO G2 prostate carcinoma and a patient with BPH are compared in Fig. 3. The patient with carcinoma exhibited a much lower phosphomonoester concentration, 5 versus 64, and subsequently a lower phosphomonoester/ATP ratio, 0.13 versus 0.8. The same observation was made in the whole prostate carcinoma group compared to patients with BPH.

Figure 4 shows typical ^{1}H imaging pictures of a patient with BPH. The probe is positioned in the rectum surrounded by air, stool, and lubricating jelly. Ventral to the probe the prostate is visible, with a smooth capsule and a regular inner structure. Figure 4b shows a longitudinal image with parts of the Os pubis.

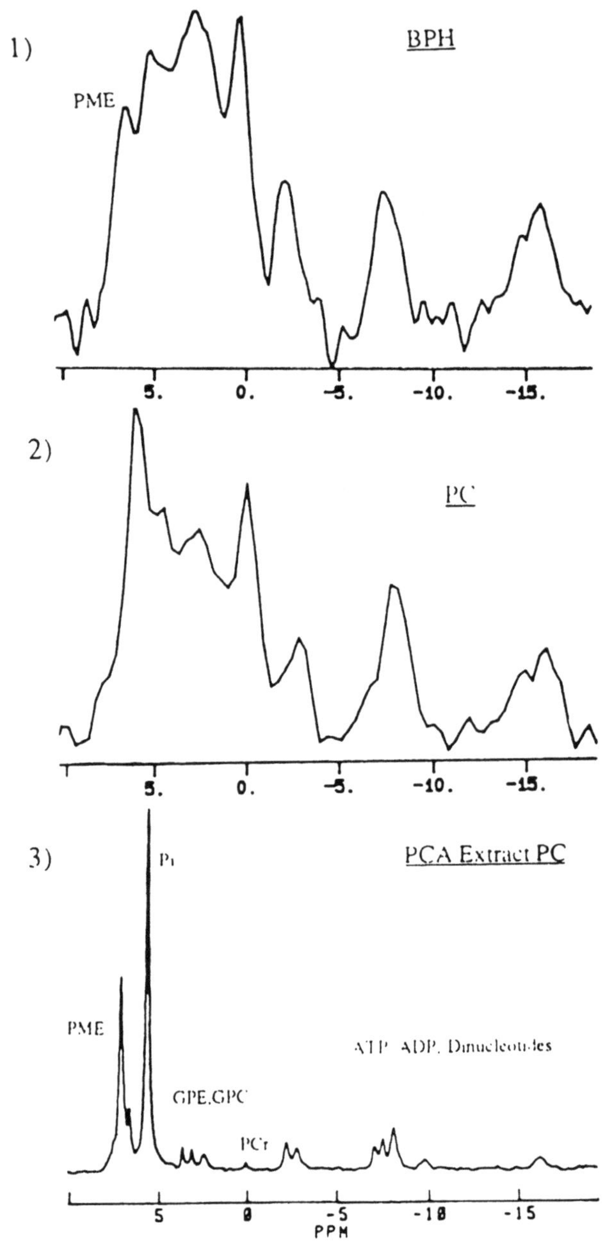

Fig. 2. Comparison of ^{31}P spectra of one patient with benign prostate hyperplasia (*BPH*), one with prostate carcinoma (*PC*), and tissue obtained after TUR-P for prostate carcinoma in a third (*PCA Extract PC*)

Figure 5 shows pictures of a patient radically prostatectomized for a pT3 pNO carcinoma. The pathohistologic report describes an infiltration of the periprostatic fat without involvement of the seminal vesicles. On both sides the border between the prostate and the capsule has been lost. Moreover, the inner structure of the gland has a somewhat irregular pattern. The hole in the prostate corresponds to the urethra.

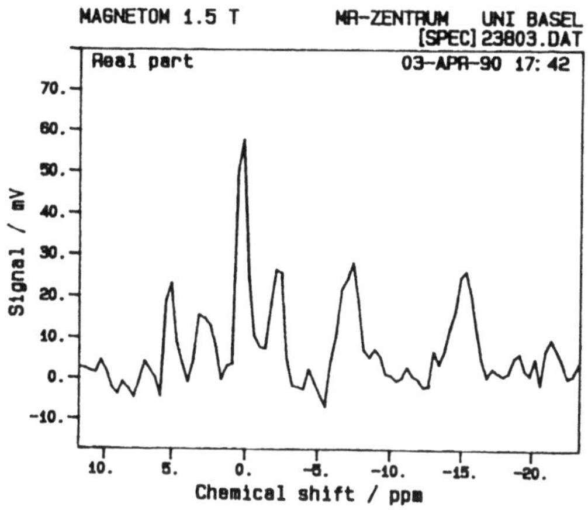

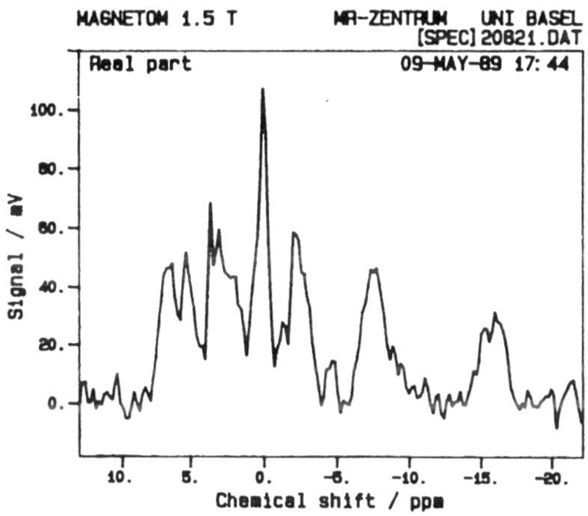

Fig. 3. Comparison of ^{31}P spectra of a patient radically prostatectomized for prostate carcinoma stage pT3 pNO G2 MO and a patient with benign hyperplasia

Summary

The differences between phosphomonoester/ATP ratios in BPH and carcinomas may help in distinguishing between different prostatic diseases.

In the planning of radical prostatectomy, ^{1}H imaging can help to detect infiltration of the seminal vesicles or capsular penetration. The inhomogeneous structure in cases with carcinoma, again in combination with the spectrogram, can help to establish the diagnosis.

References

Narayan P, Hricak H (1987) Promising areas of research explored at Veterans Administration Center. VA medical center, vol 5, no 1, pp 11

Thomas et al. (1989) ^{31}Phosphorus MR spectroscopy of human prostate in vivo. Proc SMRM, Amsterdam, p 297

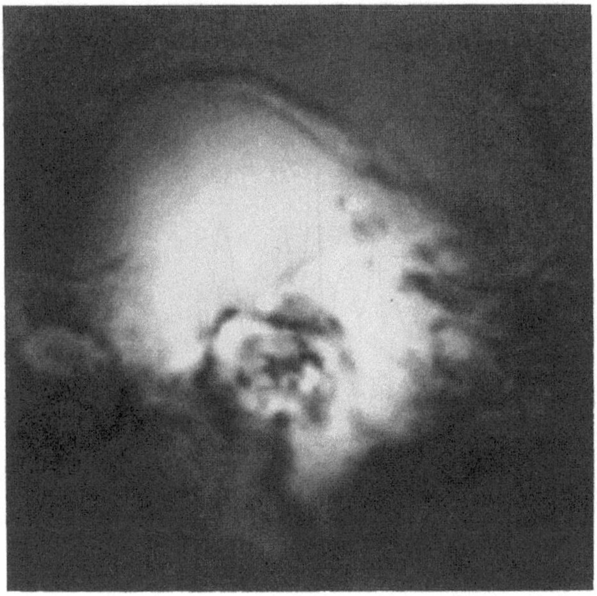

a

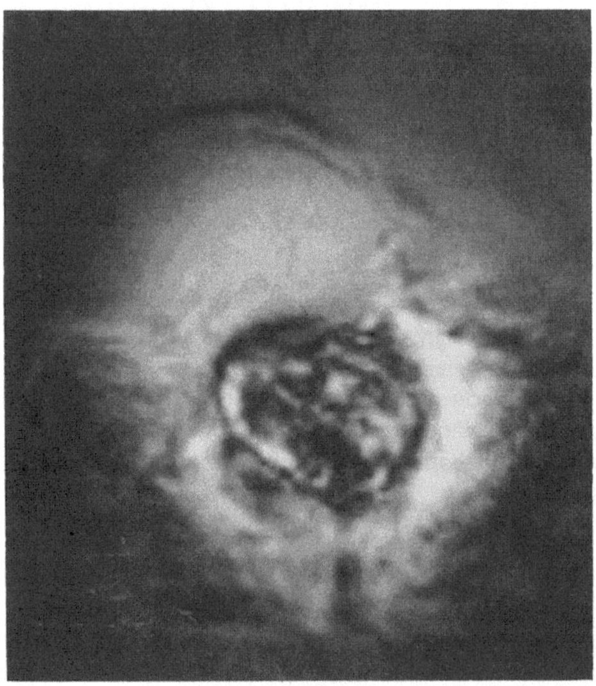

b

Fig. 4a, b. ^{1}H Imaging of prostates with benign hyperplasia

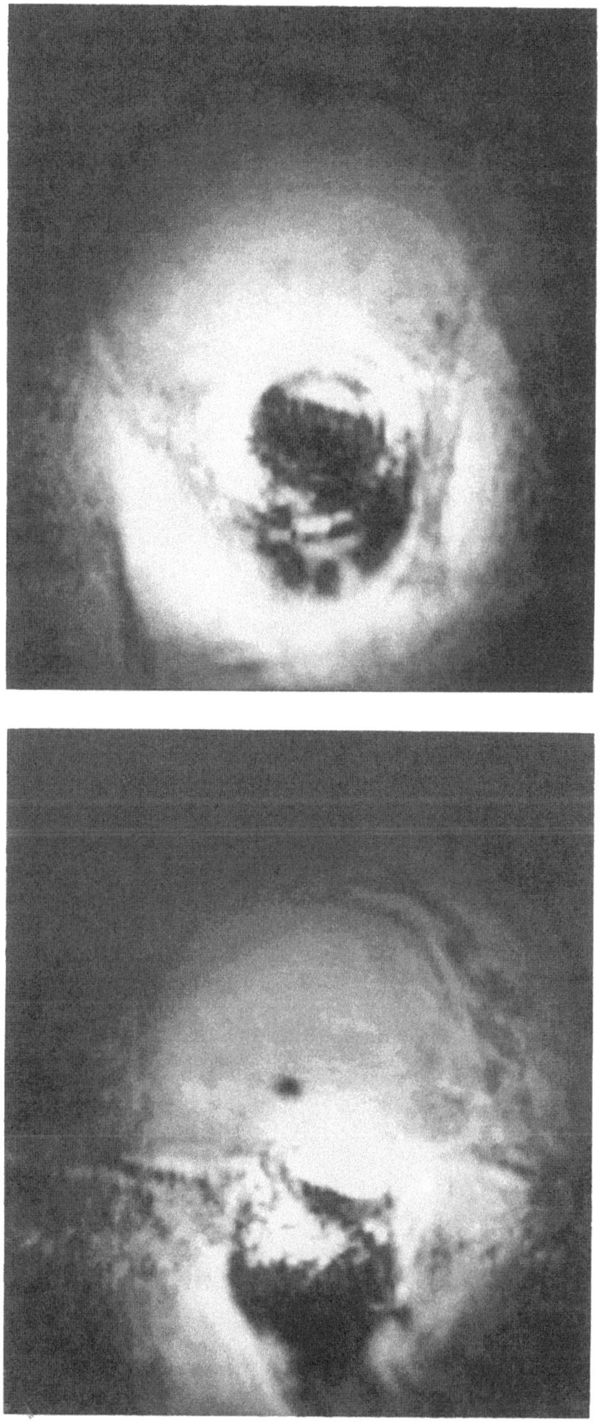

a

b

Fig. 5a, b. ^{1}H Imaging of a prostate radically excised for a tumor stage pT3

IV. Bladder, Bladder Cancer

Evaluation of Acute-Phase Proteins for Clinical Monitoring of Urinary Tract Infections and Postoperatively

D. M. WILBERT, C. SCHAERFE, W. L. STROHMAIER, and K.-H. BICHLER[1]

Introduction

The classical and laboratory signs of inflammation such as elevated body temperature, blood sedimentation rate or serum leucocyte count, do not always provide accurate information on the status of an inflammatory disease. The same is true when these variables are used to monitor patients immediately postoperatively, particularly after major surgery.

Measurement techniques available today for several types of acute-phase proteins constitute interesting diagnostic tools for the monitoring of bacterial infectious diseases (Behr 1989). C-reactive protein (CRP) is the best known acute-phase protein, in addition to complement 3 (C3) or haptoglobin. CRP is a glycoprotein with a molecular weight of 105 500 Daltons. Its production by hepatocytes is initiated by infections, inflammatory reactions and tissue traumatization and mediated by interleukin 1. Activation of CRP by components of bacterial or cellular membranes leads to precipitation of soluble ligands, activation of the complement cascade, interaction with lymphocytes and aggregation of thrombocytes. Significant elevation of CRP serum levels are demonstrable 6 h after the initial stimulus (Behr 1989; Kushner 1978). After cessation of stimulation, CRP levels decline with a half-life of approximately 48 h, until a normal value below 0.6 mg/100 ml is reached.

In a prospective study the acute-phase proteins CRP, haptoglobin and C3c were compared with the above-mentioned classical indicators of inflammation to determine their value for monitoring of inflammations with particular respect to urinary tract infections and urological surgery.

Material and Methods

There were a total of 30 patients in three groups. Group 1 consisted of 10 patients with infections of the urogenital tract such as epididymitis or septicaemia secondary to pyelonephritis. The second group consisted of 10 patients who had undergone minor urological surgery like inguinal orchiectomy, penile surgery or prostate biopsy. The third group was of a further 10 patients who had had major surgery, such as lymphadenectomy, cystectomy, nephrectomy or radical prostatectomy.

In all patients the following were measured every other day for at least 9 days: CRP, haptoglobin, C3c, blood sedimentation rate, leucocyte and thrombocyte

[1] Urologische Universitätsklinik, Hoppe-Seyler-Str. 3, W-7400 Tübingen, FRG.

count, body temperature, prothrombin time, antithrombin and partial thromboplastin time. CRP was determined by three different methods: radial immunodiffusion with LC-partigen plates, enzyme-linked immunosorbent assay (Melisa, Elias-Company, Freiburg, FRG) (Martinez and Coll 1987), and photometric measurement of opalescence (turbidimetry, Turbitimer, Behringwerke, Marburg, FRG). All other measurements were made by routine laboratory methods. The results are given as percentage variation from the normal values.

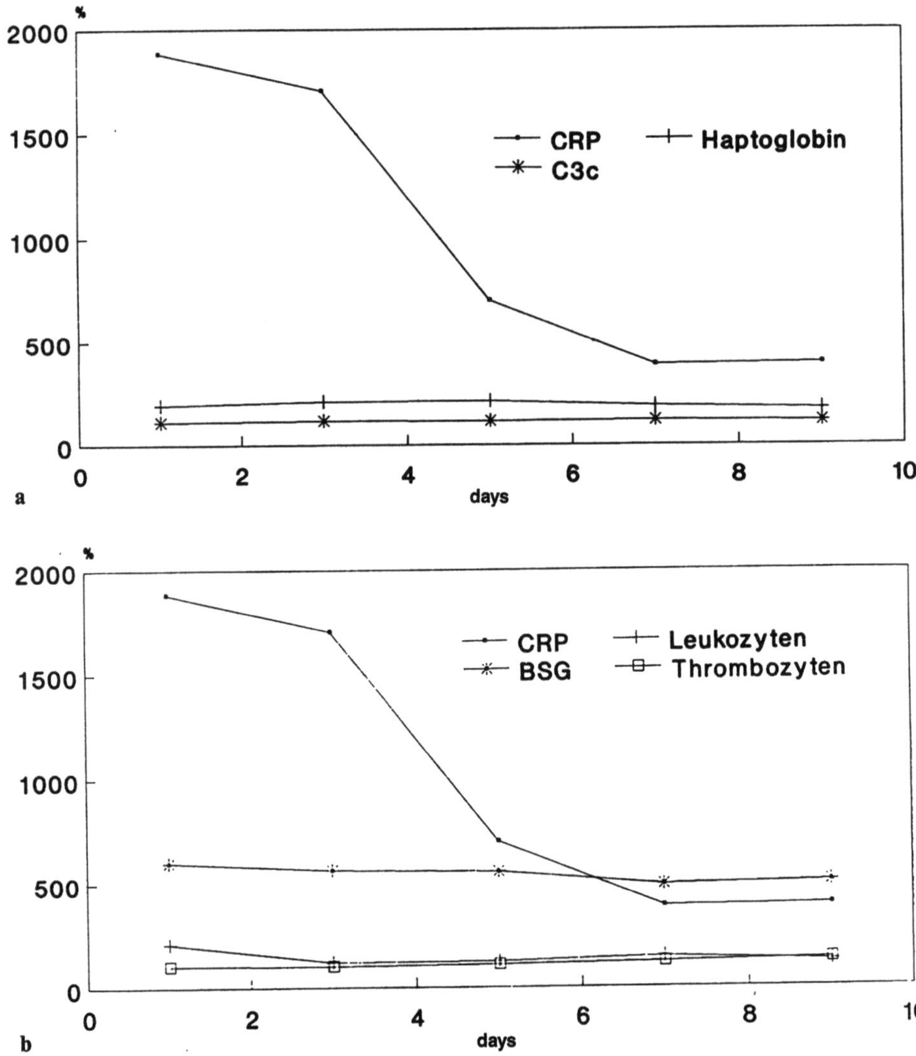

Fig. 1. a Serial determinations of CRP, haptoglobin and C3c in group 1 patients (urogenital infections, $n = 10$). Means of ten measurements expressed as percentage variation from normal value. **b** Serial determinations of CRP, leucocytes, blood sedimentation rate and thrombocytes in group 1 patients (urogenital infections, $n = 10$). Means of ten measurements expressed as percentage variation from normal value

Results

Group 1: At day 1 CRP was elevated 1805% above normal, declining towards normal values within 7 days after initiation of appropriate antibiotic therapy. Haptoglobin increased from day 1 (197%) to day 5 (213%) and declined thereafter to 175% of normal on day 9. C3c showed only minor variations from 112% to 105% between day 1 and 9. The blood sedimentation rate was substantially elevated to 601%, on day 1. In the following days it declined very little, to 508% on day 9. The leucocyte count, initially elevated at 211%, fell back to 125% on day 9 (see Fig. 1a and b).

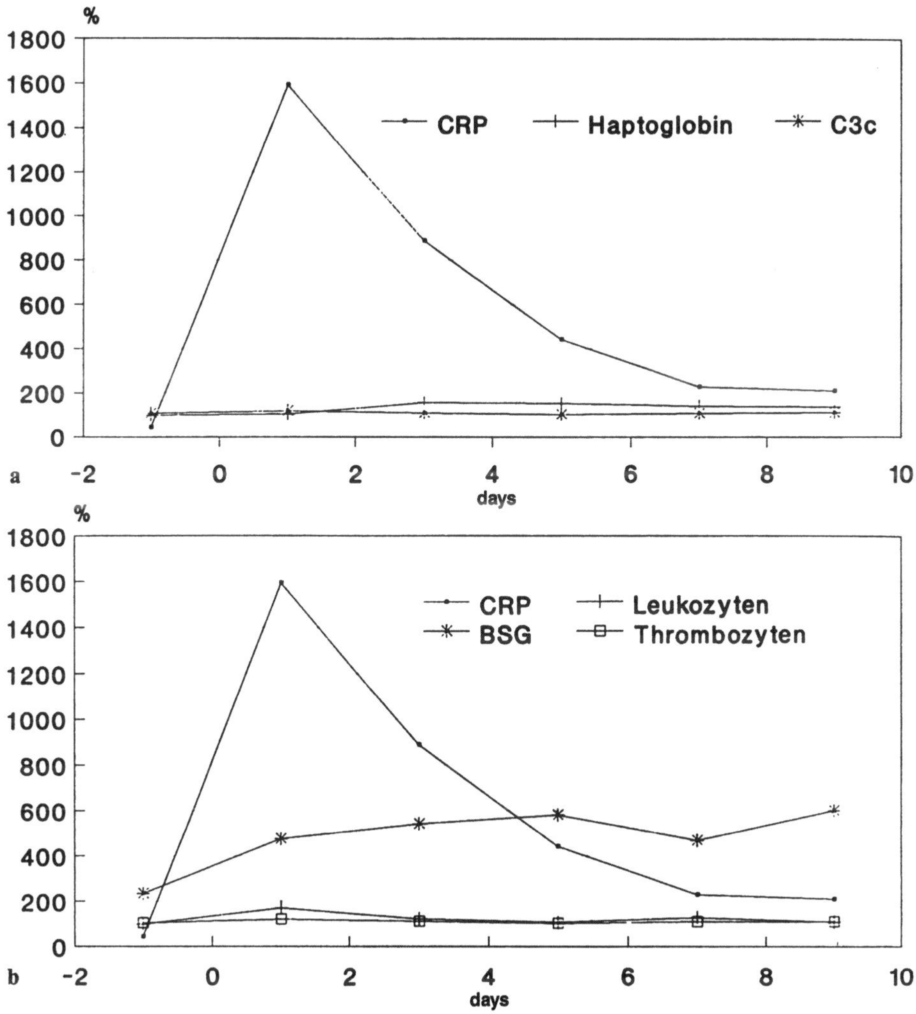

Fig. 2. a Serial determinations of CRP, haptoglobin and C3c in group 3 patients (major surgery, $n = 10$). Means of ten measurements expressed as percentage variation from normal value. **b** Serial determinations of CRP, leucocytes, blood sedimentation rate and thrombocytes in group 3 patients (major surgery, $n = 10$). Means of ten measurements expressed as percentage variation from normal value

Group 2: All preoperative tests were within normal limits. On postoperative day 1, CRP levels were increased to 435% and gradually declined to normal values by day 7. Haptoglobin reached its maximum on day 3 and did not reattain the normal limits by day 9. C3c was highest on day 7, being only slightly elevated (113%). The increase in blood sedimentation rate reached its maximum on day 3 (271%). The leucocyte count was raised to 140% on postoperative day 1, declining to normal values on day 5.

Group 3: Except for the blood sedimentation rate, all tests produced findings within normal limits preoperatively. On postoperative day 1 CRP rose to 1593%, thereafter declining with a half-life of 48 h. Haptoglobin was only moderately elevated on day 3 (158%). C3c decreased slightly. The blood sedimentation rate reached its maximum on day 9, at 600%. The leucocyte count was elevated to 170% on postoperative day 1, declining over the next 5 days, rising on day 7, and resuming normal values on day 9 (see Fig. 2a and b).

No results of any coagulation tests are shown, as they did not demonstrate any significant changes except for the thrombocytes, which were slightly reduced in group 1.

Looking at results of the various tests for determination of CRP, the radial immunodiffusion test had an inter-assay coefficient of variation of 7.28% as compared to 8.5% with the ELISA test and 4.8% with the turbidimetry. The intra-assay coefficient of variation was 3.9% with turbidimetry and 3.1% with the ELISA test.

Discussion

Because of the rapid and significant rise in its levels, CRP appears to be the most distinctive test for the evaluation of infectious or traumatizing stimuli of all the acute-phase proteins and all other laboratory variables measured (Hellerstein 1982; Maury 1984). By determining serial CRP levels, it is possible to assess ongoing infections and their response to antimicrobial therapy or complications after surgery, such as abscess formation. When the stimulation of acute-phase proteins subsides, CRP rapidly resumes normal levels, due to its short half-life of 48 h. CRP levels are not elevated by viral infections or tumors. It is therefore used in pediatric patients to differentiate viral from bacterial infections (e.g., meningitis).

The test results of the MELISA assay and turbidimetry were comparable; however, for small series turbidimetry is more rapid and less expensive. With the new tests available, namely CRP-ELISA and turbidimetry, CRP determination should be used routinely to monitor patients with severe infections of the urinary tract and patients undergoing major urological surgery.

References

Behr W (1989) Nach Infektionen fahnden – die CRP-Bestimmung: Möglichkeiten und Grenzen. Diagn Lab 39:95–106

Hellerstein S, Duggan E, Welchert E, Mansour F (1982) Serum C-reactive protein and the site of urinary tract infections. J Pediatr 100:21–25

Kushner I, Broder ML, Karp D (1978) Control of the acute phase response. J Clin Invest 61:235–242
Martinez JA, Coll JM (1987) Preliminary clinical studies of C-reactive protein quantified by enzyme-linked immunoassay. Clin Chem 33:2185–2190
Maury CPJ, Teppo AM (1984) Comparative study of serum amyloid-related protein SAA, C-reactive protein and β-2-microglobulin as markers of renal allograft rejection. Clin Nephrol 22:284–292

Lysosomal Enzymuria in the Diagnosis of Upper versus Lower Urinary Tract Infections

C. Skrezek, H. Bertermann, and H. Wand[1]

Introduction

For following the progress of renal infections, particularly when there is a question whether the cause of a kidney infection can be corrected surgically, it is important to be able to differentiate between urinary tract infections in which the renal parenchyma is involved and those in which it is not. The classical symptoms, such as fever and flank pain, can occur in bladder and kidney infections, according to findings by Busch and Huland 1984, just as antibody-coated bacteria have been found in both cases (Stamey 1980).

The lysosomal enzyme *N*-acetyl-β-D-glucosaminidase (NAG) is localized selectively in proximal tubular cells of the kidney and is excreted when the function of these cells is impaired. With the methodological progress made in the preanalytic phase and the optimization of the colorimetric test, NAG has meanwhile become a highly sensitive marker of occult renal dysfunction. It is simple to be measured by a photometer after a few pipetting steps. In a clinical study we therefore tested the value of NAG as a diagnostic index for demonstrating or excluding a renal infection.

Material and Methods

54 patients, 28–68 years old, with acute urinary tract infections were investigated prospectively. Clinical status, laboratory findings, bacteriology, sonography, urography, and renal functions were evaluated in order to try to identify two patient groups: those with (A) and those without (B) renal infections, i.e., acute pyelonephritis.

Urine was collected as follows: the first micturition was discarded and each subsequent micturition in 3-h or 24-h periods was measured for volume and aliquot portions centrifugated and cooled to 4 °C. Urinary NAG (for method see Skrezek et al. 1990) and creatinine (Jaffé method) were measured by colorimetry. Urinary excretion of sodium and potassium (flame photometry) and clearance of endogenous creatinine were determined simultaneously.

[1] Urologische Universitätsklinik, Arnold-Heller-Str. 7, W-2300 Kiel, FRG.

Results

In 12 men between 20 and 23 years of age with healthy kidneys, the daily NAG excretion profile was measured in urine samples taken at 3 h intervals. The average values ranged from 1.3 to 2.2 Θ/g creatinine, with maximum levels occurring in the early morning hours (6–9 a.m.) and minimum levels in the early evening (6–9 p.m.; Fig. 1). Similar studies on older patients revealed the same circadian rhythm at slightly higher levels. The mean of all control groups was 2.5 U/g creatinine. Taking into account the standard deviation, we set the upper limit of the normal range at 2.8 U/g creatinine (not shown).

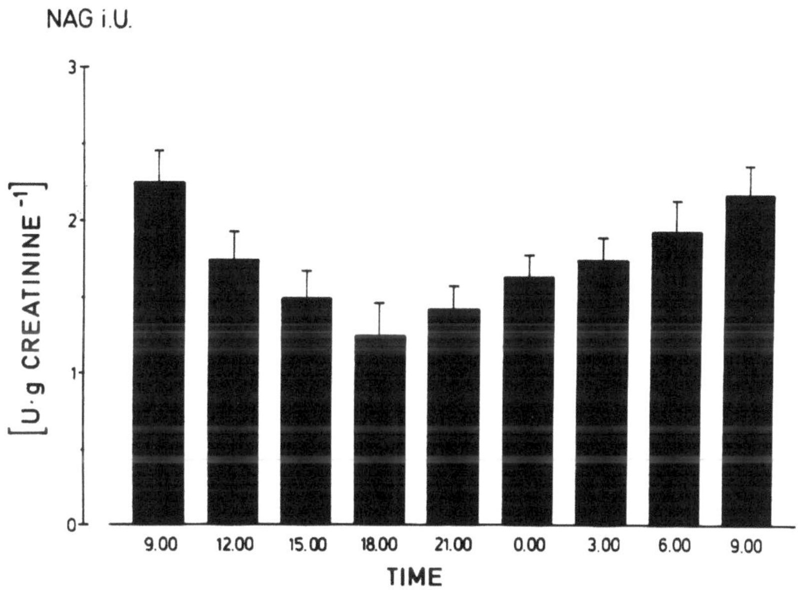

Fig. 1. Circadian variation in NAG excretion in urine collected from a group of young men ($n = 12$) with healthy kidneys ($\bar{X} \pm$ SEM)

In 20 patients with acute pyelonephritis, NAG excretion was measured at the time of diagnosis and subsequently during 14 days of antibiotic therapy. Figure 2 shows the results. The highest values measured averaged 50 U/g creatinine. When treatment was successful, NAG excretion dropped dramatically, but it did not reach normal levels again until the 2nd week. In distal urinary tract infections, such as cystitis, urethritis, or epididymitis, no increased release of NAG was found.

Prolonged increased enzyme release or a renewed rise indicated protracted or recurrent infection. Figure 3 shows a dramatic renewed increase in NAG excretion in 7 patients, in whom enzyme excretion did not return to normal until 1 week after a change to a different antibiotic. Bacteriological investigation showed a change in pathogens and/or development of resistance to antibiotic therapy. The

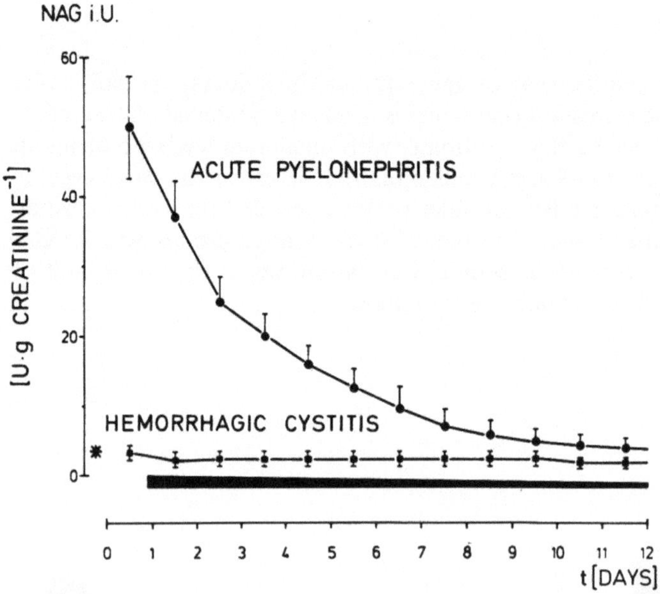

Fig. 2. NAG excretion in the urine of patients with urinary tract infections during antibiotic therapy. *Bar*, antibiotic therapy; ● acute pyelonephritis; ■ hemorrhagic cystitis; * upper limit of the normal range ($n = 16$; $\bar{X} \pm$SEM)

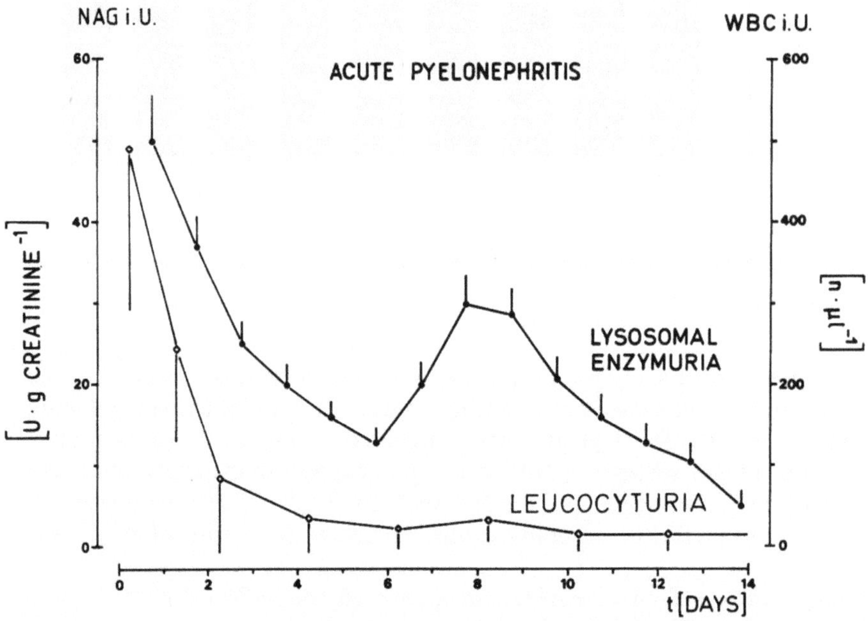

Fig. 3. Time courses of lysosomal enzymuria (NAG, *closed circles*) and leucocyturia (white blood cells, *open circles*) in recurrent kidney infections (relapse, reinfection) during antibiotic therapy ($n = 7$; $\bar{X} \pm$SEM)

open diamond symbols illustrate the white blood cell count in the urine measured simultaneously, which is indicated on the right ordinate: it can be clearly seen that this index stagnated, compared with NAG excretion.

Figure 4 shows the percentage of patients with pathological urinary findings, comparing the two indices, in 27 patients with acute pyelonephritis. In the 1st week white blood cells are detectable in the urinary findings of 25 patients (93%). Twenty-six patients (96%) show pathologically elevated NAG excretion. The situation is completely different in the 2nd week: only 18 patients (66%) still show leucocyturia while 24 (89%) have a pathological level of NAG excretion.

At the same time as evaluating the rate of enzyme release, we assayed the renal K^+ excretion rate in all 27 patients with acute pyelonephritis. When the NAG excretion rate was normal, the K^+ excretion rate was about 60 μM/min; with increasing NAG excretion rate the K^+ excretion rate dropped to 15 μM/min. Calculations showed the regression to be linear. The correlation coefficient was −0.98 (Fig. 5). The K^+ measured in the urine originates primarily in secretion processes in the distal segment of the tubule. It is therefore evident that renal infection damages both the proximal tubules and the distal tubules equally.

In all patients with acute pyelonephritis, daily measurements of the clearance of endogenous creatinine were taken as a measure of the glomerular filtration rate (GFR). When the NAG excretion rate was normal, a GFR of about 110 ml/min was found. As the NAG excretion rate rose, the GFR dropped to 40 ml/min. There was a linear correlation between the NAG excretion rate and the GFR in patients with acute pyelonephritis in one or both kidneys; the correlation coefficient was −0.95 (Fig. 6). No substantial differences were found between NAG excretion rates based on 3-h vs 24-h urine-collecting periods.

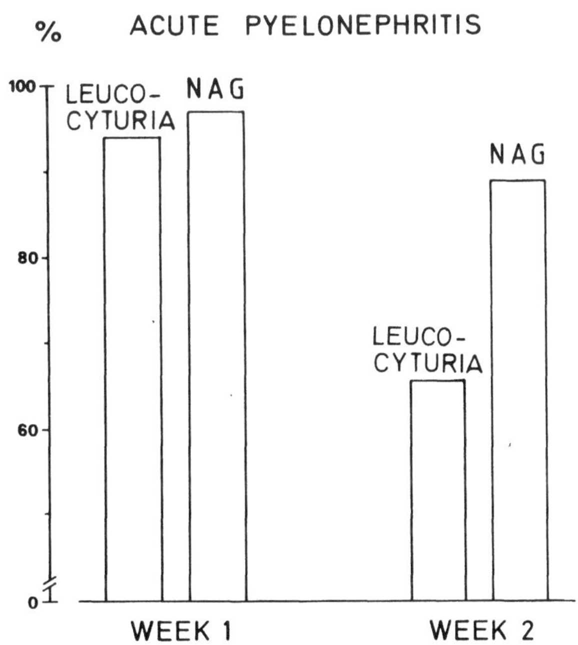

Fig. 4. Percentage of increased urinary NAG excretion and leucocyturia in acute pyelonephritis. Comparison of the 1st and 2nd weeks of antibiotic therapy ($n = 27$)

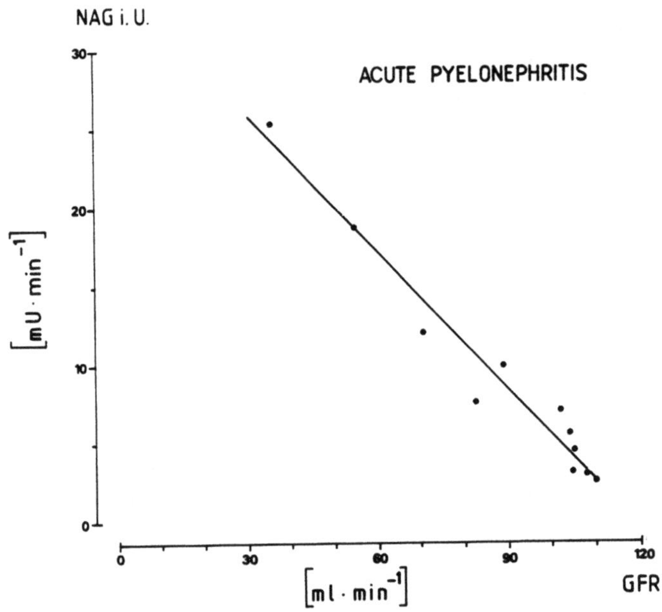

Fig. 5. Correlation between the renal K^+ excretion rate and the rate of urinary NAG release in patients with acute pyelonephritis in one or both kidneys ($n = 27$; $r = -0.98$)

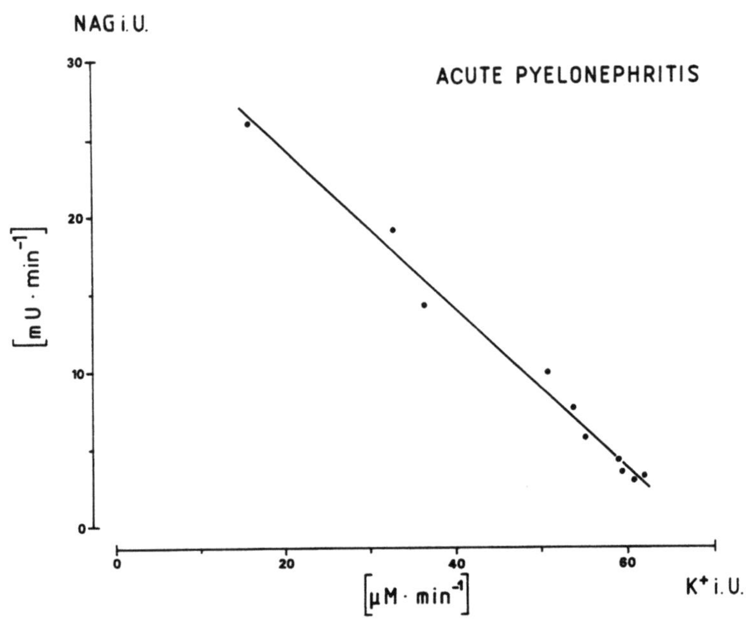

Fig. 6. Correlation between glomerular filtration rate (GFR) and the rate of urinary NAG release in patients with acute pyelonephritis in one or both kidneys ($n = 27$; $r = -0.95$)

Conclusions

NAG enzymuria (optimized method) provides an objective, quantitative, and sensitive measure of damage to the renal parenchyma in urinary tract infections. This makes it a simple and certain method of differentiating between upper and lower urinary tract infections and following the progress of renal infections.

References

Busch R, Huland H (1984) Correlation of symptoms and results of direct localization studies in patients with urinary tract infections. J Urol 132:282

Stamey TA (1980) Pathogenesis and treatment of urinary tract infections. Williams & Wilkins, Baltimore

Skrezek C, Bertermann H, Schulz FP, König B (1990) NAG – Ein sensitiver Marker für Nierenfunktionsstörungen. Urologe [A] 29:27

The Caeco-appendiceal Junction: A Urologically Applicable Sphincter Mechanism?

W. HÜBNER[1] and R. HARTUNG[1]

Introduction

Reliable urine drainage is essential for the social integration of patients after undergoing bladder removal. As early as 1911, Coffey (1911) described a method of implanting the urethra into the intact colon, successfully achieving continent, stoma-free drainage. Although this procedure frequently leads to electrolyte irregularities, a high incidence of pyelonephritis and, compared to the general population, a 500 times greater risk of carcinoma at the point of implantation, its implementation can be correctly indicated in suitable cases (Goldwasser and Webster 1986).

The ileum conduit, described in 1950 by Bricker (1950), is associated with a considerably lower complication rate than ureterosigmoidostomy (Goldwasser and Webster 1986). Despite the social and psychological disadvantages of urine drainage into an external reservoir, this method is still a standard procedure today. Drawing on the work of Kock et al. (1982) and Skinner et al. (1984), great interest is nowadays being shown in surrogate bladders using detubularised sections of the intestine (Benchekroun et al. 1989; Hinman 1988; Issa et al. 1989; Kock et al. 1989; Rowland et al. 1987; Skinner et al. 1984; Thüroff et al. 1986). The creation in these operations of a low-pressure reservoir with sufficient capacity and an anti-refluxive implantation of the ureters ensures continence over long periods without putting the upper urinary tract at risk. After initial difficulties with the efferent nipple of these surrogate bladders, this problem was solved both functionally and cosmetically with the development of new stoma techniques: continent appendix-navel stoma, tapered ileum, reinforcing the efferent nipple etc. (Benchekroun et al. 1989; Issa et al. 1989; Kock et al. 1989; Riedmiller et al. 1990; Rowland et al. 1987). For male cystectomy patients, or female patients with supratrigonal cystectomy, the original aim of achieving continent, stoma-free drainage after bladder removal has been achieved by attaching low-pressure intestinal pouches into the urethra (Davidsson et al. 1990; Hautmann et al. 1987, 1988; Kock et al. 1989; Light and Engelmann 1986; Melchior et al. 1986). This present paper sets out to investigate whether the circle of patients receiving a micturating surrogate bladder after cystectomy can be widened through the use of the caeco-appendiceal junction (CAJ) as an additional continence mechanism.

[1] Urologische Klinik und Poliklinik der Technischen Universität, Klinikum rechts der Isar, Ismaninger Str. 22, W-8000 München 80, FRG.

Theory

Since a continent micturating surrogate bladder is already available for male patients, the following remarks are mainly directed at the case of female patients. They are therefore for the most part applicable to male patients who have had to undergo urethrectomy due to tumor infiltration of the bladder neck/prostatic urethra, or because of CIS in the course of a cystectomy. In male patients with surrogate bladders, continence is ensured by the following:

1. Low-pressure reservoir with sufficient capacity
2. Remaining intrinsic urethral sphincter
3. Pelvic floor.

Re. point 1: Concerning pressure readings in pouches, we may refer to the literature (Benchekroun et al. 1989; Davidsson et al. 1990; Goldwasser and Webster 1985, 1986; Hautmann et al. 1987, 1988; Hinman 1988; Kock et al. 1982, 1989; Light and Engelmann 1986; Melchior et al. 1986, 1988; Persson and Melchior 1986; Rowland et al. 1987; Skinner et al. 1984; Thüroff et al. 1986). In natural pouches taken from the small intestine, pressures of 15–35 cm H_2O can be expected. When using the caecum, pressure peaks of up to 60 cm H_2O can occur under provocation (rapid filling of the pouch during the "cystometry"); basic pressures are around 30–45 cm H_2O, according to the degree of filling.

Re. point 2: In men, sufficient original urethral sphincter capable of long-term contraction remains after radical cystoprostatectomy (consisting of smooth muscle fibres and striated slow-twitch fibres), so that continence is assured.

Re. point 3: The striated muscle of the pelvic floor, in conjunction with abdomino pelvic pressure transmission, is responsible for stress continence. Under stress, there are additional muscle contractions of the external sphincter and the pelvic floor. After the smooth and striated slow-twitch muscle fibres around the proximal urethra and the bladder neck have been removed, the replacement sphincter mechanism must fulfil the following criteria:

1. Circular muscle (smooth), capable of long-term contraction
2. Surgical applicability
3. Urine-compatible mucosa.

The CAJ appears to fulfill these requirements. We have investigated whether the CAJ is suitable for use as a substitute bladder neck after cystectomy.

Method

The three taenias of the large intestine converge in the region of the CAJ, reinforcing the circular muscle. To determine the sphincter-like characteristics of this muscle ring, five postmortem specimens of unremarkable appendices were examined histologically. Measurement of the circular muscle was carried out at the caecum, at the CAJ and at the vermiform appendix under magnification by a factor of 250 (Fig. 1).

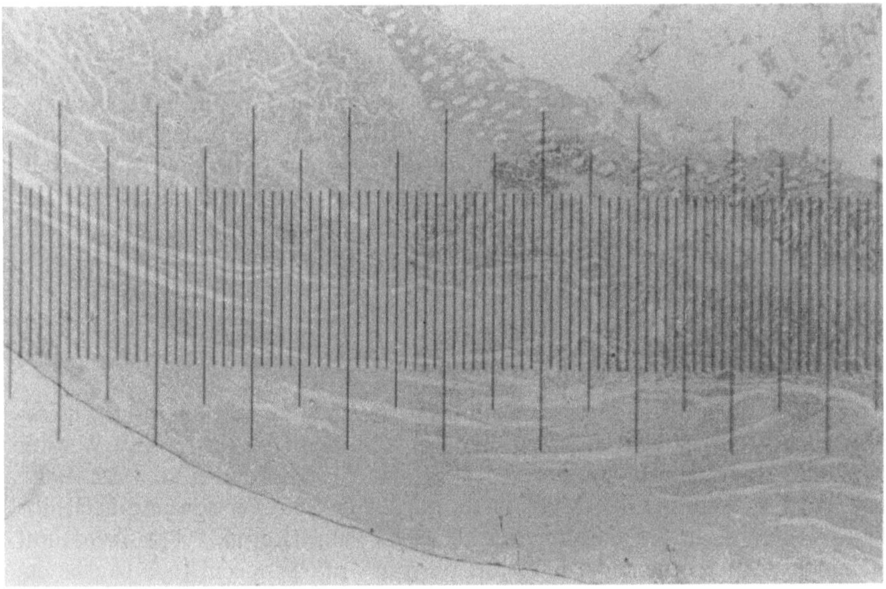

Fig. 1. Caeco-appendiceal junction. HE staining, ×250

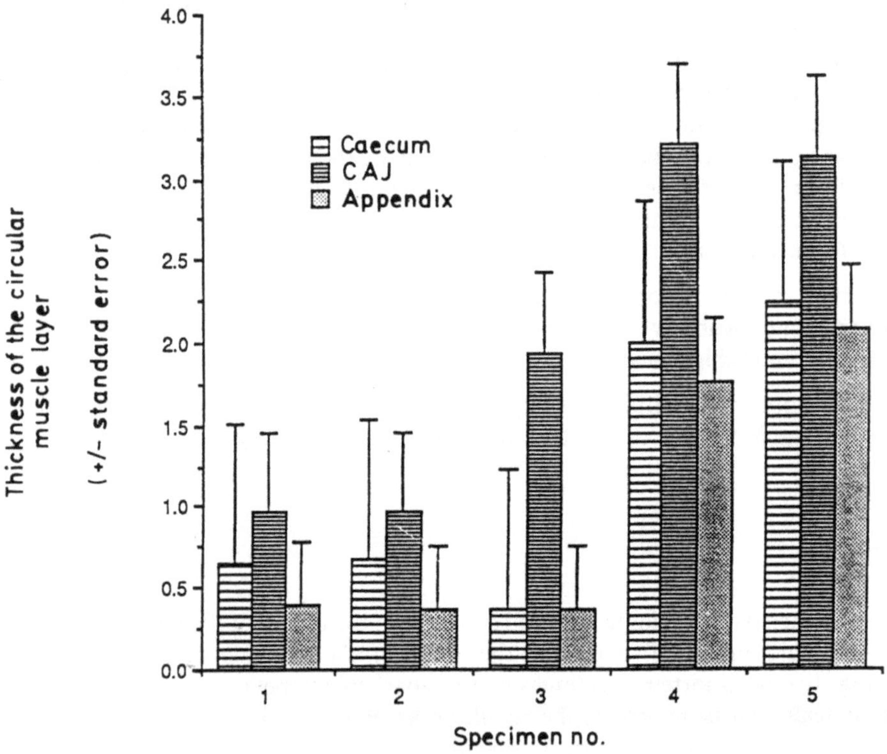

Fig. 2. Thickness of circular muscle layer in millimetres

As a functional test of the CAJ we performed pressure profiles on seven appendices intraoperatively before routine appendectomy in cases of cystectomy (four cases), hemicolectomy (two cases) and bladder augmentation (one case). The caecum was mobilised and after opening of the appendix at the distal end pressure was measured using a microtip catheter. To test operability we performed two trial operations on female cadavers. After mobilisation of the caecum the veriform appendix was drawn through the urethral channel.

Results

Histology

In all the specimens examined, a thickening of the circular muscle layer was apparent at the CAJ. The individed data can be gathered from Fig. 3. These findings confirm the presence of a sphincter-like muscle ring of smooth muscle in the region of the CAJ.

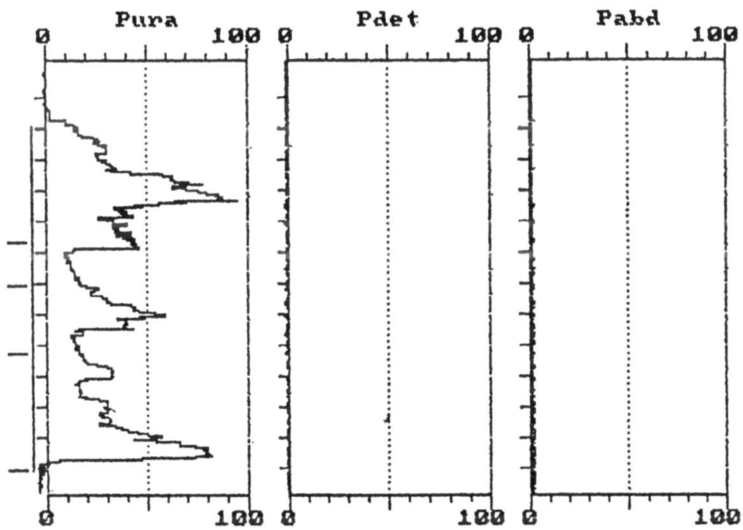

Fig. 3. Pressure profile appendix in patient no. 1
Test start: 10:04:08,
test end: 10:06:14,
maximum detrusor pressure (cm H_2O): 0,
maximum urethral pressure (cm H_2O): 95,
functional urethral length (cm): 5.1

Pressure Profiles

The results of the pressure profiles are summarised in Table 1. Except for one case (3) all readings are comparable with pressure profiles of continent women and also correlate to the pressure profiles of continent men with surrogate bladders.

Table 1. Pressure profiles at the CAJ ($n = 7$)

Patient no.	P_{max} (cm H_2O)
1	95
2	49
3	37
4	109
5	46
6	80
7	67

In case 3 the appendix was slightly inflamed, but even the reading of 37 cm H_2O should, together with the muscle tone of the pelvic floor, ensure continence.

Example

Figure 3 shows an appendix pressure profile (case 1). After low pressure in the caecum, pressure increases in the CAJ to 95 cm H_2O (sphincter). The second peak can be ascribed to a reflex contraction at the opened tip of the appendix; this phenomenon was registered in all specimens.

Trial operation

During the trial operation on the cadavers it was possible, after mobilising the ascending colon and the mesentery, to transfer the caecum smoothly into the true

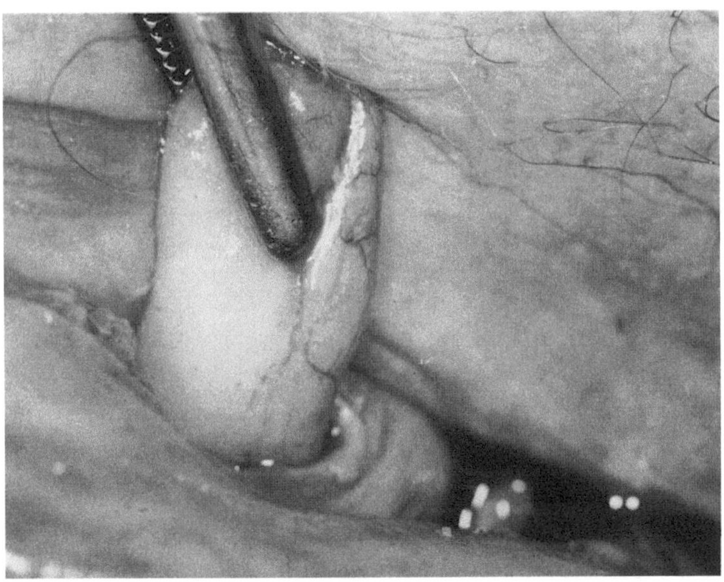

Fig. 4. Appendix pulled through the urethral channel

pelvis. During the cystectomy, the urethral mucosa was disengaged using submucosal saline injection, care being taken to preserve the adventitia. The appendix could then be pulled through the resulting channel and was finally secured with mucocutaneous stitches (Fig. 4).

Discussion

Continence in women depends on the following factors:

1. The so-called mucosal sphincter
2. The smooth bladder neck and urethra muscle with striated slow-twitch fibres
3. The elastic fibres of the urethral wall
4. The striated muscle of the pelvic floor.

The first three factors, which are responsible for basic continence, cease to be effective after cystectomy in female patients, so that bladder replacement for women was only possible if the trigone, or parts thereof, were intact, or using an artificial sphincter. In addition, women have weaker pelvic floor muscles than men. In the CAJ with appendix we find smooth muscle suitable for long-term contraction, as well as elastic fibres, so that basic continence would seem to be ensured by this mechanism.

For bladder replacement in men where the urethra is attached, a urethral resistance of at least 45 cm H_2O is required. The recorded readings from the CAJ therefore lead us to expect continence; in vivo the pelvic floor muscle contributes an additional continence factor.

Micturition in cases of bladder replacement is brought about by abdominal strain. Although a co-ordinated process of micturition can naturally no longer take place after such operations, a certain learning process seems feasible, consisting of an conscious relaxation of the pelvic floor. This is substantiated by the extremely variable micturition pressures between 30 and 120 mg H_2O recorded in surrogate bladders (Davidsson et al. 1990; Frohneberg 1988; Hautmann et al. 1987, 1988; Kock et al. 1989; Light and Engelmann 1986; Persson and Melchior 1986). Apparently, conscious relaxation can reduce urethral resistance to such an extent that sufficient flow of urine occurs, even with low micturition pressures. The question why, on the other hand, stress continence occurs with simultaneous intact abdomino pelvic pressure transmission and micturition pressures of under 40 cm H_2O, can be adequately explained by the intact reflex of the pelvic floor muscle over the pudendal nerve (Thüroff et al. 1982). The pressure readings recorded by us at the CAJ lead us to expect micturition using abdominal strain to be possible, at least after conscious relaxation of the pelvic floor has been mastered.

In both the trial operations on the cadavers it was possible to mobilise the caecum into the true pelvis. This agrees with data in the literature concerning attachment of an (ileo-) caecal pouch to the membranous urethra (Davidsson et al. 1990; Gilchrist et al. 1950; Goldwasser and Webster 1985, 1986; Light and Engelmann 1986). After careful disengagement of the urethra, the appendix can be drawn through the urethral channel. Since it is not necessary to perform an anastomosis in the true pelvis when using this method, the procedure appears comparatively straightforward, and the continence mechanisms of the pelvic floor can be preserved to the maximum degree. The ureters can be implanted into the caecum in an antirefluxive manner.

According to our results, the CAJ provides, both anatomically and functionally, a sphincter mechanism which could serve as a substitute bladder neck in cases of bladder replacement. Such a procedure would be conceivable for the following groups of patients:

1. Female patients who have undergone cystectomy due to invasive bladder tumor or interstitial cystitis affecting the trigone and urethra.
2. Male cystectomy patients with tumor infiltration of the bladder neck/prostatic urethra.
3. Male cystectomy patients with CIS.

As with all methods in which the vermiform appendix is employed for urological operations (Issa et al. 1989; Lipsky and Melchior 1988; Mitrofanoff 1980; Riedmiller et al. 1990), a macroscopically suitable appendix is a necessary precondition of the operation. In addition an intra-operative test of function ability (pressure profile) and calibration would be required. Under these circumstances it seems possible to employ the CAJ as a substitute bladder neck.

References

Benchekroun A, Essekalli N, Faik N, Marzouk M, Hachimi M, Abakka T (1989) Continent urostomy with hydraulic ileal valve in 136 patients: 13 years of experience. J Urol 142:46–51

Bricker EM (1950) Bladder substitution after pelvic evisceration. Surg Clin North Am 30:1511–1516

Coffey RC (1911) Physiologic implantation of the severed ureter or common bile-duct into the intestine: JAMA 142:397–399

Davidsson T, Mansson W, Colleen S (1990) Continent urinary diversion and bladder replacement using the right colon. Eur Urol 18:345

Frohneberg D (1988) Personal communication

Gilchrist RK, Merricks JW, Hamlin MH, Rieger IT (1950) Construction of a substitute bladder and urethra. Surg Gynecol Obstet 90:752–760

Goldwasser B, Webster GD (1985) Continent urinary diversion. J Urol 134:227–236

Goldwasser B, Webster GD (1986) Augmentation and substitution enterocystoplasty. J Urol 135:215–224

Goodwin WE, Harris AP, Kaufman JJ, Beal JM (1953) Open, transcolonic ureterointestinal anastomosis: a new approach. Surg Gynecol Obstet 97:295–298

Hautmann RE, Egghart G, Frohneberg D, Miller K (1987) Die Ileum-Neoblase. Urologe [A] 26:67–76

Hautmann RE, Egghart G, Frohneberg D, Miller K (1988) The ileal neobladder. J Urol 139:39–44

Hinman FJ (1988) Selection of intestinal segments for bladder substitution: physical and physiological characteristics. J Urol 139:519–523

Issa MM, Oesterling JE, Canning DA, Jeffs RD (1989) A new technique of using the in situ appendix as a catheterizable stoma in continent urinary reservoirs. J Urol 141:1385–1387

Kock NG, Nilson AE, Nilsson LO, Norlén LJ, Philipson BM (1982) Urinary diversion via a continent ileal reservoir: clinical results in 12 patients. J Urol 128:469–475

Kock NG, Ghoneim MA, Lycke KG, Mahran MR (1989) Replacement of the bladder by the urethral Kock pouch: functional results, urodynamics and radiological features. J Urol 141:1111–1116

Lieskovsky G, Boyd SD, Skinner D (1987) Management of late complications of the Kock pouch form of urinary diversion. J Urol 137:1146–1150

Light JK, Engelmann VH (1986) Le bag: total replacement of the bladder using an ileocolic pouch. J Urol 136:27–31

Lipsky H, Melchior H (1988) Uretersatz durch Appendix. Verh Dtsch Ges Urol 40:56–57

Melchior H, Spehr CH, Knop-Wagemann J, Persson MC, Juenemann KP (1988) The continent ileal bladder for urinary tract reconstruction after cystectomy: surgery in 44 patients. J Urol 138:714–719

Melchior H, Spehr CH, Persson CH (1986) Die kontinente Ileum-Blase: Ein erster Bericht über 5 Patienten. Akt Urol 17:256–260

Mitrofanoff P (1980) Cystostomie continente trans-appendicularie dans le traitement des vessies neurologiques. Chir Ped 21:297–303

Persson C, Melchior H (1986) Ileozystodynamik: Urodynamische Untersuchungen der kontinenten Ileumblase. Urologe [A] 25:259–266

Riedmiller HF, Steinbach H, Köhl V, Hohenfellner R (1990) Kontinentes Appendix-Stoma – Modifikation der Mainz-Pouch Technik. In: Hartung, Hübner (Hrsg) Chirurgie des Kleinen Beckens. Springer, Berlin Heidelberg New York Tokyo (in press)

Rowland RG, Mitchell ME, Bihrle R, Kahnoski RJ, Piser JE (1987) Indiana continent urinary reservoir. J Urol 137:1136–1139

Skinner DG, Boyd SD, Lieskovsky G (1984) Clinical experience with the Kock continent ileal reservoir for urinary diversion. J Urol 132:1101–1106

Skinner DG, Lieskovsky G, Boyd SD (1987) Continuing experience with the continent ileal reservoir (Kock pouch) as an alternative to cutaneous urinary diversion: an update after 250 cases. J Urol 137:1140–1145

Thüroff JW, Bazeed MA, Schmidt RA, Tanagho EA (1982) Mechanisms of urinary continence: an animal model to study urethral responses to stress conditions. J Urol 127:1202–1206

Thüroff JW, Alken P, Riedmiller H, Engelmann U, Jacobi GH, Hohenfellner R (1986) The Mainz pouch (mixed augmentation ileum and caecum) for bladder augmentation and continent diversion. J Urol 136:17–26

DNA/Cytokeratin Flow Cytometry in Bladder Lavage: An Improvement in the Diagnosis of Bladder Tumors?

T. LIEDL[1], M. PROSINGER[1], B. GANZMANN[1], and D. JOCHAM[2]

Introduction

Flow cytometry is expected to be a valuable adjunct to clinical staging and morphological grading in the assessment of the malignancy potential of neoplasm (Barlogie et al. 1983). By now, DNA measurement in specimens taken from solid genitourinary tumor tissue has become a promising prognostic tool. The low tumor identification rate in bladder lavage, however, has prevented flow cytometry from becoming part of the routine diagnostic procedure. The main problems are unsolved questions of quantification and standardization and the failure to exclude disturbing subpopulations (Tribukait 1987) by means of physical cell properties.

The aim of our study is to gate the urothelial cells as the region of interest by employing an antibody against cytokeratin (Achtstätter et al. 1985) and to perform a selective cell cycle analysis. After a more accurate characterization of tumor biology has been achieved, the clinical applications of this method should be investigated.

Material and Methods

Material

Between July 1987 and September 1989, 402 bladder lavage specimens obtained during cystoscopy were submitted to routine cytology and flow cytometric DNA determination. Of these cases, 164 were evaluated histologically at the time of lavage.

Preparation

Each specimen was obtained by irrigating the bladder with 100 cm^3 normal saline via several pulses with a syringe and then divided into aliquots.

1. For cytology the slides were evaluated after staining with a modified Papanicolaou technique.
2. In flow cytometry specimens, the erythrocytes were removed by a lysing buffer.

[1] Urologische Klinik und Poliklinik der Universität Klinikum Großhadern, Marchioninistr. 15, W-8000 München 70, FRG.

[2] Urologische Klinik der Medizinischen Universität, Ratzeburger Allee 160, W-2400 Lübeck, FRG.

After fixation with 70% methanol, the cells could be stored at −20 °C for months. Following filtration through a 70 µm nylon mesh and washing, the cells were adjusted to a concentration of 10^6/ml and prepared according to the protocol shown in Fig. 1. In brief, an indirect antibody labeling technique for cytokeratin immunofluorescence was followed by staining with propidium iodide as DNA dye. Kept in a refrigerator, the samples were stable for several days.

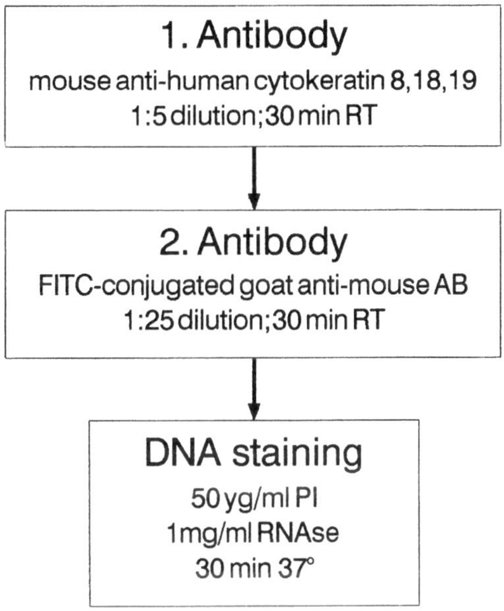

Fig. 1. Protocol for indirect antibody labeling and DNA staining of bladder lavage

Measurement

The samples were analyzed using an FACS Analyzer (Becton-Dickinson, Mountainview, Calif, USA). After calibration, the flow cytometer was standardized with monosized FITC-labeled test beads. Before each test series a "cocktail" containing cytokeratin-negative chicken red blood cells, human leukocytes, and proliferating cytokeratin-positive HeLa cells served as a control for the accuracy of labeling and gating. Ten thousand cells per specimen were examined by simultaneous measurement of volume, scatter, and green (cytokeratin) and red (DNA) fluorescence.

Data Evaluation

The results were plotted as a two-dimensional display of the fluorescences (Fig. 2): along the abscissa is the cytokeratin content in a logarithmic scale, along the ordinate is the DNA content in a linear scale. Cell cycle analysis of the gated region of interest was performed using the sum of broadened rectangle (SOBR) algorithm.

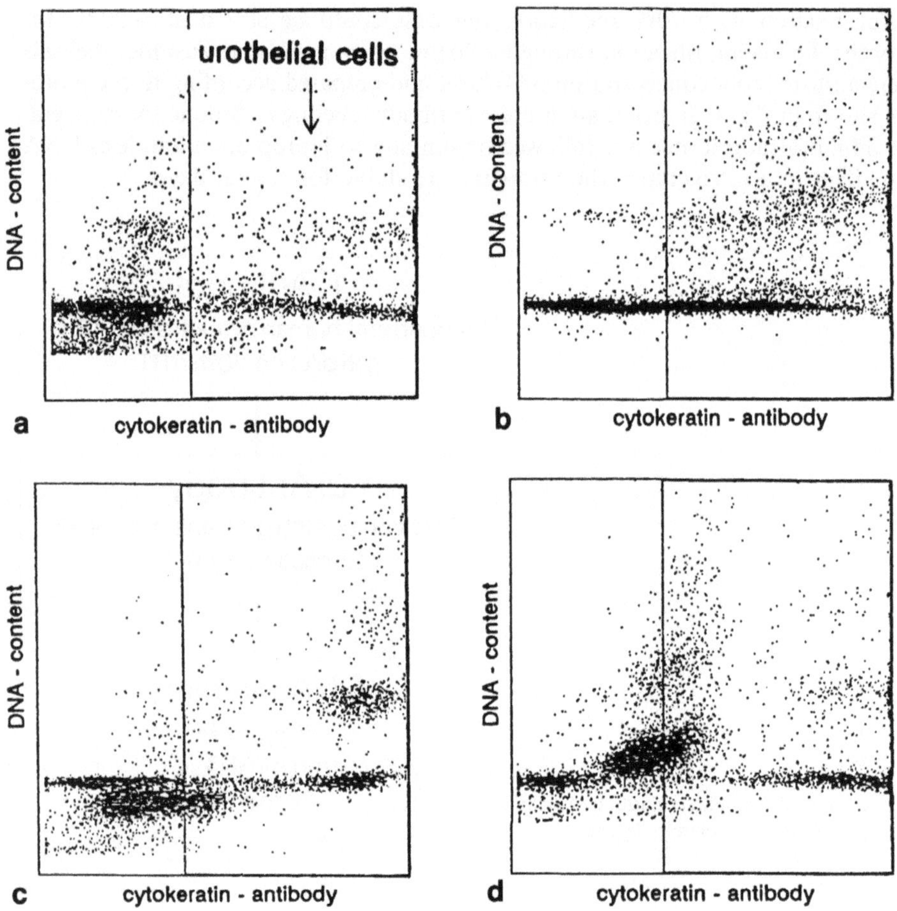

Fig. 2a–d. Identification of subpopulations in bladder lavage using the fluorescence dot plot. **a** Cystitis, **b** near-diploid tumor, **c** pyknosis, **d** squamous cells

Results

In the fluorescence dot plot (Fig. 2), the horizontal lines represent cells with the same DNA content; the first line is the G_{01} phase, followed by the S and G_2M phase, which is twice as high as the resting G_{01} cells. The cytokeratin content increases from left to right; based on standardization, a definite gate between cytokeratin-negative cells and cytokeratin-positive urothelium can be set in the fluorescence dot plot.

Identification of Subpopulations

As a result of cytokeratin-antibody labeling, distinct subpopulations can be identified:

a) Specimens in which more than 35% of the cells were cytokeratin-negative inflammatory cells, are considered as showing cystitis (Fig. 2a) by flow cytometry. The agreement of cytological and flow cytometric results increased from 67% in cases of chronic to 78% in cases of acute inflammation.
b) By using the inflammatory cells as internal reference, near-diploid carcinomas (Fig. 2b) with only slight changes of DNA content can be demonstrated. Tetraploid-aneuploid neoplasms and small tumor clones are detected by selective cell cycle analysis of the urothelium.
c) Pyknotic cells (Fig. 2c), sometimes appearing like hypoploid tumor cells in the DNA histogram, are identified by their cytokeratin-negative property.
d) Squamous cells (Fig. 2d), which are able to simulate aneuploidy or high proliferation by staining the cytoplasmic RNA, are recognized in the fluorescence dot plot as a distinct population, cut by a standard gate and clearly separated from urothelial and inflammatory cells.

Comparison of Flow Cytometry and Cytology

Seventy-three percent of the cases of histologically confirmed bladder tumor (Fig. 3a) were detected by cytology. Aneuploid stem lines were demonstrated by flow cytometry in 47% of the cases. This percentage of tumor diagnosis could be increased using the urothelial proliferation as a second parameter: more than 25% of the urothelium in $S+G_2M$ phase may indicate the presence of tumor. The SOBR algorithm, however, is too sensitive to perturbations of the early S phase (broad CV of the G_{01} peak) and late S phase (physiological urothelial cells with two nuclei) and does not yield reliable results: no difference in proliferation between tumor and normal specimens could be determined.

Twenty-five percent of the specimens from patients with histologically tumor-free biopsies (Fig. 3b) at the time of specimen collection were identified as malignant by cytology, versus 8% aneuploid by flow cytometry. Since all of these aneuploid samples were cytologically positive, it is assumed that in these cases the bladder lavage was superior to histological material.

Correlation of Aneuploidy and Cytological Grading

The percentage of aneuploid tumors (Fig. 4) increased with the degree of anaplasia: from 26% in G_1 to 78% in G_3 tumors. Seventeen percent of the specimens judged as "normal" or "suspicious" by cytology, showed DNA histograms with aneuploid stemlines. Within 9 months on average, half of these patients developed a tumor or tumor recurrence, which was confirmed by biopsy or cytology.

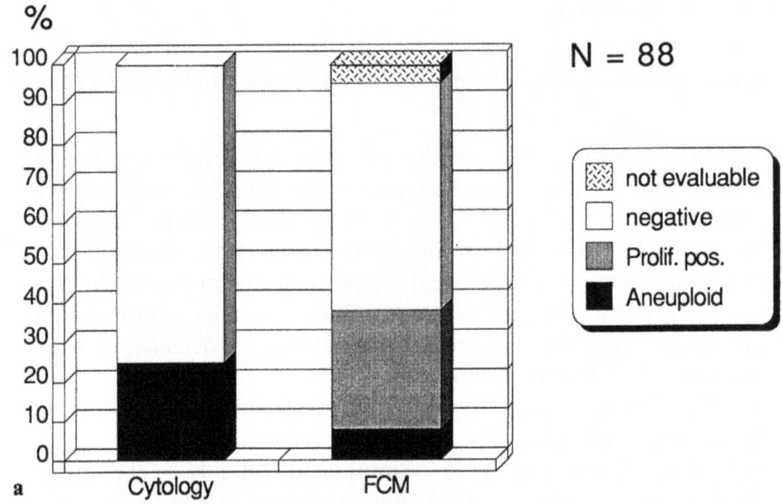

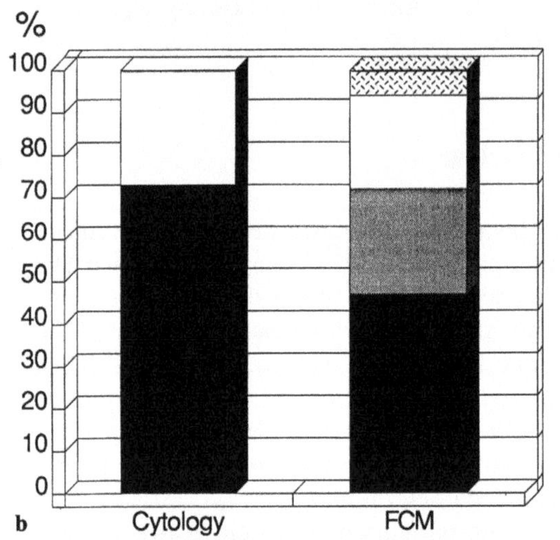

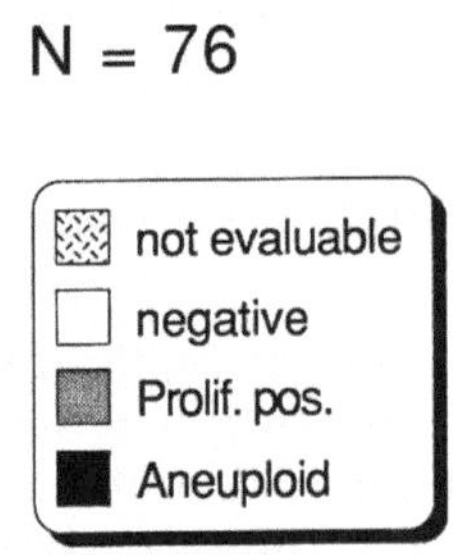

Fig. 3a, b. Comparison of cytology and flow cytometry. **a** Histologically confirmed bladder tumors, **b** histologically tumor-free biopsies

Discussion

Method

Aneuploid is a prognostically reliable indicator of malignancy (Barlogie et al. 1983). A variety of staining techniques have been used in previous studies to develop DNA flow cytometry for clinical application. However, the main problem in bladder lavage is the mixture of various subpopulations, which cannot be gated by physical cell properties because of overlap in cell size (Ratliff et al. 1985). Large amounts of inflammatory or squamous cell contamination interfere with the

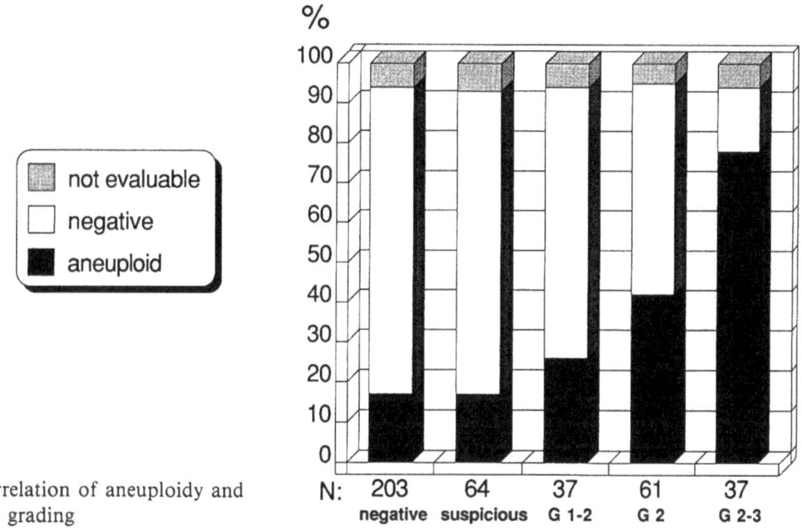

Fig. 4. Correlation of aneuploidy and cytological grading

analysis of epithelial cells, leading to false-negative and false-positive results. The usefulness of flow cytometry may be considerably improved by measuring a second variable in addition to DNA, e.g., biochemical cell characteristics for which tumor cells differ from normal cells, or Lewis A/B cell surface antigens (Leyh et al. 1989).

Flow cytometric analysis of bladder biopsies has shown that the expression of cytokeratin 18 epitopes in tumor cells correlates quantitatively with higher grade and stage (Feitz et al.). In the present approach an antibody against cytokeratin 8, 18, 19 was employed to exclude disturbing subpopulations like cytokeratin-negative pyknosis and slightly cytokeratin-positive squamous cells. By determining the proportion of cytokeratin-negative inflammatory cells in a specimen, a statement about the presence and severity of cystitis can be made. Using the inflammatory cells as internal reference, the quality of preparation and measurement can be checked retrospectively. By investigation of selective histograms of the cytokeratin-positive urothelial cells, the recognition of small tumor clones, tetraploid-aneuploid and near diploid carcinomas is considerably improved. Standardized measurement and definite criteria for the evaluation of data would allow the routine employment of the DNA/cytokeratin method in the diagnostic procedure and long-term follow-up of patients.

Clinical Assessment

There is currently no agreement among investigators as to whether flow cytometry or cytology yields better results, which may also depend on differences between preparation techniques. In our study, using histology as a reference, flow cytometric aneuploidy seems to be less sensitive than conventional cytology, but to have a much higher specifity in the diagnosis of bladder tumors. It might be possible to improve the sensitivity in the near future by re-evaluation of urothelial proliferation using a more accurate algorithm.

In agreement with other study groups (Tribukait 1987), we found a clear correlation between aneuploidy and grading. We want to stress that flow cytometry offers another means of diagnosing, characterizing, and monitoring patients having or suspected of having bladder tumors: aneuploidy can precede cytological and histological evidence of tumor or tumor recurrence and provide additional information about prognosis. In future, flow cytometry may help to distinguish between cell alterations caused by tumor and cytostatic treatment, and to monitor patients receiving intravesical chemotherapy.

Cytology and flow cytometry should not be seen as competing but as complementary tests and should both be an integral part in the management of bladder cancer.

Summary

More than 400 bladder lavage specimens were analyzed by multiple-parameter flow cytometry. The presented standardized DNA/cytokeratin-AB labeling method allows reliable identification and gating of interfering subpopulations such as inflammatory, pyknotic, and squamous cells. In this way, a separate cell cycle analysis of the urothelium is possible and small tumor clones become considerable easier to detect.

Our results showed an increased incidence of aneuploid tumors with the degree of anaplasia. To date, half of the patients in whom flow cytometry showed aneuploidy, although the cytological diagnosis was either "normal" or "suspect", have developed tumor recurrence.

Since flow cytometry appears to anticipate cytological evidence of tumor recurrence and to provide additional information about prognosis, we use the method routinely for diagnosis and follow-up care.

References

Achtstätter T, Moll R, Moore B, Franke W (1985) Cytokeratin polypeptide patterns of different epithelia of the human male urogenital tract. Immunofluorescence and gel electrophoretic studies. J Histochem Cytochem 33:415–426

Barlogie B, Raber M, Schumann J et al. (1983) Flow cytometry in clinical cancer research. Cancer Res 43:3982–3997

Feitz W, Beck H, Smeets A, Debruyne F, Vooijs G, Herman C, Ramaekers F (1985) Tissue-specific markers in flow cytometry of urological cancers: cytokeratins in bladder carcinoma. Int J Cancer 36:349–356

Leyh H, Valet G, Lehmer A (1989) Automatic identification of bladder tumor cells by multiple parameters in flow cytometry. In: Rübben H, Jocham D, Jacobi G (eds) Investigative Urology 3. Springer, Berlin Heidelberg New York Tokyo, pp 115–119

Ratliff J, Klein F, White F (1985) Flow cytometry of ethanol-fixed versus fresh bladder barbotage specimens. J Urol 133:958–960

Tribukait B (1987) Flow Cytometry in assessing the clinical aggressiveness of genito-urinary neoplasms. World J Urol 5:108–122

First Clinical Experiences with Photodynamic Fluorescence Diagnosis in Urology

R. BAUMGARTNER [1,2], A. BUSER [1], M. KRIEGMAIR [2], H. LENZ [1], H. STEPP [1], E. UNSÖLD [1], and D. JOCHAM [3]

Introduction

The diagnosing of early stage cancer on the basis of detection of systemically applied fluorescing porphyrin compounds is attracting growing interest. Porphyrin derivative-induced fluorescence was initially used for visualization of mainly experimental tumors and highly proliferating neoplasms (Figge et al. 1948). Improved tumor markers and sensitive fluorescence detection devices allow endoscopic administration to various hollow organs such as lung (Kato et al. 1990; Lam et al. 1990) and esophagus (Monnier et al. 1990). In regard to the bladder, histopathologic examination of resected specimens confirmed the correlation of fluorescence intensity with tumorous sites (Benson et al. 1982). In this paper, first clinical experiences with fluorescence imaging of cancerous lesions of the bladder are reported.

Material and Methods

The fluorescent component of the porphyrin derivative Photofrin II (QLT Inc., Vancouver, Canada) is used as a tumor marker. Photofrin II, which is the most active substance in photodynamic therapy (Manyak et al. 1988), has a strong photosensitizing capability. It is responsible for side effects like superficial photodynamic processes during fluorescence excitation with violet light and photosensitization of the patients' skin. To avoid these two effects the drug dosage has been reduced for diagnostic purposes to 0.15 – 0.5 mg/kg bodyweight, i.e., to 10% – 20% of the dose currently used for photodynamic treatment.

On the other hand, reduction of the concentration of the tumor marker leads to competing effects between the porphyrin fluorescence and background signals, mainly due to fluorescence of dyes intrinsic to tissue, such as melanin and hemoglobin. To suppress this background level, a new method has been developed based on excitation of tissue with light at two different wavelengths and subsequent digital image processing (Baumgartner et al. 1987).

Figure 1 shows the fluorescence spectra from Photofrin II in a patient's bladder tissue after excitation with violet and blue light. Because of the low tumor marker

[1] Zentrales Laserlaboratorium der GSF, Ingolstädter Landstraße 1, W-8042 Neuherberg, FRG.
[2] Urologische Klinik und Poliklinik der Universität Großhadern, Marchioninistr. 15, W-8000 München 70, FRG.
[3] Urologische Klinik der Medizinischen Universität, Ratzeburger Allee 160, W-2400 Lübeck 1, FRG.

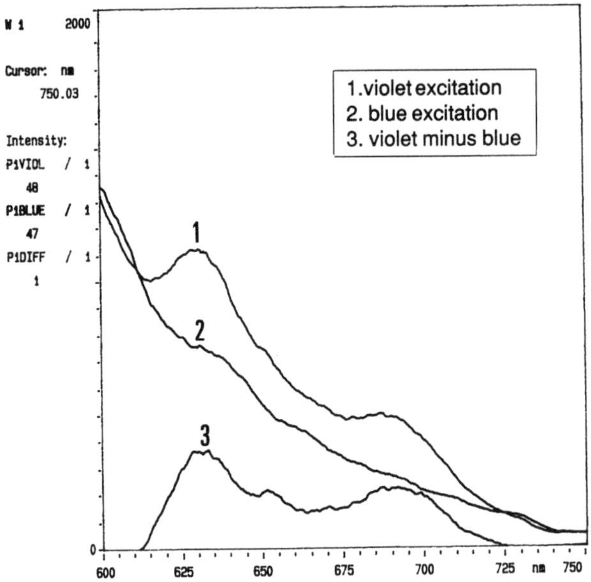

Fig. 1. Fluorescence emission spectra endoscopically detected after violet (*1*) and blue (*2*) laser excitation from a human bladder tumor and the differential tumor marker spectrum (*3*) after computer-assisted subtraction

dose, the characteristic emission bands at 630 and 690 nm after violet excitation are superposed by the tissue's own fluorescence. Excitation of the same tissue area with blue light around 470 nm is still effective in exciting autofluorescence, but with a negligible contribution from Photofrin II fluorescence. Computer-assisted subtraction of the blue-excited spectrum from the violet-excited spectrum results in a spectrum free of background signals. This contrast-enhancing method, demonstrated on fluorescence spectra, can also be performed with video images using digital image-processing techniques.

To optimize a detection system for this purpose, the low fluorescence quantum yield of Photofrin II of approx. 2% has to be considered. In addition, Photofrin II is chemically unstable, which results in a rapid decrease of fluorescence intensity after excitation of the tissue with irradiances exceeding 100 mW/cm^2. Further reduction of the excitation light dose is necessary, since photobleaching has indicated superficial phototoxic effects on the tissue under examination. Sensitive light detection devices are necessary, especially for endoscopic applications.

A Krypton ion laser was used as an excitation light source. It delivered violet and blue light to excite the fluorescence of the tumor marker incorporated in the bladder tissue. Multiline emission in the violet and blue spectrum ranges is achieved by a modified laser resonator, mounting four standard resonator mirrors in a collinear configuration. The output power at each wavelength range can be tuned separately by fast computer-assisted tilting of the piezo-mounted resonator mirrors. In addition, the wavelength range can be switched alternately with video frequency in order to display difference images every 80 ms. The intensity of light levels necessary for optimum autofluorescence subtraction is preset and controlled on an electronic circuit. On-line registration of fluorescence spectra using an optical multichannel analyzer alternately at violet and blue excitation permits exactitude of intensity at both wavelengths.

Laser light is coupled into a single-core plastic fiber (core diameter 500 μm) inserted into the endoscope. The fiber tip is modified to achieve homogeneous illumination of the area of tissue observed through the endoscope. The video signal obtained from the intensified CCD camera is fed into an image-processing computer that performs storage and subtraction of the fluorescence images. The images are taken at a maximum repetition rate of 16 Hz and displayed on a monitor in a steady state mode. A colour TV camera is used for visual survey of the surface of the bladder tissue, illuminated with white light. Switching between the cameras takes place electromechanically with a mirror inserted in the endoscope. The frequency of mirror switching is computer-controlled, which allows biopsies to be taken from tissue with enhanced fluorescence intensity.

The fluorescence detection device used in the operating theatre is a modular system integrating the various controlling and presentation components in moveable racks (Fig. 2). On the left in Fig. 2, the optical multichannel analyzer (OMA)

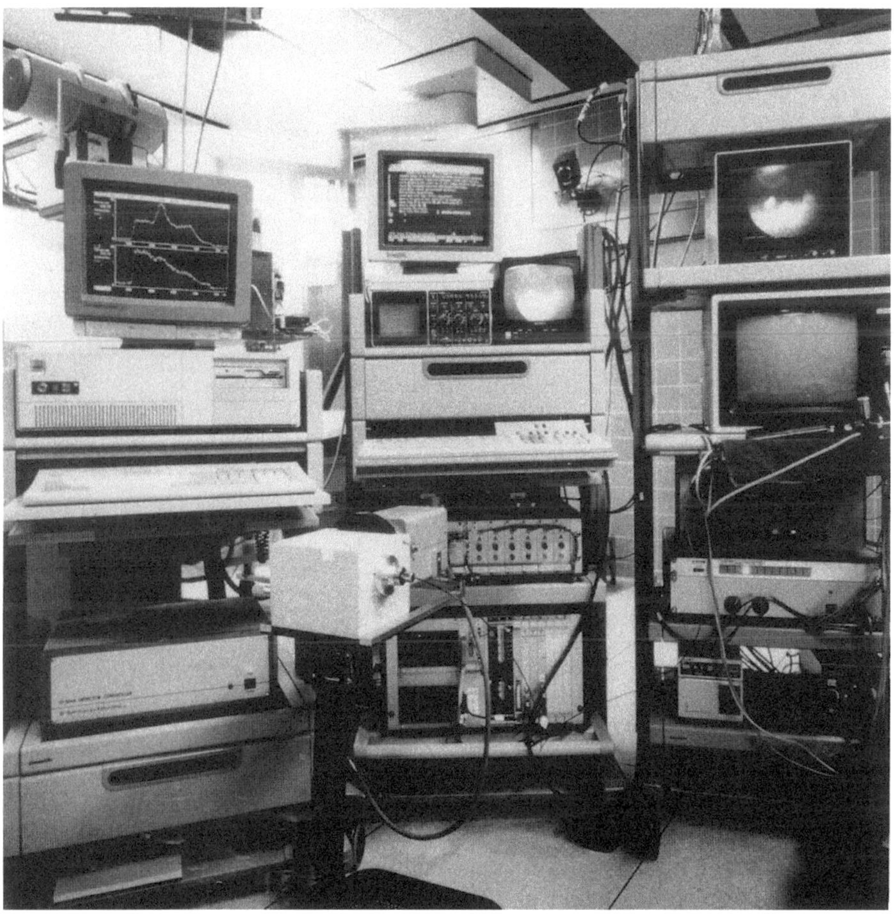

Fig. 2. Detection and documentation unit of the fluorescence diagnosis system in the urological operating theatre

is shown, used for registration and display of fluorescence spectra after violet and blue excitation. The optical detection head of the spectrum analyzer is placed in front of the racks. The rack in the middle contains the image processing unit and the electronic circuits for laser and operation. On the right, the fluorescence and colour images are displayed on two video monitors.

For endoscopic application, a conventional cystoscope was coupled to the video image detection systems. This instrument, shown in Fig. 3, is modified by integration of optical channels for laser light transfer and spectrum registration. The image intensifier camera (ICCD) and the colour CCD camera are mounted in a rectangular configuration. By means of a moveable mirror, described above, the optical pathway of the endoscope can be switched between the two cameras in just a few milliseconds. This ensures almost complete overlap of the conventional view and the corresponding fluorescence image.

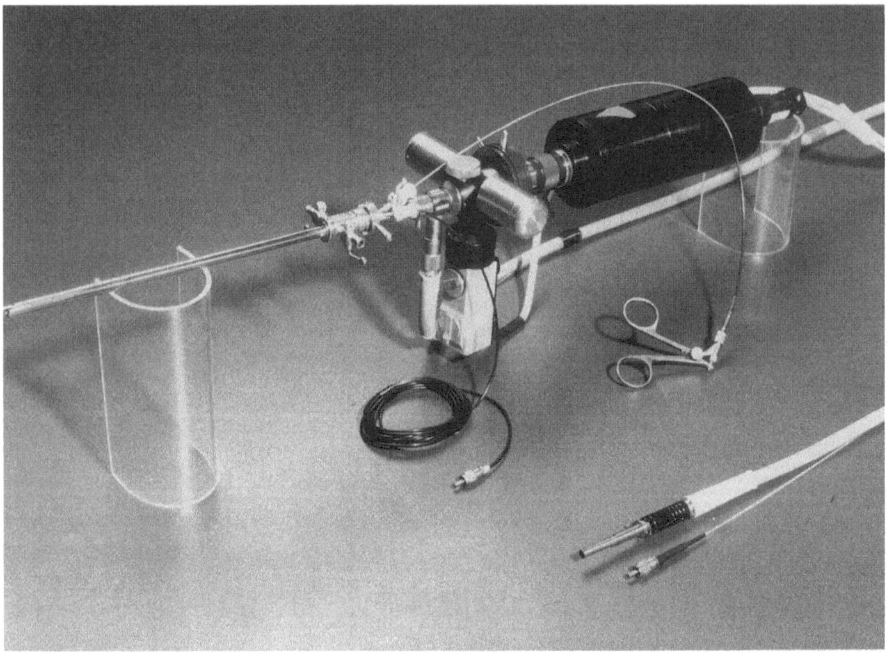

Fig. 3. Fluorescence cystoscope with adapted colour and intensified video cameras

Results

So far, ten patients with confirmed or apparent bladder tumors have been treated using the photodynamic fluorescence technique. The endoscopic view of a part of the bladder wall is shown on the left in Fig. 4; the corresponding digitally processed fluorescence image of the same tissue area is shown on the right. Although details cannot be discerned, bright tumor marker fluorescence is visible. By image

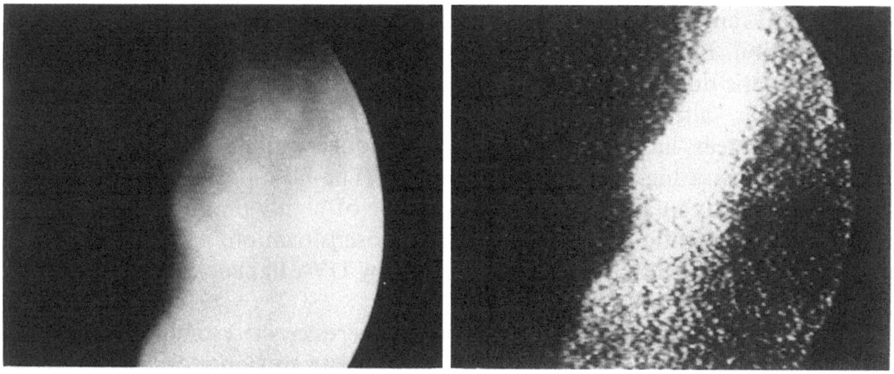

Fig. 4. Endoscopic view of a tumor-bearing bladder surface: TV display of the site (*left*) and the contrast-enhanced fluorescence image (*right*)

subtraction and the elimination of background signals, healthy tissue areas in the foreground appear dark. Histopathological examination showed superficial tumors at the site of enhanced fluorescence emission.

The clinical date relating to the correlation of fluorescence intensity and histological findings in the ten patients is summarized in Tables 1 and 2. The dose

Table 1. List of patients

	Sex	Age	Photofrin II-dose (mg/kg bw)	Number of biopsies
1	Male	61	0.4	8
2	Male	59	0.15	2
3	Male	64	0.4	3
4	Male	78	0.4	13
5	Male	79	0.5	7
6	Female	79	0.4	4
7	Male	67	0.4	5
8	Female	65	0.4	3
9	Female	83	0.4	7
10	Male	75	0.4	4
Total				56

Table 2. Correlation of fluorescence contrast with histological findings

	Biopsies	%
True positives	10	18
True negatives	29	52
False positives	17	30
False negatives	0	0
Total	56	100

of Photofrin II ranged from 0.15 to 0.5 mg/kg bodyweight and was given 48 h before examination. Eight of the patients were given 0.4 mg/kg bodyweight, 20% of the therapeutic dose. As shown in Table 2, no false-negative results have been obtained so far, although biopsy mapping of the entire organ, including nonfluorescing areas, has been performed. Additionally, all histologically proven malignancies show a high fluorescence contrast. The false-positive fluorescence findings were mostly in areas noted visually to be of highly proliferating inflammatory tissue or necrotic. In regard to skin photosensitization, patients reported negligible discomfort. This was also confirmed by UVA light sensitivity tests on their skin.

Further fluorescence diagnostic procedures are necessary to establish the device in clinical routine. Valuable information is expected from fluorescence mapping and histological examination of human bladders after cystectomy. This procedure will allow correlation of fluorescence intensity with different grades of malignancy over the entire surface of the organ. An extension of the use of the technique to other organs is in preparation. Detection two-wavelength-excited fluorescence in photomarked tumors promises to be a valuable tool, especially for delineation of malignancies of the skin and endoscopic detection of occult tumors in the lung, gastrointestinal organs, and others.

Acknowledgement. The authors thank Karl Storz KG, Tuttlingen for developing and providing endoscopic equipment, and W. Dietz for technical assistance. The project is supported by the Federal Ministry of Research and Technology (BMFT), Bonn, under grant no. 0706903.

References

Baumgartner R, Fisslinger H, Jocham D, Lenz H, Ruprecht L, Stepp H, Unsöld E (1987) A fluorescence imaging device for endoscopic detection of early stage cancer – instrumental and experimental studies. Photochem Photobiol 46:5

Benson RC Jr, Farrow GM, Kinsey JH et al. (1982) Detection and localization of in situ carcinoma of the bladder with hematoporphyrin derivative. Mayo Clin Proc 548–555

Figge FHJ, Weiland GS, Manganiello LOJ (1948) Cancer detection and therapy. Affinity of neoplastic, embryonic, and traumatized tissues for porphyrins and metalloporphyrins. Proc Soc Exp Biol Med 68:640–641

Lam S, Hung J, Palcic B (1990) Detection of lung cancer by ratio fluorometry with and without Photofrin II. SPIE Optic Fibers Med 1201:561–568

Manyak MJ, Russo A, Smith PD, Glatstein E (1988) Photodynamic therapy. J Clin Oncol 6:380–391

Monnier P, Savary M, Fontolliet C, Wagnieres G, Chatelain A, Cornaz P, Depeursinge C, Van den Bergh H (1990) Photodetection and photodynamic therapy of "early" squamous cell carcinomas of the pharynx, oesophagus and tracheo-bronchial tree. Lasers Med Sci 5:149–169

Kato H, Imaizumi T, Aizawa K, Iwabuchi H, Yamamoto H, Ikeda N, Tsuchida T, Tamachi Y, Ito T, Hayata Y (1990) Photodynamic diagnosis in respiratory tract malignancy using an excimer dye laser system. J Photochem Photobiol B6:189–196

Analysis of Tumor Heterogeneity in Monolayers and Tumor Spheroids of a Transitional Cell Carcinoma Cell Line

F. A. OFFNER[1], G. OTT[1], L. FÜZESI[1], V. PREISLER[1], J. HUNDECK[1], B. KLOSTERHALFEN[1], F. HOFSTÄDTER[2], St. HAUPTMANN[1], H. RÜBBEN[3], and C. J. KIRKPATRICK[1]

Introduction

The concept of the heterogeneity of tumor subpopulations has a major impact on research in basic and clinical oncology. In human cancer, the cell population within a single neoplasm is often heterogeneous. Tumors which appear homogeneous by light microscopy may contain cells with very different abilities to invade or metastasize, or with varying degrees of sensitivity to cytotoxic agents and irradiation. There is increasing evidence that tumor heterogeneity is at least partially a consequence of the positions of the tumor cells in relation to each other and to normal tissue elements (Heppner 1984).

In transitional cell carcinoma of the bladder, glandular or squamous metaplasia is a common event (Hofstädter 1986). However, to date only one report has been published of a bladder cancer cell line expressing this phenotypical heterogeneity in vitro (Russell et al. 1988; Brown et al. 1990). We have recently established a new bladder cancer cell line with a mixed, i.e., adenosquamous differentiation pattern (Offner et al. 1990). Since we considered the possibility that cells grown in two-dimensional monolayers did not show the behavioral repertoire of cells in situ, we additionally used the multicellular tumor spheroid (MCTS) model as a culture model of intermediate complexity. MCTSs grown systematically from single cells exhibit defined three-dimensional structural characteristics and in regard to differentiation have been shown to reflect the in vivo situation more closely (Sutherland et al. 1986; Sutherland 1988). In the present paper we report our comparative analysis of tumor heterogeneity in monolayers and MCTSs of the transitional cell carcinoma cell line HOK-1.

Materials and Methods

Tissue Culture

The transitional cell carcinoma cell line HOK-1 was used between passage 30 and 40. Tumor cells were grown as monolayers in 25-cm^2 plastic tissue culture flasks

[1] Institut für Pathologie der RWTH, Pauwelsstr. 30, W-5100 Aachen, FRG.
[2] Institut für Pathologie der Universität, W-8400 Regensburg, FRG.
[3] Urologische Klinik der Universität/Gesamthochschule, Hufelandstr. 55, W-4300 Essen 1, FRG.

in a 1 : 2 mixture of Dulbecco's modified Eagle's medium (DMEM, Seromed) and MCDB-151 (Sigma) supplemented with 5% fetal calf serum (Boehringer) and penicillin/streptomycin (100 IU/ml, 100 mg/ml, Seromed), phosphoethanolamine (10^{-4} *M*), bovine insulin (0.5 μg/ml) and EGF (2.5 ng/ml; all Sigma). To culture tumor spheroids, cells were detached with 0.05% trypsin-EDTA, washed once in medium, and plated on agarose-coated (1% agarose, Serva) wells in 96-microwell cluster plates at a cell density of 4000 cells/200 μl. Within 4 days of incubation at 37 °C, the cells formed solid cell aggregates. Medium was changed every 2nd day.

Immunohistochemistry

Indirect immunofluorescence was used to analyze cytokeratin expression. Monolayers were grown on glass slides fixed in precooled (−20 °C) methanol, rinsed in acetone, and stained with monoclonal antibodies against different cytokeratin species (see Table 1). A fluorescein-conjugated goat anti-mouse immunoglobulin (1/50) was used as a second antibody. Cryostat sections of MCTSs were briefly fixed in acetone and thereafter treated in the same manner.

Light and Electron Microscopy

For light microscopy cells were grown on glass slides until confluent, fixed in methanol/ethanol (1 : 2) and stained with periodic acid-Schiff (PAS) and Alcian blue for mucin. MCTSs were fixed in 10% formalin embedded in paraffin and sections were stained in the same way. For electron microscopy, monolayers and MCTSs were fixed in cacodylate-buffered 3% glutaraldehyde, postfixed in osmium, dehydrated in EtOH, and embedded in epon. Ultrathin sections were examined with a Philips EM 400T transmission electron microscope. Scanning electron microscopy was conducted with a Philips SEM 515.

Results

Monolayers of HOK-1 cells showed a wide range of morphological features (Fig. 1 a). Most cells formed closely opposed clusters of polygonal epithelial cells varying in size. A considerable proportion of these cells showed active mucin production, as demonstrated by positive staining with PAS and Alcian blue (Fig. 1 a, inset). In addition, there were a few spindle-shaped cells and cells which developed long dentritic extensions. Ultrastructurally, three cell types could be distinguished. First, there were cells which showed intracytoplasmic lumina with short blunt microvilli. They contained secretory material and correspond to mucin droplets seen by light microscopy. Many cells showed numerous electron-dense tonofibrils (Fig. 1 b, *arrowhead*). Occasionally, bundles converging perpendicularly onto desmosomes were seen. Finally, there were cells displaying no special differentiation features, consistent with a transitional phenotype. Immunohistochemically all cell

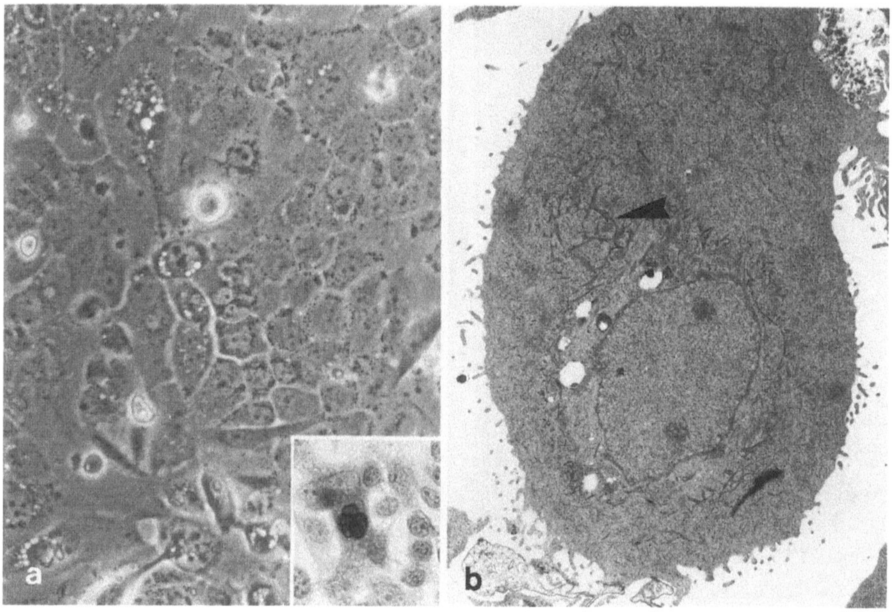

Fig. 1a, b. Phase contrast microscopy and transmission electron microscopy of cells grown as a monolayer

types stained positively for the antibody KL-1. Moreover, some cells reacted with 8.60 which detects the cytokeratin subtypes 10 and 11. Moll et al. (1988) have shown that these cytokeratin types are predominantly expressed in squamous epithelial cells.

Four days after initiation of MCTSs, almost round tumor cell aggregates developed. However prolonged culture (days 8–20) led to grossly irregular tumor cell clusters (Fig. 2a). Sections of these aggregates revealed two segregating cell populations (Fig. 2b). One population (A) consisted mainly of large cells. Numerous cells within this area produced mucin as demonstrated by Alcian blue and PAS stain. The second population (B, *arrowhead* in Fig. 2) was formed by small tightly packed cells. Ultrathin sections revealed that in population A, cells with either squamous (tonofibrils) or glandular differentiation characteristics dominated. By contrast, cells in population B showed mainly undifferentiated cells with moderate quantities of rough endoplasmic reticulum. Immunohistochemically, MCTSs on day 4 were positive for several cytokeratins including CK 10 and CK 11 (Table 1). There was no detectable expression of vimentin. In MCTSs with the two distinct populations, cells in area A showed essentially the same characteristics. However, in area B there was only occasional positivity for cytokeratins but moderate expression of vimentin.

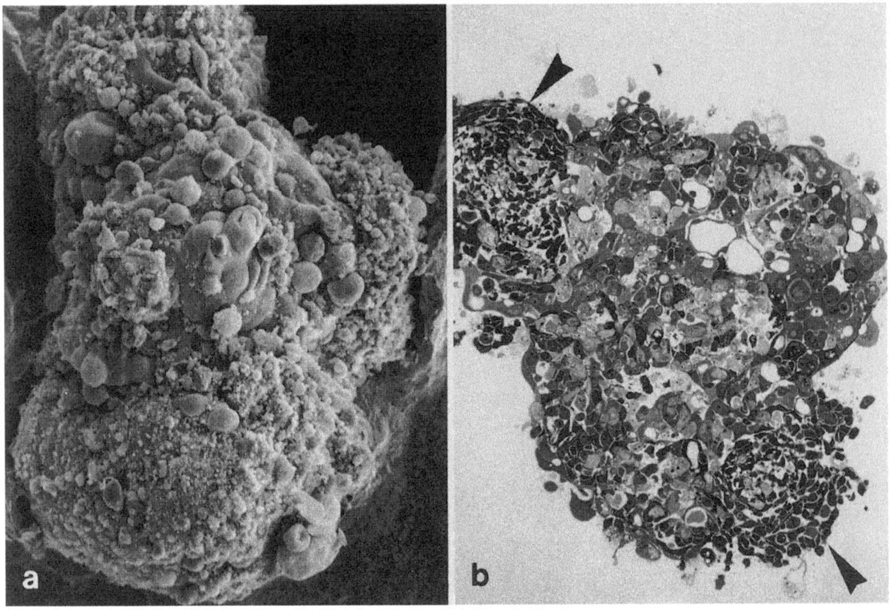

Fig. 2a, b. Scanning electron microscopy and semithin section of MCTS (cultured for 16 days)

Table 1. Cytokeratin expression of HOK-1

Mab designation	Specificity	Immunofluorescence microscopy		
		Monoplayer (P31)	MCTS (P31)	
			Area A	Area B
KL-1[a]	Human keratins, MW 56 kD	+ + +	+ + +	+
8.12[b]	CK 13, 16	+	+ +	−
4.62[b]	CK 19	+ + +	+ + +	+
8.60[b]	CK 1, 10, 11	+ +	+ +	−
RGE 53[c]	CK 18	+	+ +	+
VIM-3B4[d]	Vimentin	−	−	+

[a] Immunotech, France.
[b] Biomakor, Israel.
[c] Eurodiagnostics, Netherlands.
[d] Progen, FRG.

Discussion

Tumor heterogeneity is one of the major factors limiting therapeutic success. It is therefore particularly desirable to establish experimental models which meet the needs of studying the phenomenon of tumor heterogeneity in vitro.

As demonstrated, the cell line HOK-1 in vitro expresses squamous as well as glandular and transitional differentiation characteristics. However, in monolayer cultures these cell types are randomly distributed. In MCTSs, on the other hand, there seem to exist cell-segregating forces which allow the detection of two areas consisting mainly of two distinct cell types, namely, differentiated and undifferentiated. Boyer et al. (1989) have recently shown that, upon changes of the microenvironment, the rat bladder carcinoma cell line NBT-II is able to undergo a transition from an epithelial to a mesenchymal state of differentiation associated with a decrease in cytokeratin expression and an onset of vimentin expression. They hypothesized that single cell infiltration of carcinoma tumors is accompanied by the acquisition of a fibroblastic-like morphology and acquired locomotory capabilities, and that this conversion between epithelial and mesenchymal morphologies (similar to the epithelium-to-mesenchym transition found in embryonic development) could be mimicked in vitro in appropriate conditions of culture. However, the epithelial-to-mesenchymal transition may be an intrinsic property of certain tumor subpopulations. In this context it is interesting to note that in MCTSs cultured in a standard medium (RPMI-1640) we were unable to observe cell separation with the appearance of vimentin-positive cells. However, the latter was clearly seen when the cells were switched back to the medium described, indicating that a subpopulation of HOK-1 cells requires certain culture conditions for segregation. Possibly a mechanism like the one mentioned above is involved in the differentiation and segregation of different cell populations in HOK-1 MCTSs. A detailed clonal analysis and an evaluation of the mechanisms of the tumor cell-to-cell interaction would be of great interest.

Summary

We describe in detail the growth pattern and differentiation of the transitional cell carcinoma cell line HOK-1 grown as monolayers and tumor spheroids. In monolayers, cells with transitional, glandular, and squamous differentiation characteristics are randomly distributed. In tumor spheroids, a sorting out of different cell subpopulations associated with different expression of cytoskeletal proteins is observed. The cell line HOK-1 may serve as an interesting model for the analysis of cell-to-cell interaction in human bladder cancer.

References

Boyer B, Tucker GC, Valles AM, Franke WW, Thiery JP (1989) Rearrangements of desmosomal and cytoskeletal proteins during the transition from epithelial to fibroblastoid organization in cultured rat bladder carcinoma cells. J Cell Biol 109:1495–1509

Brown JL, Russell PJ, Philips J, Wotherspoon J, Raghavan D (1990) Clonal analysis of a bladder cancer cell line: an experimental model of tumor heterogeneity. Br J Cancer 61:369–376

Heppner G (1984) Tumor heterogeneity. Cancer Res 44:2259–2265

Hofstädter F (1986) Tumors of the urogenital system. Verh Dtsch Ges Pathol 70:172–183

Moll R, Achtstätter T, Becht E, Balcarova-Ständer J, Ittensohn M, Franke WW (1988) Cytokeratins in normal and malignant transitional epithelium. Am J Pathol 132:123–144

Offner FA, Ott G, Füzesi L, Preisler V, Hundeck J, Klosterhalfen B, Hofstädter F, Rübben H, Kirkpatrick CJ (1990) Tumorheterogenität: Etablierung und Charakterisierung einer neuen humanen Harnblasenkarzinomzellinie mit adenosquamöser Differenzierung. Z Urol Post 3:206–208

Russell PJ, Jelbart M, Wills E, Singh S, Wass J, Wotherspoon J, Raghavan D (1988) Establishment and characterisation of a new human bladder cancer cell line showing features of squamous and glandular differentiation. Int J Cancer 41:74–82

Sutherland RM (1988) Cell and environment interactions in tumor microregions: the multicell spheroid model. Science 240:177–184

Sutherland RM, Sordat B, Bamat J, Gabbert H, Bourrat B, Mueller-Klieser W (1986) Oxygenation and differentiation in multicellular spheroids of human colon carcinoma. Cancer Res 46: 5320–5329

Tumour Induction at Ureterosigmoid Anastomosis without Faecal Stream: An Experimental Study *

W.-D. E. MIERSCH [1] and J. VOGEL [2]

Introduction

To date there have been more than 100 case reports describing the occurrence of malignant tumours after ureterosigmoidostomy performed after benign primary disease. It is beyond doubt that this kind of supravesical urinary diversion may lead to tumour induction (Bristol and Williamson 1981; Miersch et al. 1989; Miersch 1990; Urdameta et al. 1966). However, induction of malignant tumours has also been observed after other forms of urinary diversion with bowel segments. Tumours have been found in colocystoplasties, ileocystoplasties, in a rectal bladder, and also in colon and ileal conduits (Chiang et al. 1982; Shousha et al. 1978). Here, in these urinary diversions without faecal stream, postoperative care with regard to the possible induction of tumour is by no means general. To determine the possible risk, we decided to examine whether induction of tumour at the site of anastomosis is possible without faecal stream, and, if so, to what extent it is possible.

Materials and Method

Male Han: Wistar rats weighing approx. 200 g were chosen, because in earlier close studies no relevant spontaneous incidence of intestinal tumours was found (Deerberg et al. 1980). They were operated under Rumpun-Ketanest anaesthesia. Using microsurgical techniques, the left ureter was antirefluxively implanted into a rectal bladder according to Mauclaire (Miersch 1988). The faeces were excluded from the rectal bladder by an anus praeter. Before the implantation the intestinal segment which was used to form the rectal bladder was carefully cleaned and disinfected with polyvinyl iodine (Fig. 1). The right ureter was left in situ because we wanted to avoid the development of hyperchloremic acidosis in order to eliminate the possible influence of the metabolic process on carcinogenesis. Six to 8 weeks after the operation urography was performed to check the patency of the anastomosis (Fig. 2). Animals with open anastomoses were kept under observation. As standard diet they received Altromin R. Administration of carcinogens was completely avoided. Rats showing a sign of disease were selected and killed by an overdose of anaesthetic. After section the animals were examined macroscopically and with magnifying lenses. If tumour formation was seen, a longitudinal section was

---

* Supported by a grant from the Dr. Mildred Scheel Foundation for Cancer Research, FRG.

[1] Urologische Universitätsklinik, Sigmund-Freud-Str. 25, W-5300 Bonn 1, FRG.
[2] Institut für Pathologie der Universität, Sigmund-Freud-Str. 25, W-5300 Bonn 1, FRG.

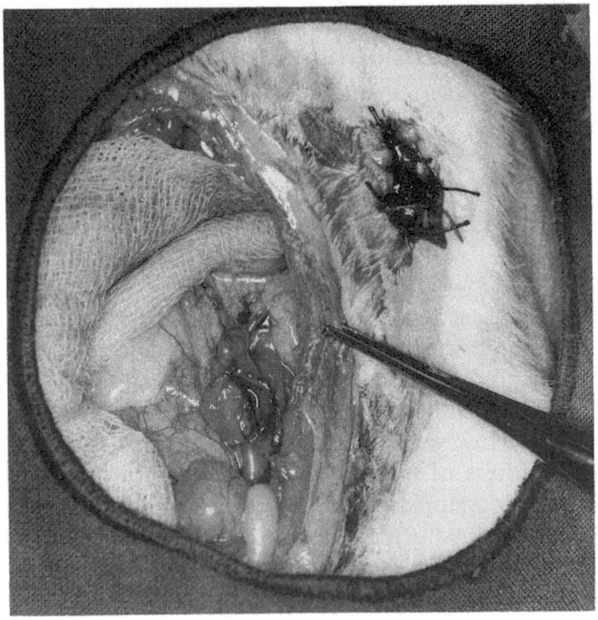

Fig. 1. Site of operation; ureterocolic anastomosis marked by thread. Faeces are excluded by anus praeter

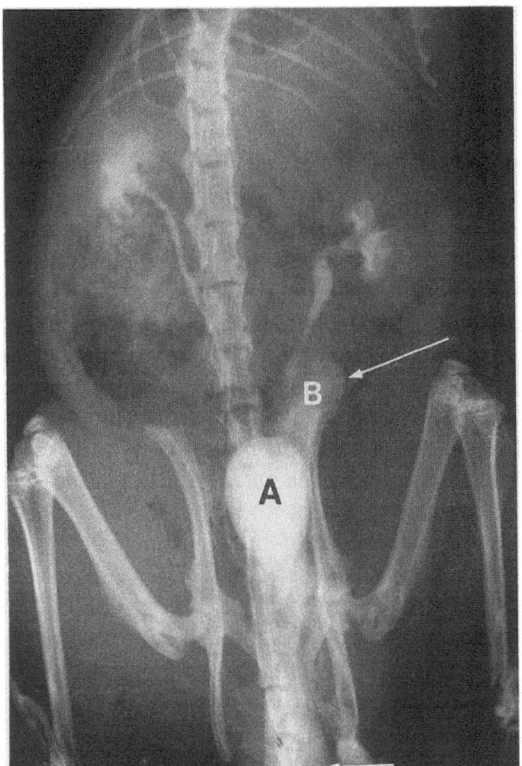

Fig. 2. Urogram; right kidney fills the urinary bladder (*A*), left kidney fills the rectal bladder (*B*), whose border is indicated by the *arrows*

taken from the region of the ureterocolic anastomosis, embedded in paraffin, and later on worked up by many different sections. The histological examination was performed with routinely stained sections. The observation period was limited to 2 years. In a control group ($n = 80$) the colon was irritated in the same way as by implantation of the ureter.

Results

After an average observation period of 19.9 months 76 Han: Wistar rats were evaluable. In 30 of these rats, the appearance of a tumour was found macroscopically. In 19 cases (25%) histological examination revealed a real neoplasm. Six malignant tumours (7.9%) could be diagnosed, all of them polypous transitional cell carcinomas (Fig. 3) which had developed directly at the site of the anastomosis and showed a clear intermixture of mucosa and urothelial parts, especially in their base. In all cases the artificially produced borderline between urothelium and intestinal mucosa was somewhat unstable. Surplus repairs and extremely high inflammatory activity were seen (Fig. 4). The benign neoplasms (17.1%) consisted of 1 adenoma (Fig. 5) of the intestinal type and 12 urothelial papillomas (Fig. 6). These tumours were also located directly at the site of the anastomosis. All the other apparent tumours ($n = 11$) proved to be mucosal hyperplasia or foldings of the intestinal mucosa or the intestinal wall.

After an average observation period of 19.1 months no intestinal tumour was identified in the control group.

Discussion

Among urologists it is generally agreed that regular follow-up examinations, particularly by endoscopy, should be performed after ureterosigmoidostomy with combined diversion of both urine and faeces (Amis et al. 1981; Martinez et al. 1986; Starling et al. 1984; Uehling et al. 1982). Our results reveal evident induction of carcinoma at the site of the implantation even without faecal stream. This precept should therefore be extended to all supravesical urinary diversions using bowel, especially colon. Although in our experiment only one adenoma was induced, it is to be expected that, following the adenoma-carcinoma sequence, adenocarcinomas may develop (Hill 1978; Morson 1974). Overall, the induction of malignant tumours (7.9%) is similar to tumour induction in experimental ureterosigmoidostomies with constantly balanced metabolism (Miersch and Vogel 1989).

All tumours developed directly at the site of the anastomosis. Here we discovered an extremely unstable borderline of transitional cell epithelium and intestinal mucosa, with regenerating activity raised to a maximum. The mucosa of the colon often tried to coat the ureter, while the transitional cell epithelium often extended beyond the implantation site and protruded into the colon. All the other parts of the rectal bladder were found to be tumour-free. This emphasizes the importance of a local factor in the induction of tumour.

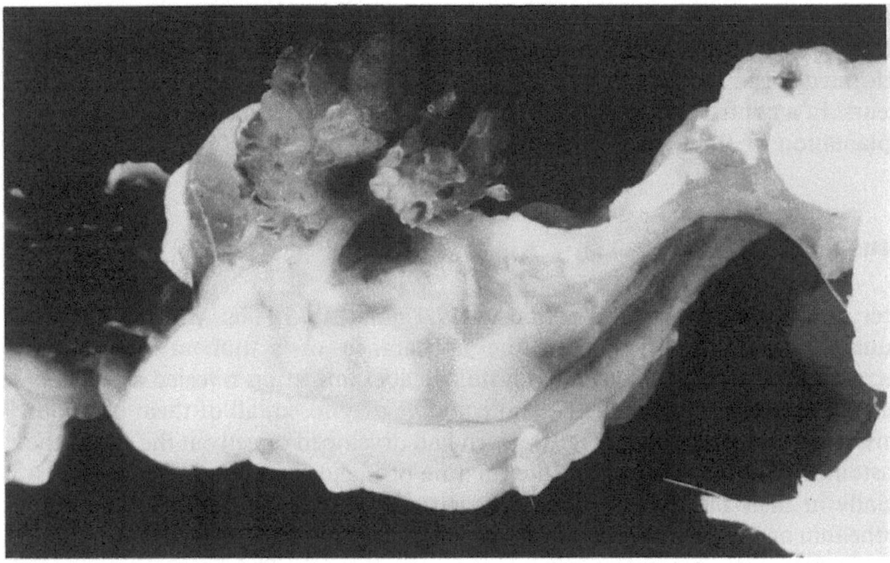

a

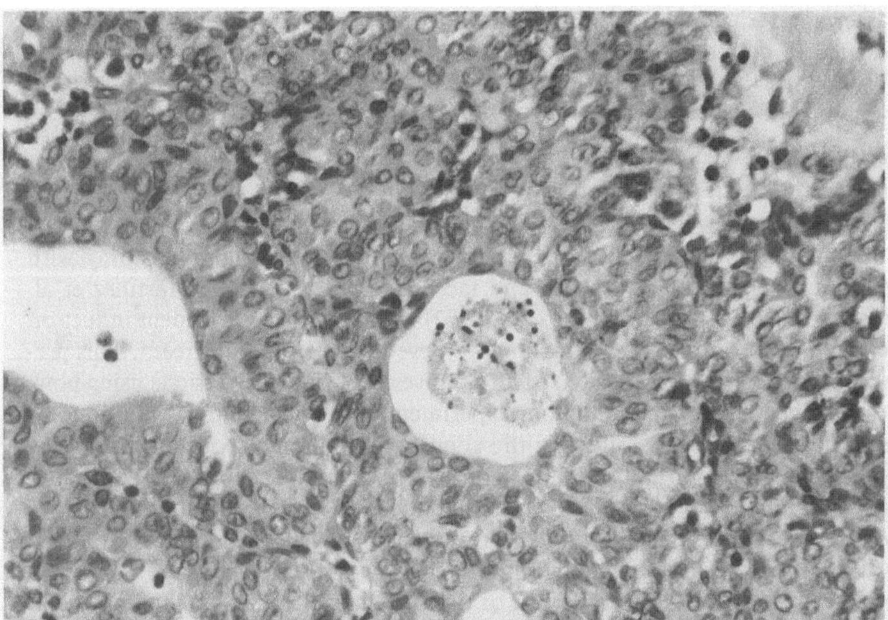

b

Fig. 3 a. Macroscopic view of transitional cell carcinoma at the site of ureter implantation; **b** Histological view of transitional cell carcinoma at the site of ureter implantation (×450); **c** Histological view of lymphnode metastasis of transitional cell carcinoma at the site of ureter implantation (×250)

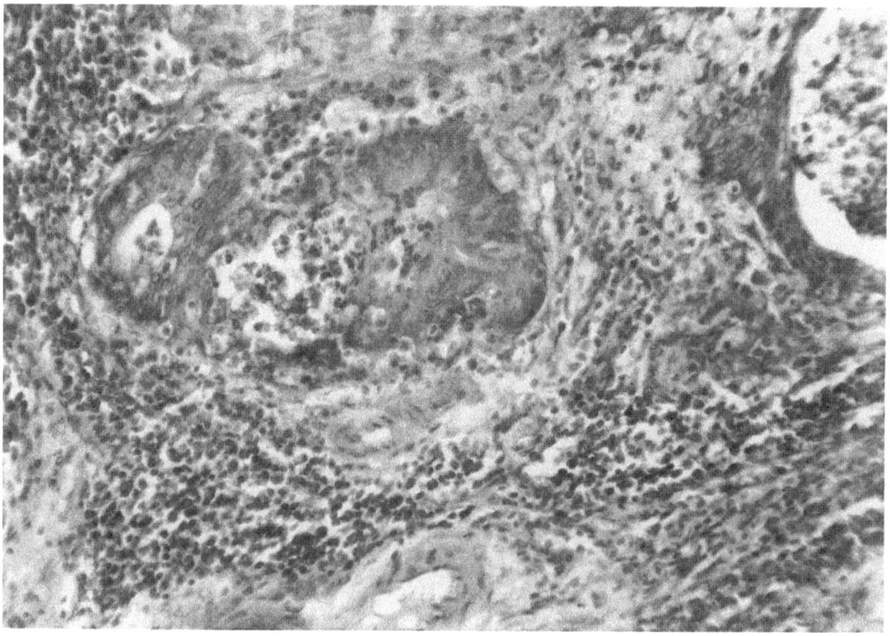

Fig. 3c

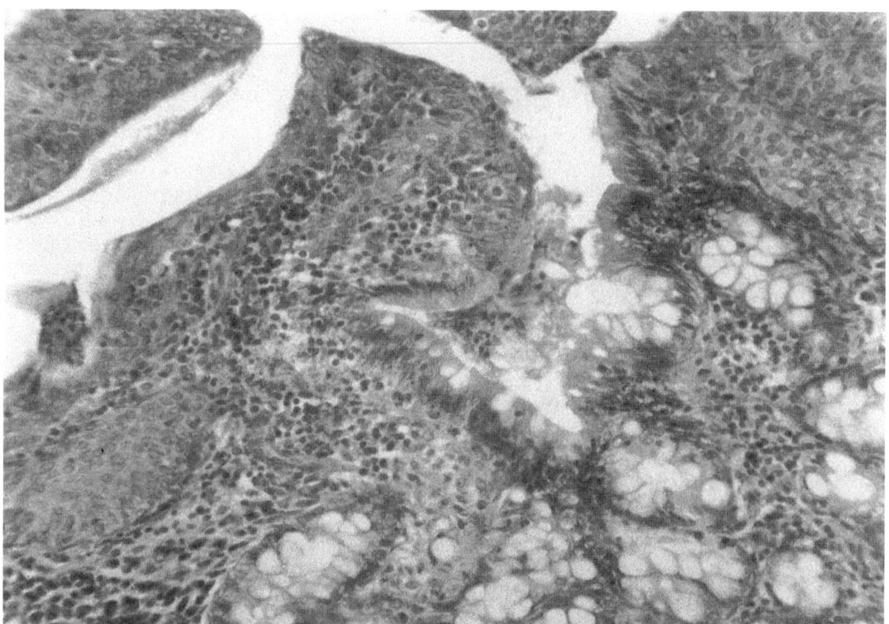

Fig. 4. Unstable artificially produced borderline between urothelium and mucosa of the colon (×250)

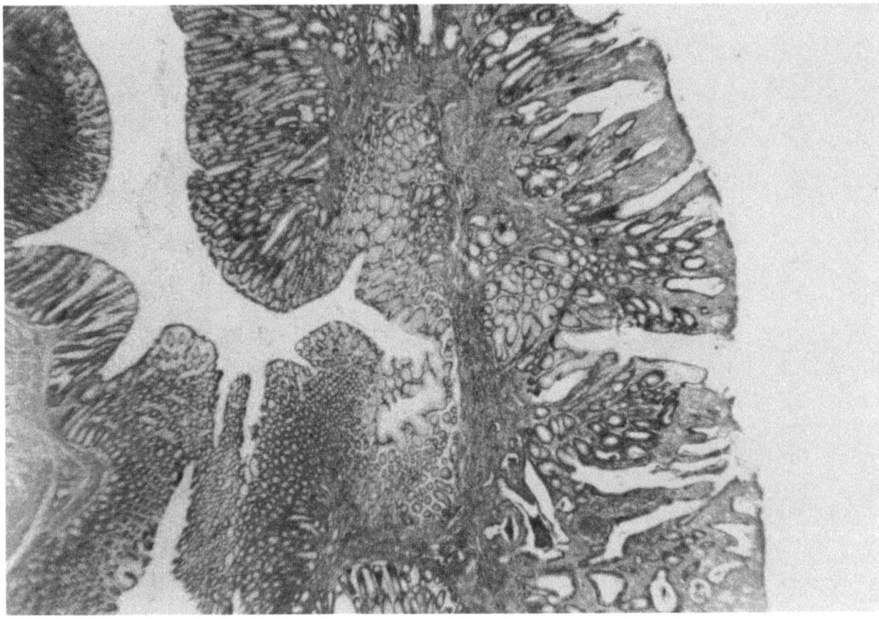

Fig. 5. Histological view of adenoma at the site of ureter implantation (×80)

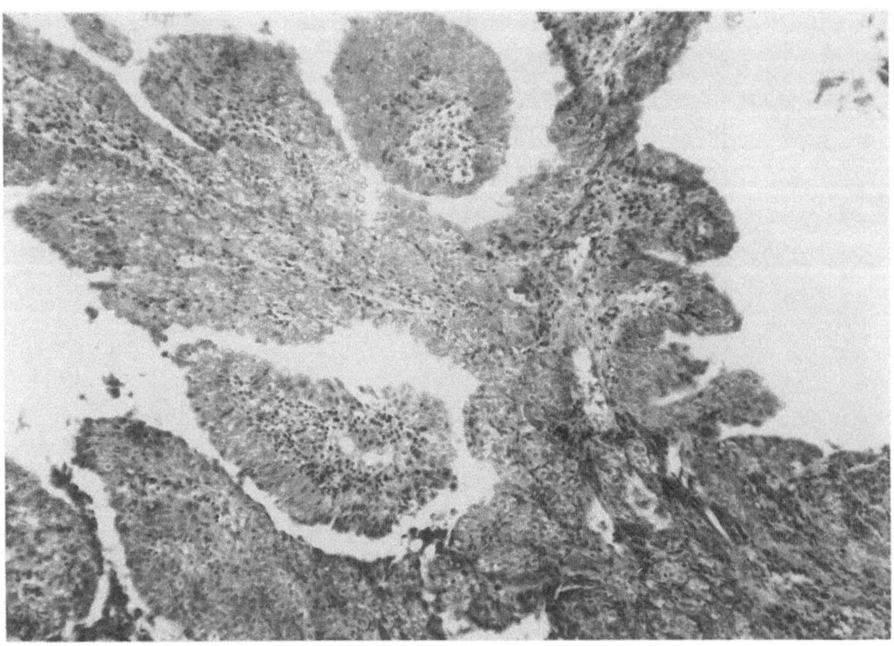

Fig. 6. Histological view of urothelial papilloma at the site of ureter implantation (×80)

The old theory of tumour induction, which postulated development of carcinogenous *N*-nitrosamines (Crissey et al. 1980; Stewart 1986), from the mixture of urine and faeces, must be regarded very critically. It should further be considered that, compared to the high level of nitrate in our food, the amount of absorbable nitrate discharged with the urine may be quite small, so that even without ureterosigmoidostomy, development of *N*-nitrosamines should be possible with the existence of faeces, nitrate, and a mixed bacterial flora. Facts relating to this theory, especially those taking diet and nitrate level into account, have not yet been published and are to be the subject of further research. Kälble et al. (1990), despite using a very precise method, did not find a significant difference between the formation of *N*-nitrosamines in the faeces of rats operated after Crissey's model (Crissey et al. 1980) and that in rats without urinary diversion.

References

Amis ES, Cronan JJ, Pfister RC (1981) Filling defects in small bowel urinary conduits. Am J Roentgenol 137:787–792

Bristol JB, Williamson RCN (1981) Ureterosigmoidostomy and colon carcinogenesis. Science 214:351

Chiang MS, Minton JP, Clausen K, Clatworthy HW, Wise HA (1982) Carcinoma in a colon conduit urinary diversion. J Urol 127:1185–1187

Crissey MM, Steele GD, Gittes RF (1980) Rat model for carcinogenesis in ureterosigmoidostomy. Science 207:1079–1080

Deerberg F, Rapp KG, Pittermann W, Rehm S (1980) Zum Tumorspektrum der Han:Wist-Ratte. Z Versuchstierkd 22:267–280

Hill MJ (1978) Epidemiology and etiology of colon cancer. In: Grundmann E (ed) Colon cancer (Cancer Campaign, vol 2). Fischer, Stuttgart, pp 15–27

Kälble T, Tricker AR, Möhring K, Berger MR, Geiss H, Staehler G (1990) The role of nitrate, nitrite and *N*-nitrosamines in carcinogenesis of colon tumours following ureterosigmoidostomy. Urol Res 18:123–129

Martinez E, Viladoms JM, Roca M, Vida F, Riello H, Zungri E (1986) Fiberendoscopy in the diagnosis of the pathology of the ileal conduit. Urol Int 41:260–262

Miersch W-D (1988) A new microsurgical model for the study of carcinogenesis of colonic urinary diversion in rats. Urol Int 43:269–271

Miersch W-D, Vogel J, Molitor D (1989) Spätergebnisse nach Harnleiter-Darm-Implantation: Morphologische Veränderungen der Darmschleimhaut. In: Verhandlungsbericht der Deutschen Gesellschaft für Urologie, 40. Tagung, Saarbrücken 1988. Springer, Berlin Heidelberg New York Tokyo, pp 206–207

Miersch W-D, Vogel J (1989) Tumors experimentally produced in a rat model for carcinogenesis in ureterosigmoidostomy. Invest Urol 3:135–142

Miersch W-D (1990) Dünn- oder Dickdarm als Blasenersatz? TW Urol Nephrol 2:318–329

Morson BC (1974) Evolution of cancer of the colon and rectum. Cancer 34:845–849

Shousha S, Scott J, Polak J (1978) Ileal loop carcinoma after cystectomy for bladder exstrophy. Br Med J 2:397–398

Starling JR, Uehling DT, Gilchrist KW (1984) Value of colonoscopy after ureterosigmoidostomy. Surgery 96:784–787

Stewart M (1986) Urinary diversion and bowel cancer. Ann R Coll Surg Engl 68:98–102

Uehling DT, Starling JR, Gilchrist KW (1982) Surveillance colonoscopy after ureterosigmoidostomy. J Urol 127:34–36

Urdaneta LF, Duffell D, Creevy CD, Aust JB (1966) Late development of primary carcinoma following ureterosigmoidostomy: report of three cases and literature review. Ann Surg 164:503–513

Endogenous Nitrosation and Induction of Sigmoid Carcinoma Following Ureterosigmoidostomy in a Rat Model

T. KÄLBLE[1], A. R. TRICKER[2], W. SCHREIBER[1], K. MÖHRING[1], and G. STAEHLER[1]

Abstract

In former investigations no increased nitrosamine excretion in urine/feces mixtures of rats was found following ureterosigmoidostomy, despite an incidence of colon tumors of 31.4%. Therefore, further experiments have been performed to clarify the role of endogenous nitrosation in the rectosigmoid following ureterosigmoidostomy. After gavage of 20 mg nitrate and 100 mg proline there was no significant difference in nitrosoproline (NPRO) excretion between 10 operated and 10 control rats. The lack of difference between the two groups in regard to NPRO excretion following gavage of 50 µg NPRO showed that there is no NPRO absorption or metabolism in the rectosigmoid. Analysis of rectosigmoid contents from 20 ureterosigmoidostomized rats and 10 control rats showed *N*-nitrosodimethylamine (NDMA) concentrations at the limit of detection.

Endogenous nitrosation seems to play no role in colon carcinogenesis in rats following ureterosigmoidostomy. Our results suggest that other factors such as increased proliferation at the urointestinal anastomosis are more important in humans as well.

Introduction

One of the most recognized theories concerning the development of colon carcinoma following ureterosigmoidostomy is bacteria-catalyzed formation of *N*-nitrosamines from bacterially reduced urinary nitrate and endogenous amines in feces and urine [2, 10]. In former investigations significantly increased *N*-nitrosamine excretion was found in 28 ureterosigmoidostomized patients [6] but not in a rat model for ureterosigmoidostomy [5], despite a colon tumor incidence in these animals of 31.4% (unpublished data).

The nitrosamines must therefore either be absorbed or metabolized before excretion, or else no nitrosation takes place in the rectosigmoid of rats that have undergone ureterosigmoidostomy – a question which was to be answered by the following experiments.

[1] Chirurgische Universitätsklinik, Abt. Urologie und Poliklinik, Im Neuenheimer Feld 110, W-6900 Heidelberg 1, FRG.

[2] Institut für Toxikologie und Chemotherapie, Deutsches Krebsforschungszentrum, Im Neuenheimer Feld 280, W-6900 Heidelberg 1, FRG.

Materials and Methods

Experiment 1

Twenty female Wistar rats were prospectively randomized into two groups. One group was operated on according to the ureterosigmoidostomy model of Crissey [3] and Gittes [4]; the other group acted as control. The animals in both groups received antibiotic coverage with indanyl-carbenicillin 127 mg/l drinking water. Three weeks postoperatively the 24-h excretion of nitrate, nitrite, and NPRO was analyzed in urine/feces from the operated and urine from the control rats. After gavage of a single dose of 100 mg proline and 20 mg nitrate to each animal by feeding tube, the 24-h urine analysis was repeated. Seven weeks postoperatively, five animals of each group received 50 μg NPRO each by feeding tube, followed by another 24-h collection period of urine and urine/feces mixture with consecutive measurement of nitrate, nitrite, and NPRO concentration.

Experiment 2

Thirty other female Wistar rats were prospectively randomized into three groups. Ten animals were operated on according to the rat model described above (Fig. 1) with indanyl-carbenicillin prophylaxis, ten were operated on without antibiotic coverage, and ten acted as controls. Six weeks postoperatively the mesosigmoids were divided to avoid absorption of the rectosigmoid contents, the distal recta were ligated, and 30 min later the rectosigmoids including their contents were removed for analysis of volatile *N*-nitroso compounds.

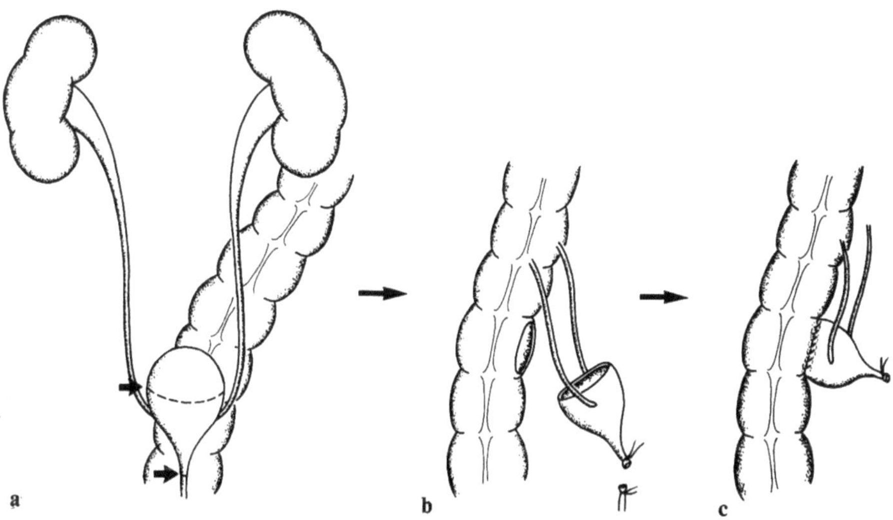

Fig. 1a–c. Rat model for ureterosigmoidostomy according to Crissey [3] and Gittes [4]. **a** Preoperative anatomy; **b** ligation of the proximal urethra, resection of the bladder dome, incision of the anterior wall of the rectosigmoid; **c** anastomosis of the remaining patch to the rectosigmoid

Analysis of Nitrate, Nitrite and *N*-Nitrosamines

Urine and urine/feces mixtures were collected in metabolic cages, the collecting box containing 2.5 *M* NaOH and 1 m*M* 2-(ethylmercurymercapto)benzoic acid for prevention of artefact nitrosamine formation and bacterial growth as well as 1 m*M* morpholine as internal control for nitrosation. For nitrosamine analysis an established gas chromatographic method with a highly nitrosamine-specific detector as described previously [5] was used.

For statistical analysis the Wilcoxon two-sample test was used.

Results

Experiment 1

The results of nitrate, nitrite, and NPRO analysis of the ten control urines and the ten urine/feces mixtures are presented in Table 1. The excretion of nitrate in ureterosigmoidostomized rats was significantly lower than in control rats, both untreated and after ingestion of nitrate and proline ($p < 0.001$). Nitrite was only detectable in the ureterosigmoidostomy group, with an increase following nitrate and proline feeding.

In regard to NPRO excretion, however, no significant difference could be found between the two groups either following gavage of nitrate and proline or after NPRO ingestion.

Table 1. Experiment 1: Urinary excretion of nitrate, nitrite, and *N*-nitrosoproline before and after gavage of 100 mg proline + 20 mg nitrate and 50 µg NPRO

	Untreated			Nitrate + proline			NPRO		
	Nitrate (mg/24 h)	Nitrite (mg/24 h)	NPRO (µg/24 h)	Nitrate (mg/24 h)	Nitrite (mg/24 h)	NPRO (µg/24 h)	Nitrate (mg/24 h)	Nitrite (mg/24 h)	NPRO (µg/24 h)
Control group ($n = 10$)									
M	0.83	0	0	13.22	0	5.05	0.86	0	48.86
SD	0.23	0	0	4.28	0	1.69	0.08	0	0.48
Ureterosigmoidostomy group ($n = 10$)									
M	0.016	0.002	0	5.79	0.34	4.61	0.013	0.003	49.25
SD	0.009	0.001	0	1.65	0.24	1.09	0.007	0.001	0.88

M, mean; SD, standard deviation.

Experiment 2

The nitrosamine analysis of the rectosigmoid contents of the ten operated animals with antibiotic coverage, the ten operated animals without antibiotic prophylaxis, and the ten operated controls is shown in Table 2. There is no significant difference between these three groups in regard to urinary NDMA concentration, the only volatile nitroso compound found, all data being at the detection limit of the analytical method of 5 ng.

Table 2. Experiment 2: Concentration of *N*-nitrosodimethylamine in the rectosigmoid contents. Median (range)

	N-Nitrosodimethylamine (ng)
Control group (n = 10)	0 (0 – 3)
Ureterosigmoidostomy with carbenicillin (n = 10)	0 (0 – 3)
Ureterosigmoidostomy without carbenicillin (n = 10)	3 (0 – 6)

Discussion

In agreement with the results of Oshima and Bartsch [7] and Chu and Magee [1], 98% of the ingested dose of NPRO was excreted by unoperated control rats in experiment 1, suggesting subtotal intestinal absorption of NPRO without metabolization. The endogenous NPRO formation of the control rats, resulting in a mean urinary concentration of 5.05 ± 1.69 µg after gavage of 20 mg nitrate and 100 mg proline, was low as expected before. The significantly decreased nitrate concentrations in urine/feces mixtures from ureterosigmoidostomized rats compared to control urines suggest absorption and/or metabolism by intestinal bacteria. The lack of significant differences between NPRO concentrations in urine/feces mixtures of ureterosigmoidectomized rats and urines of unoperated controls either following gavage of nitrate and proline or after NPRO ingestion rules out both nitrosation of proline and metabolization or absorption of NPRO in the rectosigmoid of rats.

The barely detectable NDMA concentrations of 0 – 6 ng in the rectosigmoids of operated and unoperated rats rule out the presence of significant endogenous nitrosamine formation in the rectosigmoid of rats following ureterosigmoidostomy as well. Indanyl-carbenicillin prophylaxis had no influence on NDMA concentration in urine/feces mixtures.

The lack of evidence of nitrosamine formation in the rectosigmoid of rats following ureterosigmoidostomy, despite a colon tumor incidence of 31.4% in 120 rats (unpublished data), shows that tumor growth in the colon following ureterosigmoidostomy is possible without the presence of nitroso compounds. The increased urinary nitrosamine excretion in patients with ureterosigmoidostomy [5, 6, 10] therefore probably plays only a contributory carcinogenic role. Other factors such as proliferative activity at the urointestinal anastomosis [8, 11] and the growth-stimulating effect of urine [9, 12] seem to be the most important factors in colon carcinogenesis following urinary diversions via the intestine.

References

Chu C, Magee PN (1981) Metabolic fate of nitrosoproline in the rat. Cancer Res 41:3653–3657

Cohen MS, Hilz ME, Davis P, Anderson MD (1987) Urinary carcinogen (nitrosamine) production in a rat animal model for ureterosigmoidostomy. J Urol 138:449–452

Crissey MM, Steele GD, Gittes RF (1980) Rat model for carcinogenesis in ureterosigmoidostomy. Science 207:1079–1080

Gittes RF (1986) Carcinogenesis in ureterosigmoidostomy. Urol Clin North Am 13/2:201–205

Kälble T, Tricker AR, Möhring K, Berger MR, Geiss H, Staehler G (1990) The role of nitrate, nitrite and *N*-nitrosamines in carcinogenesis of colon tumours following ureterosigmoidostomy. Urol Res 18:123–129

Kälble T, Tricker AR, Friedl P, Waldherr R, Hoang J, Staehler G, Möhring K (1990) Ureterosigmoidostomy – longterm results, risk of carcinoma and etiological factors for carcinogenesis. J Urol 144:1110–1114

Oshima H, Bartsch H (1981) Quantitative estimation of endogenous nitrosation in humans by monitoring *N*-nitrosoproline excreted in the urine. Cancer Res 41:3658–3662

Roe R, Fermor B, Williamson RCN (1987) Proliferative instability and experimental carcinogenesis at colonic anastomoses. Gut 28:808–815

Rowland RG, Henneberry MO, Oyasu R, Grayhack JT (1980) Effects of urine and continued exposure to carcinogen on progression of early neoplastic urinary bladder lesions. Cancer Res 40:4524–4527

Stewart M (1986) Urinary diversion and bowel cancer. Ann R Coll Surg Engl 68:98–102

Strachan JR, Matthews J, Rees HC, Cooke T (1987) Kinetic changes in experimental colonic urinary diversion. Br J Surg 74/11:1046–1048

Twardzik DR, Sherwin SA, Ranchalis J, Todaro GJ (1982) Transforming growth factors in the urine of normal, pregnant and tumor-bearing humans. JNCL 69/4:793–798

In Vitro Cellular Cytotoxicity Against Human Bladder Carcinoma Cell Lines

A. Böhle[1], A. J. Ulmer[2], M.-H. Wang[2], and H.-D. Flad[2]

Introduction

Clinical trials of intravesical BCG immunotherapy against superficial urothelial bladder carcinoma recurrences have yielded significant results, which seem to be superior to those of intravesical chemotherapy (Herr et al. 1987). However, the mechanisms by which BCG exerts its antitumor effects are still largely unknown. In previous immunohistological examinations we were able to demonstrate the local induction of mononuclear effector cells in the bladder wall such as helper T-cells, macrophages, and B-cells after intravesical BCG (Böhle et al. 1990a). Furthermore, a significant increase of certain cytokines in the urine, such as interleukin-1, interleukin-2, and tumor necrosis factor, has been detected after intravesical BCG therapy (Haaf et al. 1986; Böhle et al. 1990b). These findings suggest different possible effector mechanisms which might be involved in tumor rejection. In an attempt to analyse these effects in vitro and obtain more information on their cytotoxic effectiveness against human bladder carcinoma cell lines, we performed a study to evaluate in vitro the cellular cytotoxicity of different mononuclear cells and the cytokines involved.

Material and Methods

Effector Cells

Human mononuclear cells (MNC) were isolated from the peripheral blood of normal healthy donors by density-gradient centrifugation, washed repeatedly, and adjusted to a concentration of 5×10^7 cells/ml. Lymphocytes were isolated from mononuclear phagocytic cells by the carbonyl-iron phagocytosis method, resulting in a purity of lymphocytes of more than 95%.

For generation of lymphokine-activated killer (LAK) cells, lymphocytes were incubated for 4 days in the presence of 1000 U/ml recombinant interleukin-2 (rIL 2) (Glaxo, Geneva, Switzerland).

[1] Klinik und Poliklinik für Urologie der Medizinischen Universität, Ratzeburger Allee 160, W-2400 Lübeck, FRG.
[2] Institut für Experimentelle Biologie und Medizin, Forschungsinstitut Borstel, Parkallee, W-2061 Borstel, FRG.

Target Cells. Two human urothelial carcinoma cell lines, BT-A and BT-B, were kindly provided by Dr. van der Bosch, Borstel, and grown in permanent serum-free cultures (Bosch et al. 1990). K562, a human erythroleukemia cell line which is highly sensitive to natural killer cell (NK)-mediated cytotoxicity, and L929, a murine fibrosarcoma cell line with known sensitivity to monocyte/macrophage-mediated killing, served as control target cells.

Cytotoxicity Assay

An automated cytotoxicity assay was performed as described previously (Ulmer et al. 1990). Briefly, 10^7 target cells (BT-A, BT-B, K 562, or L929 cells) were labeled with 10 μM Hoechst dye H33342 for 2 h at 37 °C. After repeated washing, labeled cells were resuspended at 5×10^5/ml in U-shaped microtiter plates. Effector cells were added immediately at different concentrations, thus resulting in different effector-to-target cell (E/T) ratios. The plates were incubated for 24 h (and up to 96 h in kinetic experiments). Disintegration of DNA, resulting in the release of DNA-associated H33342, was measurable in the supernatant by a microfluor reader (Dynatech, Denkendorf, FRG), and specific release was calculated according to the formula:

$$\%\ \text{Lysis} = \frac{[\text{experiment release}] - [\text{spontaneous release}]}{[\text{maximal dye incorporation}] - [\text{spontaneous release}]} \times 100$$

Each test was performed in triplicate.

Effects of Cytokines on Bladder Tumor Cells

BT-A or BT-B cells were cultured at 4×10^4 cells per well in the presence or absence of rIL-1β (Glaxo, Geneva, Switzerland), rIL-6 (Sandoz AG, Basel, Switzerland), or rTNF (BASF/Knoll AG, Ludwigshafen, FRG). After 48 h culture, tumor cell growth was determined by the crystal violet staining method (Feist et al. 1989). Briefly, supernatants were discarded, cells were stained with crystal violet, lysed, and optical density was measured with a microplate reader at 550 nm.

Results

Effect of Recombinant Cytokines rIL-1β, rIL-6, and rTNF

Bladder carcinoma cell lines BT-A and BT-B were incubated with doses of recombinant cytokines which were in the range of levels of cytokines previously found in the urine of patients after intravesical BCG therapy (Böhle et al. 1990b) and diluted further. After a culture period of 48 h, no growth-promoting or inhibitory effect of the cytokines rIL-1β, rIL-6, or rTNF was detected in any of the cell lines (Fig. 1).

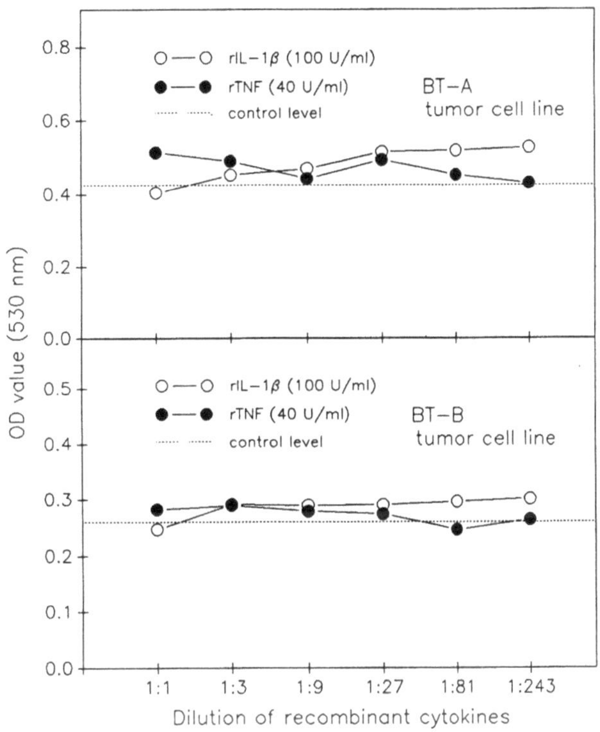

Fig. 1. Absence of effects of low doses of recombinant cytokines on growth of urothelial carcinoma cell lines

Cytotoxicity of Freshly Isolated MNC to Bladder Carcinoma Cell Lines

In order to investigate the natural cytotoxicity of freshly isolated MNC against bladder carcinoma cell lines, the effector cells were cocultured with urothelial target cells at different E/T ratios for 24 h. Bacterial LPS was added to investigate the participation of cytotoxic monocytes/macrophages that are stimulated by this antigen. The results showed that MNC had only a low cytotoxicity against BT-A or BT-B cells, even in the presence of LPS, indicating that neither NK cells nor cytotoxic monocytes/macrophages were effective in this system (Fig. 2). In contrast, coculture with control cell lines K562 and L929 exhibited a high sensitivity of these cells, which could be modulated in the case of L929 cells by addition of LPS (Fig. 3), suggesting a macrophage-related cytotoxicity. However, prolonged incubation of freshly isolated MNC with BT-A and BT-B for up to 4 days resulted in a significant increase of cytotoxicity against these carcinoma cells, apparently without a modulatory effect of LPS (Fig. 4). The rate of spontaneous dye release from BT cells was less than 15% after 96 h (data not shown).

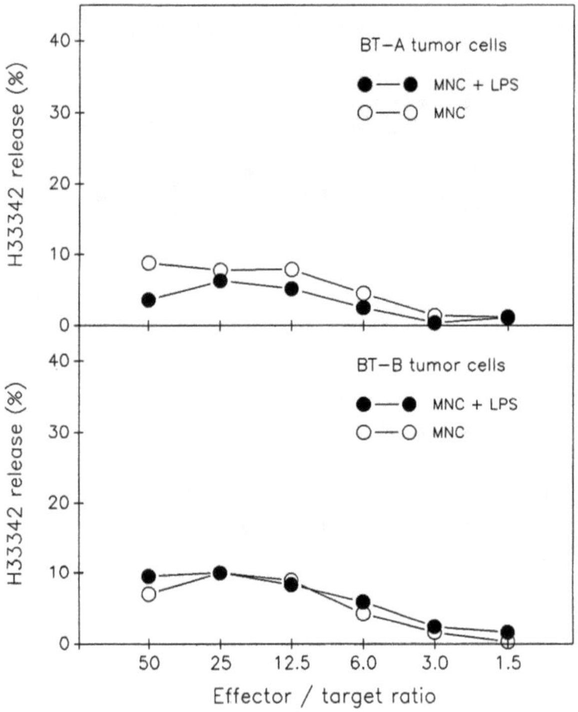

Fig. 2. Cytotoxicity of MNC against urothelial carcinoma cell lines BT-A and BT-B in presence or absence of bacterial LPS. Results are expressed as percentages of H33342 dye release

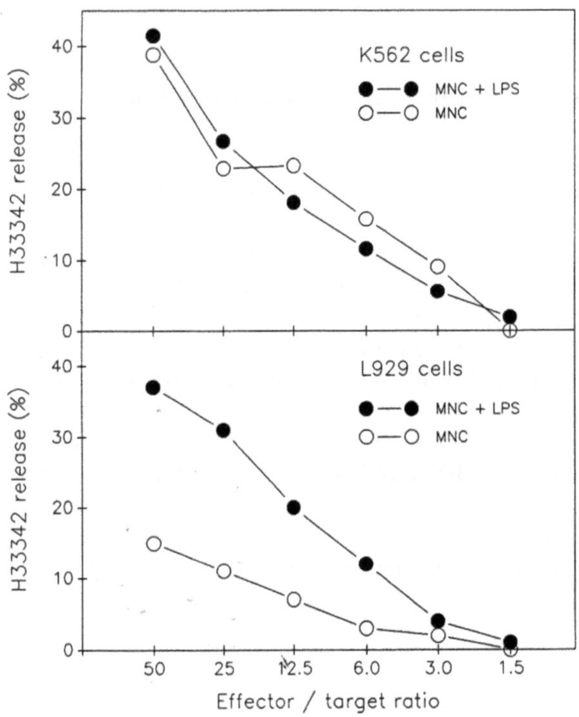

Fig. 3. Cytotoxicity of MNC against control cell lines K562 and L929

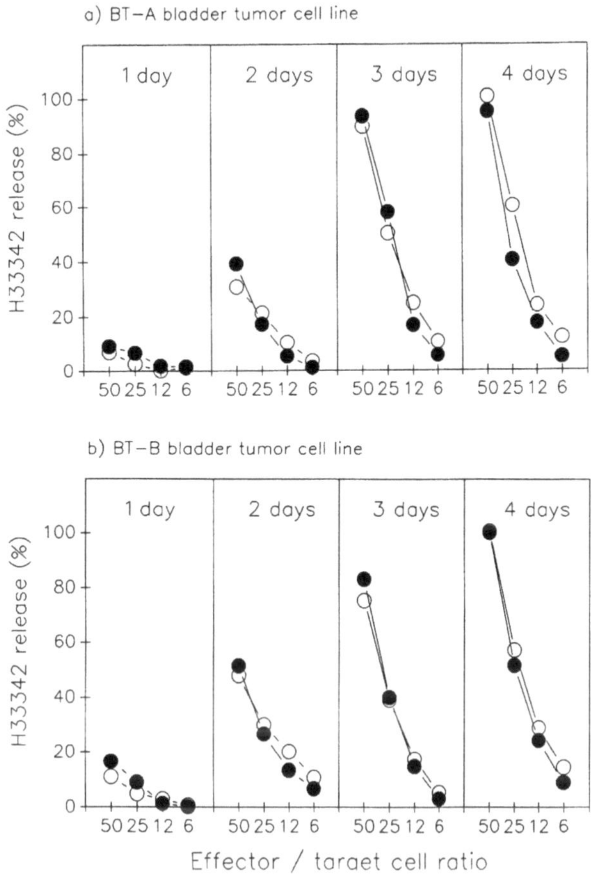

Fig. 4. Kinetics of cytotoxicity of MNC against BT-A and BT-B carcinoma cells in the presence or absence of LPS. Cells were incubated for 1–4 days

Cytotoxicity of Lymphocytes

Lymphocytes were isolated from peripheral blood and coincubated with BT cells for several days. As shown in Fig. 5, cytotoxicity increased after prolonged incubation from 6% at day 1 to 30% at day 4 at an E/T ratio of 12:1.

LAK-Cell Mediated Cytotoxicity

Incubation of lymphocytes with rIL-2 for 4 days resulted in generation LAK cells as described previously (Lotze et al. 1985). These effector cells exhibited a high degree of cytotoxicity against BT-A and BT-B within 24 h of incubation, resulting in lysis of more than 50% at an E/T ratio of 12.5 and more than 80% at an E/T ratio of 50:1 (Fig. 6).

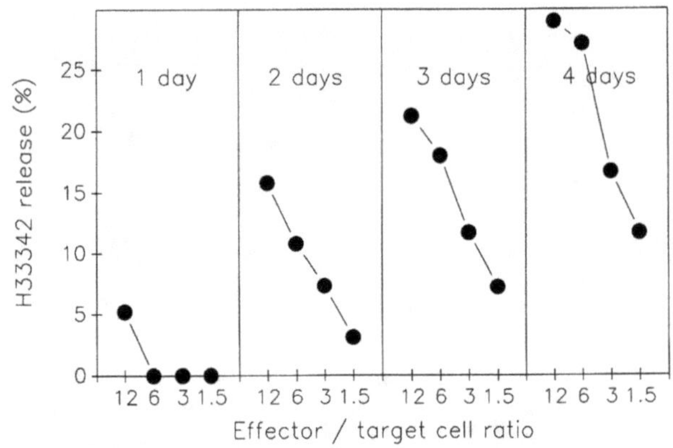

Fig. 5. Kinetics of cytotoxicity of lymphocytes (MNC depleted of phagocytic cells) against BT-A cells

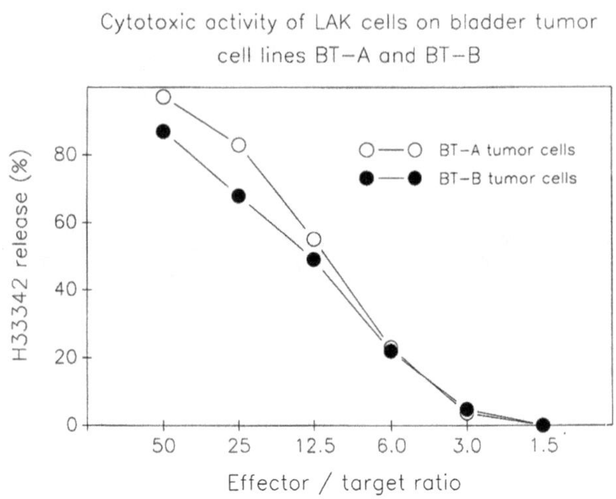

Fig. 6. Cytotoxic activity of IL-2-generated LAK cells against BT-A and BT-B urothelial carcinoma cells

Discussion

Various reports have focused on the immune effects generated by the intravesical administration of BCG (Kelley et al. 1986). In addition to the demonstration of mononuclear cells in the urine (Guinan et al. 1986), a significant accumulation of T-cells, macrophages, and B-cells was shown in the bladder wall of BCG-treated patients, aggregating to granulomas (El-Demiry et al. 1987; Böhle et al. 1990a). Furthermore, significant secretion of cytokines IL-1, IL-2, and TNF into the urine after BCG instillation was reported (Haaff et al. 1986; Böhle et al. 1990b). These findings suggest a local immune activation which is induced by

BCG, resulting in tumor rejection and a prolonged recurrence-free interval in the BCG-treated patient.

Which of the phenomena cited above play a dominant role in the therapeutic effectiveness of BCG? In the in vitro experiments presented here, we tried to answer some aspects of this question.

In our studies we found no direct inhibitory effect of the recombinant cytokines IL-1, IL-6, and TNF against bladder carcinoma cells at the concentrations examined. Although this experimental approach is highly artificial and does not reflect the immune-activating effects of cytokines in vivo, our observation seems to contradict preliminary reports by Sternberg et al. (1990), who observed a partial and a complete remission in patients with superficial bladder carcinoma treated with intravesical TNF in a phase I study. However, the doses they gave exceed the concentrations of TNF seen in the urine of BCG-treated patients and used in the experiments presented here by the factor of 10^9 and may thus reflect some other mechanism of TNF.

In further cytotoxicity assays, we found that freshly isolated MNC did not exert a significant cytolytic effect against bladder tumor cells during 24 h incubation. Increased cytotoxicity became obvious only after prolonged incubation for several days. The addition of LPS had no effect on MNC-mediated lysis, indicating that cytotoxic macrophages were not involved in the cytolytic action of the effector cells against BT-A and BT-B. Furthermore, our results show a similar kinetic of cytolysis of bladder tumor cells when MNC depleted of phagocytic cells were used as effector cells. Thus, we concluded that some form of activation of lymphocytes might take place during prolonged coincubation with allogenic bladder carcinoma cells. As coincubation of lymphocytes with carcinoma cells is known to result in IL-2 secretion and activation of the former, generation of IL-2-activated LAK cells was postulated. In a further step, therefore, bladder carcinoma target cells were incubated with IL-2-generated LAK cells, resulting in a high degree of cytotoxicity within 24 h.

Resistance of tumor cells to NK cells, but sensitivity to LAK cells, has previously been reported for fresh tumor cells of various sources (Roberts et al. 1987). Furthermore, it is known that fresh tumor cells and tumor cells in situ – in contrast to long-term cultured cell lines such as K562 or L929 – are fairly resistant to NK cells, but sensitive to LAK cells (Grimm et al. 1984). Presumably due to this mechanism, highly resistant metastatic carcinomas of various origins showed high response rates to autologous LAK cell therapy, as described previously (Rosenberg et al. 1988). Even continuous perfusion of the tumor-bearing human bladder with high doses of natural IL-2 was recently reported to stimulate local antitumor activity, which thus represents a promising new approach to infiltrating bladder carcinoma (Huland et al. 1990). These results demonstrate the effectiveness of the IL-2-induced LAK cell phenomenon in advanced carcinomas. Our results regarding the cytotoxicity of LAK cells in vitro towards bladder carcinoma cell lines suggest that this may also hold true for the localized superficial urothelial tumor cell treated prophylactically with intravesical BCG.

Since the LAK cell phenomenon is not restricted to MHC, our allogenic in vitro model may resemble well the in vivo situation in the bladder of a BCG-treated patient, and reflect the cytotoxic action of activated LAK cells against bladder carcinoma cells as one aspect of the complex mechanism of topical BCG (Fig. 7): during the BCG-induced acute inflammation of the bladder, significant amounts of IL-2 are produced locally by high numbers of infiltrating mononuclear cells and secreted into the urine. This might give a first activation of LAK cells. The further long-term recurrence-free status of the patient might depend upon continuous stimulation of LAK cells by sensitized lymphocytes with IL-2, the secretion of which has been detected within granulomas of the bladder wall more than 1 year after BCG therapy. Since direct, e.g., immunohistological detection of LAK cells is impossible as yet, further functional studies will have to confirm these assumptions.

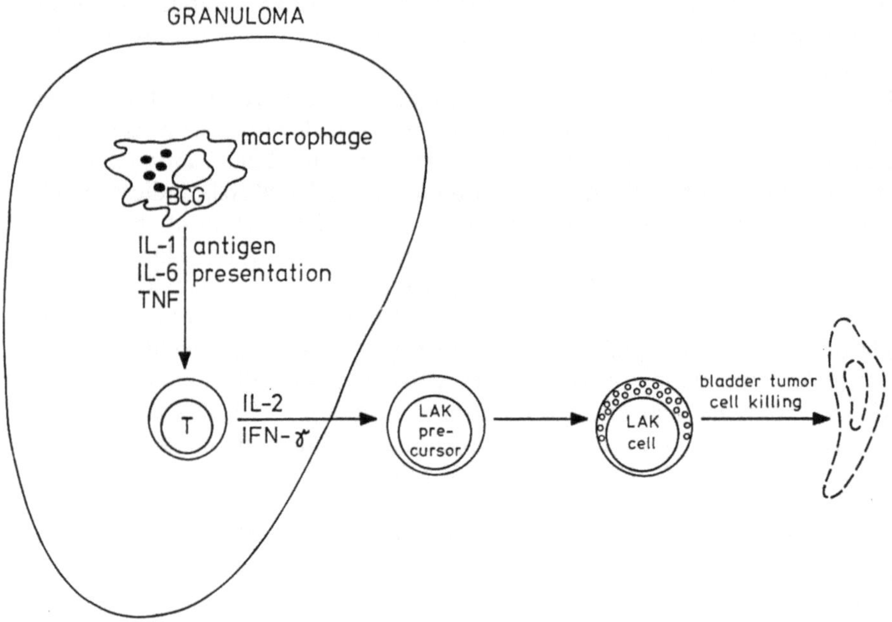

Fig. 7. Possible effector mechanism of intravesical BCG immunotherapy: BCG-induced LAK cell generation

References

Böhle A, Gerdes J, Ulmer AJ, Hofstetter AG, Flad HD (1990) Effects of local bacillus Calmette-Guérin therapy in patients with bladder carcinoma on immunocompetent cells of the bladder wall. J Urol 144:53–58

Böhle A, Nowc C, Ulmer AJ, Musehold J, Gerdes J, Hofstetter AG, Flad HD (1990) Elevations of cytokines interleukin-1, interleukin-2, and tumor necrosis factor in the urine of patients after intravesical bacillus Calmette-Guérin immunotherapy. J Urol 144:59–64

Bosch J vd, Rüller S, Horn D, Schumann R, Schlaak M (1990) Density dependent tumor cell death and reversible cell cycle arrest: mutually exclusive modes of monocyte mediated growth control. Exp Cell Res 187:185–192

El-Demiry MIM, Smith G, Ritchie AWS, James K, Cumming JA, Hargreave TB, Chisholm GD (1987) Local immune responses after intravesical BCG treatment for carcinoma in situ. Br J Urol 60:543

Feist W, Ulmer AJ, Musehold J, Brade H, Kusumoto S, Flad H-D (1989) Induction of tumor necrosis factor α release by lipopolysaccharide and defined lipopolysaccharide partial structures. Immunobiology 179:293–307

Grimm EA, Rosenberg SA (1984) The human lymphokine-activated killer cell phenomenon. Lymphokines 9:279–311

Guinan P, Shaw M, Ray V (1986) Histopathology of BCG and thiotepa treated bladders. Urol Res 14:211–215

Haaff EO, Catalona WJ, Ratliff TL (1986) Detection of interleukin-2 in the urine of patients with superficial bladder tumors after treatment with intravesical bacillus Calmette-Guérin. J Urol 136:970–974

Herr HW, Laudone VP, Whitmore WF (1987) An overview of intravesical therapy for superficial bladder tumors. J Urol 138:1363–1368

Huland E, Huland H (1989) Local continuous high dose interleukin 2: a new therapeutic model for the treatment of advanced bladder carcinoma. Cancer Res 49:5469–5474

Kelley DR, Haaff EO, Becich M, Lage J, Bauer WC, Dresner SM, Catalona WJ, Ratliff TL (1986) Prognostic value of PPD skin test and granuloma formation in patients treated with intravesical bacillus Calmette-Guérin. J Urol 135:268

Lotze MT, Matory YL, Ettinghausen SE, Rayner AA, Sharrow SO, Seipp CA, Custer MC, Rosenberg SA (1985) In vivo administration of purified human interleukin 2: II. Half life, immunologic effects, and expansion of peripheral lymphoid cells in vivo with recombinant IL 2. J Immunol 135:2865–2875

Roberts K, Lotze MT, Rosenberg SA (1987) Separation and functional studies of the human lymphokine-activated killer cell. Cancer Res 47:4366–4371

Rosenberg SA (1988) Immunotherapy of cancer using interleukin 2: current status and future prospects. Immunol Today 9:58

Sternberg C, Arena M, Pansadoro V, Calabresi F, Haas J, Defidio L, Cusumano G, Carli P, Zeuli M, Rosselli M, Cancrini A (1990) Phase I clinical trial of intravesical recombinant tumor necrosis factor (rTNF) in patients with superficial bladder cancer. Eur Urol [Suppl] 18:410

Ulmer AJ, Wang M-H, Hua Y, Flad H-D (1990) DNA fragmentation of targets by natural killer cells and cytotoxic macrophages as measured by fluorometric assay using Hoechst dye 33342. J Immunol Methods (in press)

Ultrastructural Phototoxic Effects of Sulfonated Chlorine-Aluminum-Phthalocyanine on Bladder Cancer Cell Spheroids *

K. MILLER, T. GRAU, and E. REICH [1]

Introduction

Oncological photodynamic therapy (PDT) in a clinical or in vivo experimental setting usually involves systemic administration of the sensitizing agent. Consequently, in addition to the desired phototoxic effects on the tumor, systemic side effects have to be taken into account. Despite these drawbacks, experience with topical application of photosensitizers – which theoretically would eliminate these side effects – seems still to be rather limited.

Transitional cell carcinoma (TCC) of the bladder would be an ideal target for topical PDT: instillation of therapeutic agents into the bladder is easily accomplished and has for a long time been used for chemoprophylaxis of superficial bladder cancer [4]. In an effort to establish a suitable in vitro model for topical PDT, we investigated the phototoxic effects of sulfonated chlorine-aluminum-phthalocyanine (ClAlSPc) on three-dimensional cell cultures (multicell spheroids) of a TCC cell line.

Material and Methods

Pieces of tumor harvested from a cystectomy specimen (G_2 transitional cell carcinoma) were trypsinized and cultured in a conventional monolayer technique using DMEM+20% FCS. Multicell spheroids were then drawn from 10^6 monolayer cells and seeded in 250-ml glass spinner culture flasks. Details of this technique have been described previously elsewhere [7].

The growth of the spheroids was monitored by daily measurements of 30–40 randomly selected cell aggregates under the inverse microscope. When the spheroid growth had reached its plateau phase (Fig. 1), the cultures were incubated with ClAlSPc for 4 h. The cells were then exposed to light of 675-nm wavelength supplied by an Argon-Dye laser. Energy density was 24 J/cm^2 (2-min radiation with 100 mW). For assessment under the electron microscope, the spheroids were fixed 30 min after PDT with 3.5% glutaraldehyde and 2% saccharose. In addition to conventional contrast enhancement with lead citrate, diaminobenzidine (DAB),

* Supported by Deutsche Forschungsgemeinschaft Mi 313/2-2.

[1] Urologische Universitätsklinik, Prittwitzstraße 43, W-7900 Ulm, FRG.

which specifically inhibits the cytochrome oxidase, was used to selectively stain the mitochondria of the cells.

Untreated spheroids and spheroids treated with ClAlSPc or light only were prepared in a similar fashion and used as controls.

From each group (treatment and controls), 5–7 spheroids were assessed under the electron microscope.

Results

Measurement of spheroid growth before treatment shows a plateau phase after 6 days (Fig. 1). The diameter of the cell aggregates then averaged 170 µm (range 80–300 µm). Examination under the electron microscope invariably showed normal tumor cells in the control groups, featuring large nuclei, numerous mitochondria with regular cristae, few secondary lysosomes, and regular intercellular connections (Fig. 2). By contrast, dramatic changes could be observed in the photodynamically treated spheroids: massive vacuolation of the cytoplasm, absence of normal mitochondria (in the outer cell layers of the spheroids), numerous secondary lysosomes, and dissolution of the cellular membrane (Fig. 3). Comparison of the inner and outer parts of the spheroids showed these changes to be less marked or absent in the inner layers. There is no defined borderline for these differences; photodynamic effects seem to progressively diminish towards the center of the spheroids.

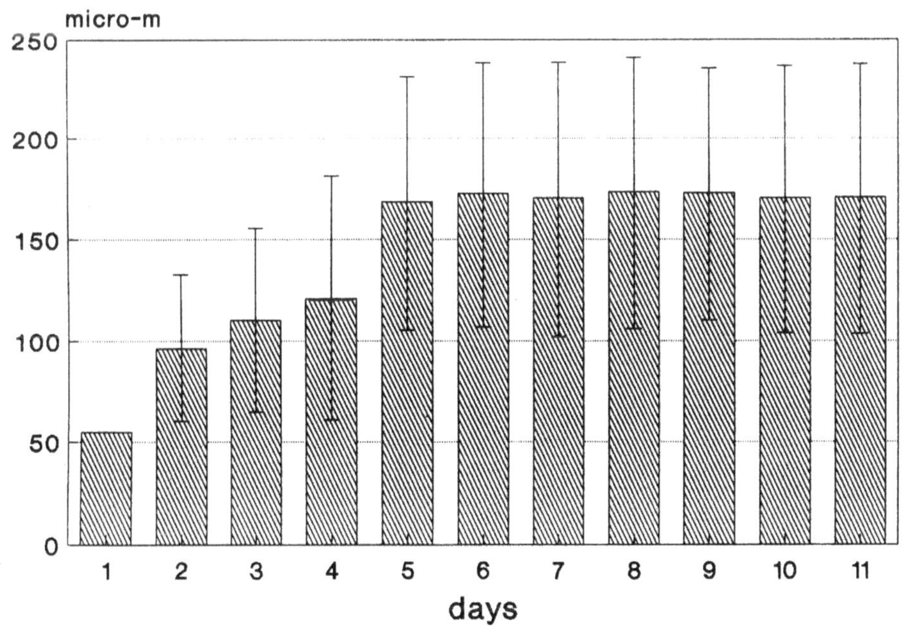

Fig. 1. Growth curve of TCC multicell spheroids (average values plus standard deviation)

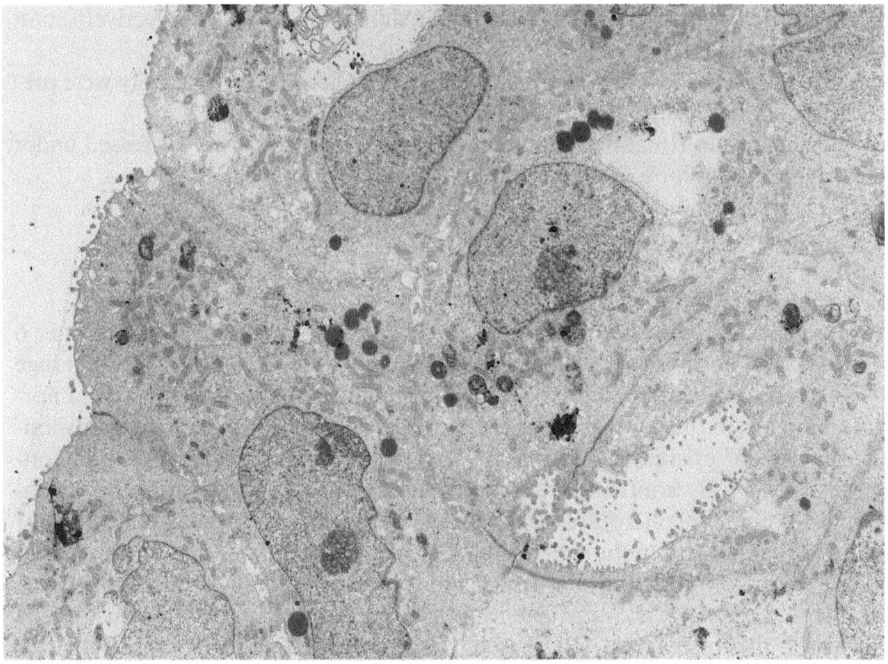

Fig. 2. Electron micrograph of the external region of an untreated TCC multicell spheroid

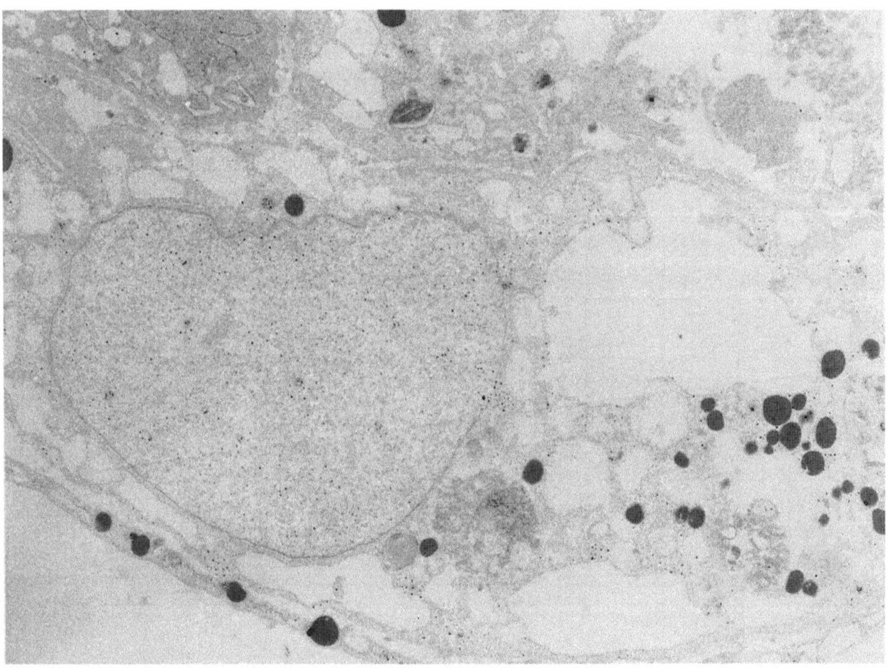

Fig. 3. Electron micrograph of the external region of a TCC multicell spheroid 30 min after PDT

Discussion

Multicell spheroids have been used as tumor models for a large number of oncological experiments and also in association with radiotherapy [7]. Compared to conventional monolayer cell cultures, the advantage is that dealing with cell aggregates is very similar to dealing with an in vivo tumor. Thus, treatment effects not only on single cells but on a complete compound of cells can be assessed. Thus, multicell spheroids should constitute a viable tumor model for a preliminary assessment of topical PDT in which, as with the in vitro setting, the tumor is directly exposed to the photosensitizing agent. Naturally, this assessment is restricted by the limited growth of the spheroids and the lack of vascularization, which may play an important role in PDT [6]. However, spheroids closely resemble in vivo tumors in regard to intercellular connections [7]. Thus, the exchange of substances between individual cells, being one of the crucial points for topical application of photosensitizers, should be similar to the in vivo situation.

The TCC tumor cell line used for our experiments produced spheroids of an average size of 170 µm, which is comparable to results reported elsewhere [7]. Control cells showed a typical pattern for the individual cell as well as for the cell compound, which indeed very much resembled in vivo tumors in a nude mouse model [5].

Subcellular phototoxic effects in the spheroids are similar to those observed in monolayer cultures [3]: the mitochondria seem to be the primary target for PDT on this level. Interestingly, morphologic changes of individual cells within a spheroid are not uniformly distributed, but decrease from the outside towards the center. As no attenuation of red light (675 nm) can be expected with a spheroid diameter of 170 µm, this effect must be attributed to

- the comparably short incubation period of 4 h,
- the comparatively short post-PDT period of 30 min, or
- lack of sensitizer in the inner cell layers.

The incubation time of 4 h was chosen to approximate a period of time which could be used in a clinical setting for topical application of a sensitizing agent. Other investigators have found a similar distribution of PDT effects in spheroids after longer incubation periods with dihematoporphyrin ether (DHE) (16 h) [2].

In monolayer cultures the maximum effect of PDT in vitro (with another sensitizer) has been observed 12 h after application [5], suggesting that changes in the inner part of the spheroids might occur at some point later than 30 min post-PDT as observed in this experiment.

The distribution of sensitizer within a spheroid theoretically depends upon the way the particular substance in use "travels" from cell to cell: is it by pure diffusion or is it a process actively initiated by the cell? The diffusion theory is favored by other authors [1, 2], suggesting that concentration of the sensitizer in the internal parts of a spheroid is largely influenced by diffusion limitations. Certainly, further experiments with variously behaving sensitizers will be necessary for clarification of these questions.

References

1. Christensen T, Moan J, Sandquist T, Medskammer L (1984) Multicellular spheroids as an in-vitro model system for photoradiation therapy in the presence of HPD. In: Doiron DR, Gomer CJ (eds) Porphyrin localization and treatment of tumors. Liss, New York
2. Jeeves WP, Wilson BC, Smith P, Ens K, Spiegl P (1987) Growth delay studies of the response of V-79 multicell spheroids exposed to DHE and red light. Photochem Photobiol 46:723–728
3. Miller K, Reich E, Grau T (1990) Anreicherung von Al Cl SPc und zytotoxische Effekte von PDT an humanen Blasentumorzellen. Kongreßband der 6. Jahrestagung der deutschen Gesellschaft für Lasermedizin, Berlin, 19.–21. September
4. Rassweiler J, Hath U, Eisenberger F (1988) Therapie des oberflächlichen Harnblasenkarzinoms. In: Rüther U, Rassweiler J (eds) Therapie des Harnblasenkarzinoms. Tumor Diagnostik Verlag, Leonberg
5. Reich E, Miller K (1990) Comparison of in-vitro and in-vivo effects of PDT. Workshop on Photodynamic Therapy, Ulm, October 1990
6. Selman S, Kreimer-Birnbaum M, Audhuri Ch, Gargo GM (1986) Photodynamic treatment of transplantable bladder tumors in rodents after pretreatment with chloroaluminum tetrasulfophthalocyanine. J Urol 136:141–145
7. Sutherland RM, Durand RE (1976) Radiation response of multicell spheroids – an in-vitro tumor model. Curr Top Radiat Res 11:87–139

Video Fluorescence Microscopic Studies of Microcirculation in Urothelial Tumors of the Rat

M. BEER[1], A. GOETZ[2], R. RIEDL[3], and L. DERVISHI[3]

Introduction

Urothelial carcinomas are characterized by a high risk of early recurrence and multifocal disease. Unfortunately, in many respects the treatment of bladder carcinoma by replacement of the bladder is inadequate. For this reason, conservative treatment with early endoscopic follow-up and intravesical chemoprophylaxis is the treatment of choice in stage TIS-T1 bladder cancer. The main diagnostic and therapeutic problem in this form of maintenance therapy is that early-stage cancers are macroscopically undetectable.

Compared with carcinomas of other tissues, the growth of urothelial cancer is accompanied by greater angiogenetic activity, which was found by histological examination even in early-stage urothelial cancers. Transplantation of urothelial cells into a rabbit cornea showed that the initiation of angiogenesis is associated with malignant urothelial cells only: transplantation of normal cells did not induce angiogenesis in rabbit corneas.

The aim of the first part of the study was to prove tumor-associated angiogenesis in vivo in video fluorescence angiography. We were particularly interested in testing the potential sensitivity and specificity of video fluorescence microscopy as a diagnostic tool for the detection of early-stage tumors and the differentiation of tumors from normal or inflamed urothelium.

The aim of the second part of the study was to look for an adjuvant procedure to increase the efficacy of intravesical chemotherapy by simultaneous reduction of the microcirculation in tumor capillaries in urothelium. We therefore tested the influence of physical properties of irrigation fluid on urothelial microcirculation comparing the effects of intravesical hyperthermia, pH value, and osmolality on microcirculatory parameters in tumors and normal tissue.

[1] Chirurgische Universitätsklinik, Abt. Urologie und Poliklinik, Im Neuenheimer Feld 110, W-6900 Heidelberg 1, FRG.
[2] Institut für Chirurgische Forschung der Universität, Klinikum Großhadern, Marchioninistr. 15, W-8000 München 70, FRG.
[3] Urologische Klinik und Poliklinik der Universität, Klinikum Großhadern, Marchioninistr. 15, W-8000 München 70, FRG.

Materials and Methods

Animal Model

The animals used were Sprague-Dawley rats averaging 300 g in body weight.

Induction of Carcinoma

Oral feeding with BBN (*N*-butyl-*N*-4-hydroxybutyl-nitrosamine) allows nearly selective induction of cancer of the bladder in rats. Enriching the drinking water with 0.05% BBN for 3 months induces urothelial dysplasias and carcinomas comparable to the carcinoma in situ in humans. After 4 months of oral carcinogenesis with BBN-enriched water supply, exophytic urothelial tumors can be found in the rat bladder.

Control Groups

Untreated animals were used as normal controls. For diagnostic purposes, experimental cystitis was produced in second control group. Cystitis was induced in female animals by sterile catheterisation of the bladder. After pretreatment of the bladder with 0.1 *N* xylol solution, 1 ml of *Escherichia coli* suspension (10^8/nl) was instilled and the catheter removed. The video microscopic studies were performed 2 or 3 days after this procedure.

Videomicroscopy

Via a median laparotomy, we performed a ventral longitudinal cystostomy. The examinations were carried out on the dorsal wall of the bladder in a specially developed chamber (see below). FITC dextrane (MW 150000) was injected intra-arterially as a bolus.

Videomicroscopic analysis was performed in the on-light technique using a modified fluorescence microscope (Orthoplan, Leitz GmbH, Wetzlar, FRG). A pulsed xenon lamp was used as light source for the stroboscope. The wave length of the emitted light was regulated to 490–450 nm. For image analysis emitted light of a wave length below 510 nm was excluded by filter systems. The images were obtained by a highly sensitive television camera (Hamamatsu) and recorded on video tape. Image analysis was performed in a second step with a standard video monitor off line.

The following morphological variables were studied: vascular diameter, capillary length, distance between capillaries, and capillary density.

The quality of blood flow was calculated as follows:

1. $\text{Incidence of stasis} = \frac{\text{Number of unperfused capillaries}}{\text{Total number of capillaries}}\ (\%)$

2. Incidence of sludge formation $= \frac{\text{Number of vessels with sludge formation}}{\text{Total number of vessels}} (\%)$

Vascular permeability for macromolecules (MW 150000) was analyzed semiquantitatively using the following classification:

0: No fluorescence in interstitial tissue
1: Focal perivascular interstitial fluorescence (<1/3 of image)
2: Confluent perivascular fluorescence (<2/3 of image)
3: Diffuse interstitial fluorescence (3/3 of image).

Hyperthermia and Superfusion media

The bladder was fixed by sutures and springs in a heatable chamber of plexiglass. To imitate endoscopic conditions, constant superfusion with temperature-controlled superfusion fluid was installed. This allowed examination in "under-water conditions". The temperature in the chamber and the temperature of the superfusion fluid were increased synchronously in steps from 37° to 40 °C, 43 °C, 45 °C, and 48 °C. The videomicroscopic analysis was performed 10 min after each adjustment of systemic temperature. Blood gas analysis and macrohemodynamic were monitored and corrected if necessary before analysis of the microcirculation. Animals with disturbed macrohemodynamic were excluded from the analysis.

As superfusion fluids we used NaCl 0.9%, NaCl 10%, glucose 10%, and glucose 20%. All studies of hyperthermia and the experiments with modification of pH value (pH 4.5–9 at 37 °C) were performed during superfusion with NaCl 0.9%.

Results

Morphometric Criteria

In vivo videofluorescence microscopy using the on-light technique allowed examination of the microarchitecture of the superficial submucosal urothelial vascular network in tumors, normal and inflammed tissues. Vascular density, capillary length, capillary diameter and the distances between vessels were analyzed to test the usefulness of these variables for differential diagnosis. Vascular density differed significantly between the three groups. Normal bladders showed a total vascular density of 79.2 ± 14.0 mm/mm^2, in experimental cystitis the total vascular density was increased to 101.7 ± 9.8 mm/mm^2, while tumors showed the highest vascular density with 164.3 ± 22 SD mm/mm^2 ($p < 0.01$; Wilcoxon-Mann-Whitney U test). Division of the data for total vascular density into vascular densities of arterioles, capillaries, and venules showed that differences in vascular density were caused by an increase in vascular density of capillaries only. The vascular density of arterioles and venules was similar in all groups.

Another sign of increased angiogenesis was found by analyzing mean capillary length. In normal tissue capillary length was 48.8±5.5 nm. Experimental cystitis showed a mean capillary length of 27.3±7.0 nm, while tumors showed the smallest capillary length 12.2±4.9 nm ($p<0.001$ for tumors vs normal tissue).

Changes in Microcirculation with Hyperthermia

Analyzing the mean diameters of capillaries at different temperatures, we found no significant differences between the groups at each temperature. However, in both normal tissue and tumorous tissue we found wider capillary diameters at higher temperatures (normal: 37.0 °C 5.1±0.4 nm, 43 °C 8.2±1.4 nm; tumors: 37 °C 4.1±0.9 nm, 43 °C 9.7±3.2 nm). Stasis and sludge formation correlated with intravesical temperature. At 37 °C sludge formation or stasis were seen neither in normal nor in tumor tissue. When the temperature was raised to 40 °C, we found sludge formation in 28±5% of vessels in tumors, while at temperatures of 40 °C normal tissue showed no signs of sludge formation or stasis. The incidence of stasis in tumors was 20.5±1.5% at 40 °C, while in normal tissue there was no sign of stasis at 40 °C. At 43 °C, however, tumors showed an incidence of sludge formation of 78±12%, which was significantly higher than in normal tissue. The incidence of stasis at 43 °C was 24±7% in normal and 48±6% in tumor tissue. At 45 °C we found an almost 100% incidence of sludge formation and stasis in both groups.

Analyzing the changes in vascular permeability at 37 °C we found no significant differences between tumor and normal tissue. Increasing the temperature to 40 °C, 2/12 animals with tumors showed grade 1 changes in permeability (normal: grade 0). Increasing the temperature to 43 °C, all normal animals showed grade 1 changes in vascular permeability. At 43 °C 9/12 animals with tumors showed grade 2 changes. Increasing the temperature to 45 °C, all normal animals showed grade 2 changes; at the same temperature, tumor-bearing animals showed grade 2 changes in only 7/12 cases, while the remaining 5 animals had grade 3 changes in vascular permeability.

In the same experimental set-up we also tested the influence of pH value and osmolality of superfusion fluid on the urothelial microcirculation, but no statistically significant differences were found.

Discussion

This experimental model demonstrated angiogenetic activity in urothelial carcinoma by means of in vivo analysis of the microcirculation. We found highly significant differences in the microarchitecture of blood vessels in tumors and normal tissue in regard to capillary density, capillary length, and the distance between capillaries. Similar results derived from pilot studies in humans have shown the validity of the animal model for human carcinoma of the bladder. On the basis of these highly significant differences we are now trying to develop an imaging modality to examine the microangioarchitecture of the urothelium during cystoscopy. The tumor-associated angiogenesis might be a basis for identification of early-stage tumors which can not be seen by endoscopic examination. The modification of this diagnostic tool for clinical use will require simultaneous online analysis of images and endoscopic findings.

Hyperthermia is used as an adjuvant therapeutic procedure in the treatment of many forms of carcinoma. The exact mechanism of interaction of hyperthermia with chemotherapeutics and radiotherapy is very complex and has not yet been completely eluciated. A direct cytotoxic effect of hyperthermia has been proven by in vitro studies in cell cultures. A second very important effect is the influence of hyperthermia on the capillary microcirculation. Many studies have shown that the capillary system of normal tissue tolerates an increase in temperature up to 44 °C without serious functional disturbances and harm to the vessels. In different animal models we were able to confirm these results by our study of normal bladders. In rats we found an influence of intravesical temperature on stasis, sludge formation, and vascular permeability even at temperatures below 44 °C (43 °C).

Comparing reactions to hpyerthermia, we found disturbances of microcirculation at lower levels in BBN-induced urothelial carcinomas than in normal tissue (40 °C vs 43 °C). The thermosensitivity of carcinoma cells is especially high in an acidotic environment with lack of ATP, O_2, and glucose. These results were consistent in different experimental tumors and in clinical use of hyperthermia. The differences in thermosensitivity between tumors and normal tissue is limited to temperatures of 41 °– 44 °C. There is a good correlation between temperature and therapeutic efficacy.

Our investigations showed that in cancer of the bladder, vascular sensitivity is different between tumors and normal tissue at temperatures between 40 °C and 43 °C. For clinical purposes, it would appear to be useful to combine local hyperthermia with topical or systemic thermosensitive chemotherapeutics. This may be of special interest in improving chemotherapy of cancer of the bladder. The additive effect of local hyperthermia combined with thermosensitive chemotherapeutics has also been proven in other experimental tumors and clinical situations. The results presented give reason to believe that local or systemic chemotherapy with adjuvant intravesical hyperthermia may be feasible in the treatment of bladder cancer.

V. Urodynamics

Effects of Isoprenaline, Papaverine and Verapamil on Rate Isolated Bladder Muscle

W. DIEDERICHS[1], L. HERTLE[1], and H. NAWRATH[2]

In general the mechanical activity of smooth muscles is determined by the concentration of free intracellular calcium. In relaxed smooth muscle, the intracellular calcium concentration is kept low. Two integrated membrane systems, the cell membrane and the sarcoplasmic reticulum, are involved in the control of the free intracellular calcium concentration (van Breemen). On bladder smooth muscle these conditions are still undergoing research. Of clinical importance in some urological disorders are drugs which induce relaxation of bladder smooth muscle and that means reduction of the free intracellular calcium concentration.

In the present study we evaluated the relaxing effects of verapamil and papaverine (which interacts with calcium channels of the cell membrane) and isoprenaline (which interact with the sarcoplasmic reticulum).

Materials and Methods

Strips of bladder dome (from adult Sprague-Dawley rats) were suspended in 10 ml organ baths containing Tyrode solution at 37 °C, gassed with 95% O_2 and 5% CO_2. The tension was measured under isometric conditions with inductive force displacement transducers and recorded on paper. Contractions were produced by exposing the muscle strips to carbachol (10^{-4} mol/l) and high potassium (85 mmol/l) Tyrode solution. Cumulative concentrations-response relationships of isoprenaline (10^{-10} to 10^{-5} mol/l), papaverine (10^{-7} to 10^{-4} mol/l) and verapamil (10^{-10} to 10^{-5} mol/l) were obtained as follows. First an initial contraction (control) was produced by using high-potassium Tyrode solution or carbachol (10^{-4} mol/l). After a wash-out period of 30 min the muscle strips returned to their previous resting tension. Then the muscle strips were incubated with one of the three drugs at lowest concentrations for 30 min. Afterwards a contraction was produced by high potassium or carbachol in the presence of the same drug concentration. Further responses were obtained by increasing the drug concentration in logarithmic increments.

Parallel experiments were carried out to study the effects of isoprenaline, papaverine and verapamil on net ^{45}calcium uptake in high-potassium activated muscle strips. The muscle strips were exposed for different times (1 – 100 min) to normal Tyrode solution or 85 mmol/l KCl Tyrode. Both solutions were labelled with ^{45}calcium (0.1 ml/1 l solution). The muscle strips were blotted, weighted

[1] Urologische Klinik der Universität Bochum, Widumerstr. 8, W-4690 Herne 1, FRG.
[2] Pharmakologisches Institut der Universität, Obere Zahlbacherstr. 67, W-6500 Mainz, FRG.

and incubated in tissue solubilizer. Vials were analysed for ^{45}calcium in a liquid scintillation counter.

The following drugs were used: ^{45}calcium (Du Pont), carbachol hydrochloride (Merck), isoprenaline sulphate (Boehringer), papaverine hydrochloride (Serva) and verapamil (Knoll).

Results

The smooth muscle response to high potassium and carbachol was biphasic (initial peak tension decreased in a second phase to a more sustained plateau) and transient (Fig. 1). To evaluate the calcium channel blocking property, the effects of papaverine and verapamil were studied on carbachol- and high-potassium-induced contraction. Both drugs reduced or abolished the biphasic muscle response. Compared with papaverine (EC_{50}: 0.16×10^{-4} mol/l) low concentrations of verapamil (EC_{50}: 0.14×10^{-6} mol/l) were more potent in reducing high-potassium- or carbachol-induced muscle contractions.

To study β-sympathomimetic effects on induced contractions isoprenaline was applied to muscle strips. Even high concentrations of isoprenaline (10^{-4} mol/l) inhibited only 50% at most of the peak tension. To evaluate additional effects of papaverine or verapamil the isoprenaline concentration response relationships were repeated in the presence of a nearly half maximum concentration of papaverine (10^{-5} mol/l) or verapamil (10^{-7} mol/l). As Fig. 2 clearly shows, verapamil did not influence the isoprenaline response. In contrast, papaverine significantly reduced the peak tension.

The calcium uptake was measured to provide details of calcium movements in addition to the tension effects. In contrast to isoprenaline, papaverine and verapamil reduced the calcium uptake significantly (Fig. 3).

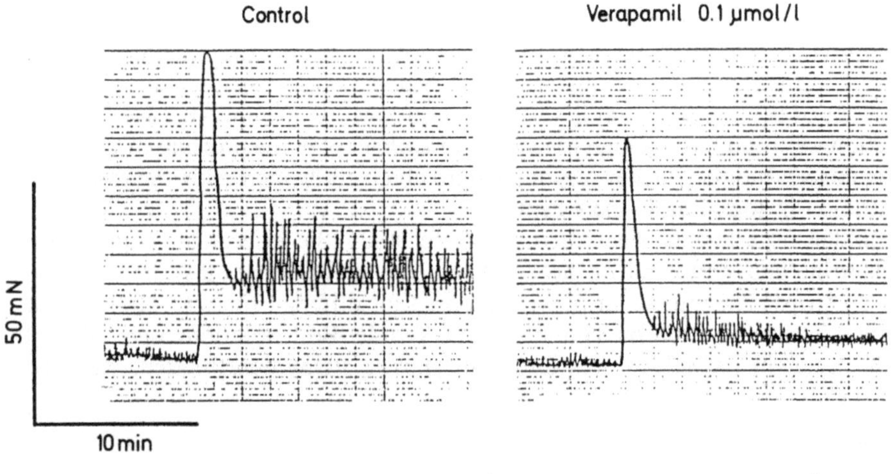

Fig. 1. Original recording of effects of carbachol 10^{-4} mol/l (control) and verapamil 10^{-7} mol/l in addition on tension of muscle strips of rat bladder dome

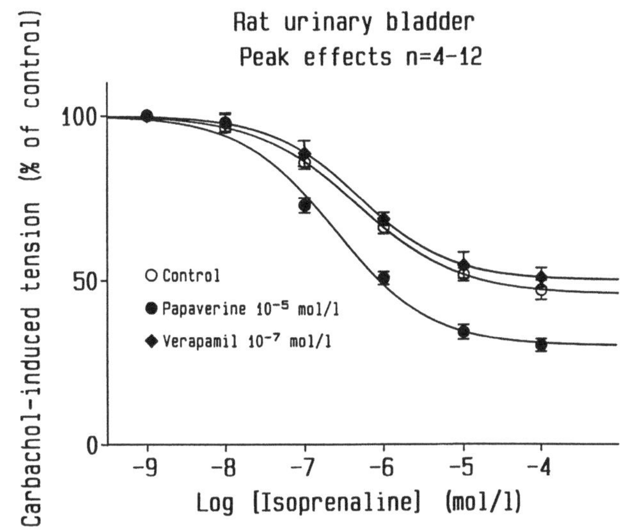

Fig. 2. Concentration-response relationship of increasing isoprenaline concentration on controls or with isoprenaline and papaverine 10^{-5} mol/l or isoprenaline and verapamil 10^{-7} mol/l on peak tension induced by carbachol on rat bladder dome

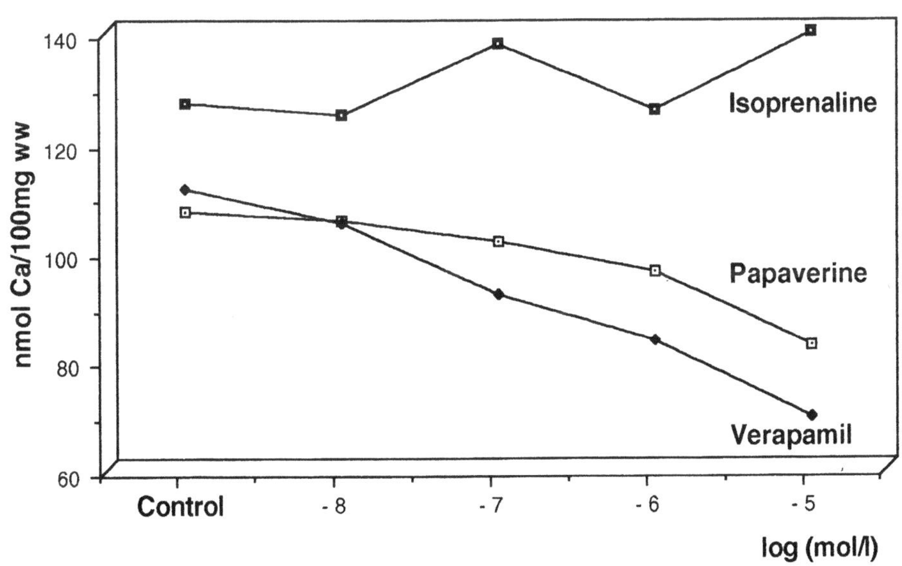

Fig. 3. Concentration-response relationships of isoprenaline, papaverine and verapamil on ^{45}calcium uptake in muscle strips of rat bladder dome contracted by 85 mmol/l extracellular potassium after 100 min

Discussion

In the present study we found that verapamil was more potent, especially at low concentrations, in reducing carbachol- or high-potassium-induced muscle contraction. These differences in potency corresponded with a decrease in ^{45}calcium uptake. However, papaverine in contrast to verapamil increased the relaxing effects of isoprenaline on carbachol-induced tension.

The contractile muscle response to high potassium or carbachol in the urinary bladder seems to be highly dependent on an extracellular source of calcium (Batra et al. 1987). However, high potassium or carbachol act on the cell membrane by different mechanism: carbachol binds to a specific receptor; high potassium exerts its effects mainly by reducing the potassium gradient across the cell membrane (Bolton 1979). On high-potassium-induced muscle contraction we observed a dose-dependent decrease in ^{45}calcium uptake with verapamil and papaverine. Both these drugs seem to reduce the calcium influx into rat bladder muscle. However, compared to verapamil, higher concentrations of papaverine were necessary to reduce the ^{45}calcium uptake. From these findings we suggest that the calcium channel blocking property of papaverine is rather non-specific. On the one hand papaverine appeared to act on the calcium influx mechanism (Huddart et al. 1984). On the other hand, papaverine is thought to be a potent inhibitor of phosphodiesterase in urinary bladder (Levin et al. 1982). Inhibition of this enzyme causes a rise in cAMP, which mediates relaxation by several mechanisms (Bolton 1979). In addition, cAMP production is increased by β-receptor activation (Bülbring and Tomita 1987). In reference to our experiments, the isoprenaline concentration response shift to the left only with papaverine on carbachol-induced contractions seems to be related to a further increase of cAMP.

We conclude that blockade of calcium channels and β-receptor stimulation are important pathways for the reduction of tension in rat bladder smooth muscle.

References

Batra S, Sjögren C, Andersson KE, Fovalus M (1987) Source of calcium for contractions induced by depolarisation and muscarinic receptor stimulation in rabbit urinary bladder. Acta Physiol Scand 130:545–551

Breemen C v, Saida K (1989) Cellular mechanisms regulating $[Ca^{2+}]_i$ smooth muscle. Ann Rev Physiol 51:315–329

Bolton TB (1979) Mechanisms of action of transmitters and other substances on smooth muscle. Physiol Rev 59:606–718

Bülbring E, Tomita T (1987) Catecholamine action on smooth muscle. Pharmacol Rev 39:49–96

Huddart H, Langton PD, Saad KHM (1984) Inhibition by papaverine of calcium movements and tension in the smooth muscle of rat vas deferens and urinary bladder. J Physiol 349:183–194

Levin RM, Einstein R, Wein AJ (1982) Phosphodiesterase activity of the lower urinary tract. J Urol 128:615–617

Effect of Trospium Chloride, Oxybutynin and Propiverine on the Interaction of Acetylcholine with Isolated Preparations of the Human Urinary Bladder

S. ALLOUSSI[1], J. BALDAUF[2], H. DEROUET[1], U. ZWERGEL[1], and S. MEESSEN[1]

Summary

The effect of trospium chloride, oxybutynin and propiverine on the interaction of acetylcholine with isolated preparations of the human urinary bladder was investigated. We were able to demonstrate the acetylcholine antagonism of these different anticholinergics. The anticholinergic action of these substances was demonstrated by a shift to the right of the dose-effect curve of acetylcholine, so that clinical use of these anticholinergics appears to be feasible in the hyperactivity type of bladder dysfunction.

Introduction

The smooth musculature of the urinary bladder can be influenced pharmacologically either by indirect action on the autonomic nervous system of by direct action on the muscle cell itself. The term "detrusor hyperactive" designates various forms of bladder dysfunction, such as reflex, unstable and hyperactive urinary bladder. In clinical terms, this condition is accompanied by pollakiuria, nycturia, as well as urge incontinence. Recently, various anticholinergics have become established in clinical pharmacotherapy of hyperactive bladder dysfunction. Trospium chloride, oxybutynin, and propiverine are substances with an anticholinergic effect. Their direct action on the smooth musculature of the human urinary bladder has not been previously investigated.

The object of our investigation was to demonstrate and compare the direct action of trospium chloride, oxybutynin, and propiverine on the isolated human urinary bladder.

Materials and Methods

The muscle strips from human urinary bladder used in our investigation were obtained in open operations on the bladder. A strip of bladder muscle (15 mm long, 5 mm wide) was excised with the scalpel at the bladder dome and transferred immediately after removal to a Krebs-Henseleit solution gassed with carbogen (95%

[1] Urologische Klinik und Poliklinik der Universität des Saarlandes, Landeskrankenhaus, W-6650 Homburg/Saar, FRG.
[2] Pharmakologisches Institut der Universität des Saarlandes, W-6650 Homburg/Saar, FRG.

O_2, 5% CO_2). After carefully dissecting away connective tissue or fat residues, the detrusor strips were gripped at both ends with a metal clip and mounted with a monofilament nonelastic thread between the attachment fixture in the organ bath and an isometric force transducer. The temperature of the organ bath was kept constant at 37 °C with a thermostat. The pH value of the solution was between 7.35 and 7.4. The preparations were then prestretched with 2 g (19.8 mN) and repeatedly readjusted to the initial tension over a stabilization period of about 1 h until the tension remained constant.

The tension curve of the muscle preparations was recorded with an electrochemical tension transducer which was connected to a compensation line plotter. The desired concentrations of acetylcholine and of the various anticholinergics investigated were prepared fresh from a stock solution by dilution with Krebs-Henseleit solution before the beginning of the experiment. The shift to the right of the cumulative dose-effect curve for acetylcholine after addition of anticholinergics was regarded as a measure of their effect. Finally, the submaximum action of the known agonist acetylcholine was established in the dose-effect curve. After pretreatment of the preparation with the antagonist, the attenuation of the action of the agonist was tested. To allow establishment of correlations between dose and effect independently of individually different organ preparations, and thus irrespective of the concentration parameters, the measurement values were normed. For this purpose, the submaximum value determined statistically in the test series was taken to be 100%. All other measurement values were related to this, i.e., they were only specified as a percentage. The concentration at which the effect fell just short of the maximum possible was designated as the submaximum dose. Damage to the organ preparation on attainment of the maximum dose is thereby prevented. This value is taken as the reference value. The shift of the dose-effect curve was tested for significance using the Wilcoxon test for pair differences, p less than 0.05 being taken as the level of significance.

Results

The dose-effect curves for acetylcholine with and without addition of anticholinergics were plotted to demonstrate the specific antagonistic action of the various anticholinergics.

The cumulative addition of acetylcholine 10^{-8} to 10^{-5} mg/ml led to a rise of the muscle tension in steps up to an average peak value of 80 mN at an acetylcholine concentration of 10^{-5} mg/ml. After addition of anticholinergics (trospium chloride 10^{-8} mg/ml, oxybutynin 10^{-7} mg/ml, and propiverine 10^{-7} mg/ml), the maximum contraction under acetylcholine fell to an average of 55 mN (equivalent to 68% of the maximum tension). The ED_{50} of acetylcholine after addition of trospium chloride was shifted by 1–2 powers of 10. An increase in the ED_{50} by 1 power of 10 for acetylcholine was also detected after addition of oxybutynin and propiverine. This specific antagonistic effect of trospium chloride, oxybutynin, and propiverine on acetylcholine action was clearly demonstrated by a shift to the right of the dose-effect curves of the various anticholinergics (Figs. 1–3).

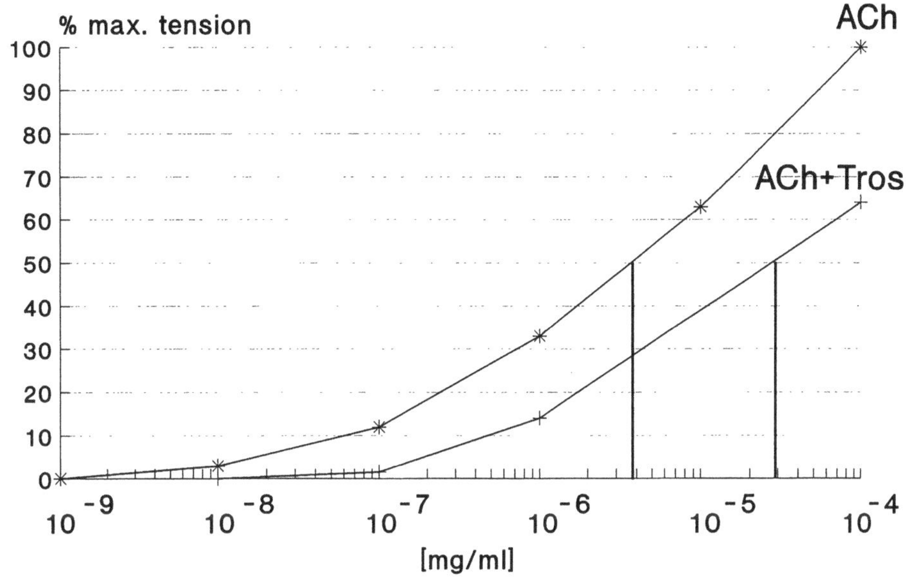

Fig. 1. Dose-effect curve of acetylcholine with and without addition of trospium chloride (10^{-x} mg/ml) (significant displacement to the right: *p* 0.05)

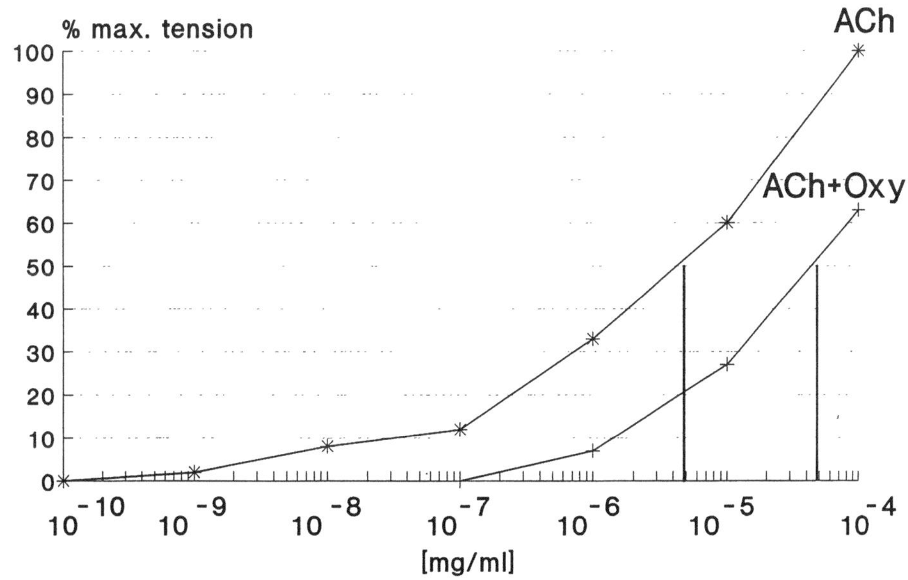

Fig. 2. Dose-effect curve of acetylcholine with and without addition of oxybutynin (10^{-x} mg/ml)

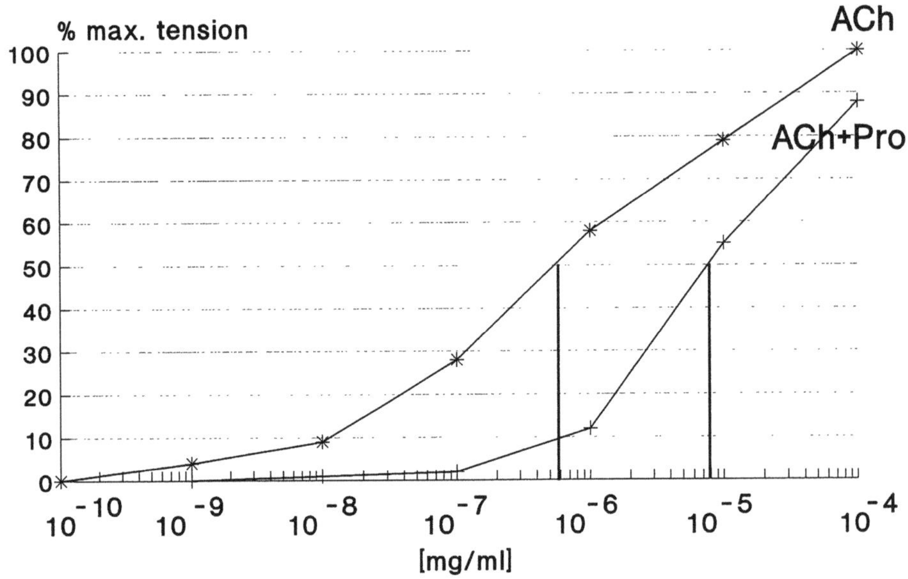

Fig. 3. Dose-effect curve of acetylcholine with and without addition of propiverine (10^{-x} mg/ml)

Discussion

Investigation of smooth muscle strips from rat, rabbit, and guinea-pig bladder carried out in vitro documented the anticholinergic action of trospium chloride oxybutynin, and propiverine (Nagai et al. 1983). After prior administration of trospium chloride, oxybutynin and propiverine, the contractions induced by acetylcholine were very much less. This was manifested in the shift of the dose-effect curve to the right. In addition, the contractions brought about by acetylcholine could be antagonized directly at any given time by trospium chloride, oxybutynin, and propiverine.

The experiment design corresponds to the conventional method for investigation of the efficacy of different drugs on smooth muscle organ preparations (Blattner et al. 1973). The selected pretest tension of 2 g (equivalent to 18.8 mN) is based on the finding that the greatest effectiveness of contractions is obtained with prior stretching to 140%–190% of the resting length (Carpenter 1968). The composition of the Krebs-Henseleit nutrient solution used here has also been tested several times and it has been used in experiments dealing with similar problems. The results reported can thus be compared with results published previously (Klarskov et al. 1983).

Since all three anticholinergics investigated could be shown to antagonize the action of acetylcholine on isolated human bladder muscle strips, our study indicates that these anticholinergics can be used to treat the hyperreflexive form of bladder dysfunction. Since these agents have equal anticholinergic action, the most suitable for clinical use would be that with the lowest side effects.

References

Blattner R, Classen HG, Dehnert H, Döring HJ (1973) Experimente an isolierten glattmuskulären Organen. Hugo Sachs Elektronik KG, D-7801 March/Freiburg, FRG
Carpenter FG (1968) Motor responses of bladder smooth muscle in relation to elasticity and fiber length. Invest Urol 6:273–283
Klarskov P, Gerstenberg T, Ramirez D, Hald T (1983) Non-cholinergic, non-adrenergic nerve mediated relaxation of trigone, bladder neck and urethral smooth muscle in vitro. J Urol 129:848–849
Nagai M, Nakajima M, Usuda S, Iriki M (1983) Inhibitory effect of diphenyl-propoxyacetic acid-L-methyl-4-piperidyl ester hydrochloride on the activity of the rat urinary bladder. 409-38 Yamanashi (Japan), May 25, 1983

Intrathecal Administration of Substance P in the Rat: Effect on Bladder and Urethral Sphincteric Activity *

A. MERSDORF[1], E. A. TANAGHO[1], and D. JONAS[2]

Introduction

In 1931 substance P was discovered in the equine intestine and brain by von Euler and Gaddum. It was identified as a peptide in 1936 by von Euler, and later studies revealed a wide, but specific, distribution pattern throughout the central nervous system (Pernow 1983). Substance P has been identified in small sensory neurons and their terminals in the dorsal horn of the spinal cord (Hökfelt et al. 1982). These substance P-like immunoreactive cells and cell fibers are present in dense concentrations in laminae I and II of the dorsal horn, notably at levels L1 – L2 and L6 – S1 (Sharkey et al. 1983). At the L6 and S1 level of the spinal cord level, these substance P-positive nerve fibers terminate in the sacral parasympathetic nucleus close to the preganglionic neurons that provide parasympathetic output to the pelvic viscera (Sasek et al. 1984).

Spinal segments L1 – L2 and L5 – S1, with minor contribution from L1 – L2, give rise in the rat to the afferents and efferents of the pudendal (somatic) and pelvic (parasympathetic) nerves, which act on visceral functions such as micturition, defecation, and copulation (McKenna and Nadelhaft 1986). The high concentration of substance P at the lumbar and sacral roots suggests that it may regulate these functions (Applebaum et al. 1980). Substance P is intensely involved in nociceptive transduction and transmission (Fields 1987); at the spinal cord level it reveals a direct excitatory effect on motor neurons (Konishi and Otsuka 1974).

In the human spinal cord, the distribution of substance P immunoreactivity is similar to that found in rats and other mammals (Pernow 1983), and thus its role in the regulation of visceral functions may also be similar. We therefore developed a rat model to investigate whether and in what way centrally evoked pain may influence bladder and sphincteric activity.

Materials and Methods

Male Wistar rats weighing between 450 and 600 g were given 100 mg/kg thiobutabarbital sodium i.p. (Inactin, Byk Gulden, Konstanz, FRG), which provided mild but sufficient anesthesia for 12 – 16 h. After tracheostomy to facilitate respiration, polyethylene-50 (PE-50) tubing was inserted into the right common carotid artery

* Supported by grant ME 902/1-2 from the Deutsche Forschungsgemeinschaft, FRG.

[1] Department of Urology, University of California School of Medicine, San Francisco, CA 94143, USA.
[2] Abt. für Urologie der Universität, Theodor-Stern-Kai 7, W-6000 Frankfurt/Main 70, FRG.

for blood pressure monitoring and PE-90 tubing into the left external jugular vein for saline infusion and drug administration. Through a ventral midline incision the urinary bladder was exposed and bladder pressure was monitored with a PE-50 catheter in the bladder dome connected to a perfusion pump and pressure transducer.

A delicate bipolar electromyography (EMG) needle electrode (Dantec) was inserted suprapubically into the external urethral sphincter, and the operating table was lowered caudally 45 °. The rats underwent serial cystometrograms during constant perfusion of 37 °C saline at a rate (21.6 μl/min) that approximated the spontaneous rate of urine formation for this species (Maggi et al. 1986). Blood and bladder pressure and sphincteric activity were measured before, during, and after bladder filling; these measurements were repeated before and after intravenous, intra-arterial, and intrathecal administration of 10 μg substance P.

Intravenous Substance P

In ten animals, 10 μg substance P (MW 1347.80; Peninsula Laboratories, Belmont, Ca., USA) was given intravenously via the PE-90 tubing in the left external jugular vein.

Intra-arterial Substance P

In three rats, PE-50 tubing was placed in the left renal artery with its distal tip in the abdominal aorta; via ligatures the blood supply was reduced to the common iliac arteries with their internal iliac arteries. The latter represent the main blood supply of the urinary bladder.

Intrathecal Substance P

In 20 rats, bilateral laminectomy at the T13 – L1 junction was performed and intrathecal PE-10 tubing was passed caudally through a slit in the dura and positioned so that the inner tip lay at the L1 level. The tubing was affixed with adhesive silicone (Silastic); the skin was sutured and the animal placed in the supine position. Substance P was delivered intrathecally via a Hamilton syringe at a dose of 10 μg per 10 μl artificial cerebrospinal fluid (CSF) (Elliott's B Solution, LyphoMed), followed by flushing with 10 μl artificial CSF (catheter volume approximately 7 μl).

Results

Intravenous Substance P

During the screening period the mean maximum amplitude of spontaneous bladder contractions was 4±2 cm H_2O; the maximum EMG activity of the external urethral sphincter was 130±50 μV. During intravesical perfusion of 21.6 μl/min saline, the bladder contractions increased to 12±8 cm H_2O and sphincteric activity rose to 330±80 μV. Shortly after intravenous administration of substance P (15±2 s), a tonic bladder contraction of 34±10 cm H_2O occurred (Fig. 1). The contraction wave was associated with the emission of several drops of urine. The sphincteric EMG activity increased to 320±50 μV. Bladder pressure and sphincteric activity returned to initial values by 5±2 min. After about 10 min, saline perfusion was repeated. Evoked bladder contractions and sphincteric activity were like the values during saline perfusion *before* substance P was given.

Intra-arterial Substance P

Although substance P reached the detrusor muscle at a much higher concentration when delivered intra-arterially, the response was similar to that after intravenous administration. However, the rise in bladder pressure was steeper and it consistently began *after* the onset of the drop in blood pressure, which, interestingly, was more pronounced.

Side effects: The first noteable reaction after intravenous/intra-arterial administration of substance P was a drop in blood pressure beginning 8±3 s after injection (Fig. 1). Mean blood pressure dropped from 176±28 to 146±20 cm H_2O by 120 s. A few minutes after substance P was given, hypersalivation occurred; it was

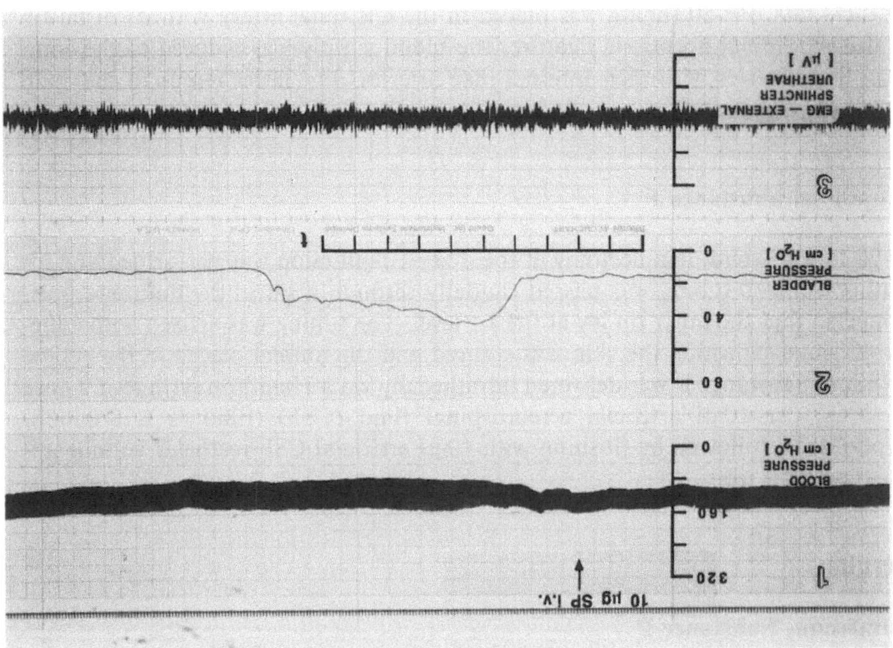

Fig. 1. A representative bladder contraction, lasting approximately 80 s, in response to intravenous substance P administration. The reaction begins 18 s after substance P injection and is paralleled by a minor increase in sphincteric activity. (*t*, 1 unit = 10 s; EMG, 1 unit = 500 μV)

mild to moderate in 2 and strong in 8 rats, producing 0.5 – 1.0 ml saliva. No other effects were detectable.

Intrathecal Substance P

The 20 rats could be classified into three groups, depending on their response to intrathecal substance P.

Group A ($n = 5$) showed immediate, strong bladder contractions. In response to 10 μg, the strong contraction wave (pressure rise 31 ± 18 cm H_2O) began at 18 ± 11 s and lasted for 112 ± 56 s. It took 11 ± 5 min for the bladder pressure to return to baseline. The EMG activity of the external urethral sphincter increased at 7 ± 4 s after substance P administration to 270 ± 140 μV. Even though sphincteric activity increased, each rat emitted a few drops of urine. When all values had returned to baseline, saline perfusion was repeated. The amplitude of bladder contractions was 7 ± 1 cm H_2O, and the sphincteric activity was 260 ± 120 μV.

In *group B* ($n = 4$), the micturition reflex was augmented after substance P administration, as indicated by strong detrusor contractions in response to intravesical perfusion. The maximum amplitude of bladder contractions without saline perfusion was 8 ± 4 cm H_2O, with a much greater increase in sphincteric EMG activity to 320 ± 60 μV at 10 ± 6 s after substance P. During intravesical perfusion, the largest contractions were recorded (25 ± 13 cm H_2O); these were paralleled by sphincteric EMG activity of 360 ± 100 μV. When the perfusion was stopped, the waves disappeared, only to reappear with renewed perfusion.

In *group C* ($n = 8$) (Fig. 2), bladder pressure increased gradually to a high, steady peak. About 30 s after intrathecal administration of substance P, bladder pressure started rising, achieving an increase of 22 ± 6 cm H_2O. In these group C rats, the mean course of the pressure rise was of noticeably longer duration than in group A. The sphincteric EMG activity was 280 ± 60 μV with substance P; the first changes in the EMG pattern were registered 17 ± 4 s after substance P administration. When the intravesical perfusion was begun after substance P, bladder pressure and sphincteric activity were distinctly higher than the corresponding values during intravesical perfusion before substance P. In four rats, perfusion induced rhythmical high-amplitude detrusor contractions (18 ± 7 cm H_2O), as it had in those in group B. Overflow voiding occurred in each rat, even though the sphincter was distinctly more active.

Side Effects. In general, blood pressure displayed the earliest visible but least homogeneous response after intrathecal administration of substance P. Nine rats demonstrated an increase, five a drop, and three mainly an increase in amplitude. These responses bore no relation to the changes in bladder pressure.

Hypersalivation, a common side effect, was most pronounced in group A, where up to 0.5 – 1.0 ml saliva was produced. Almost all animals with strong hypersalivation produced tears.

In seven rats, accumulation of mucus caused airway obstruction with audible dyspnea, necessitating suction via the tracheostomy tube. Dyspnea was reflected in the blood pressure recording (Fig. 2).

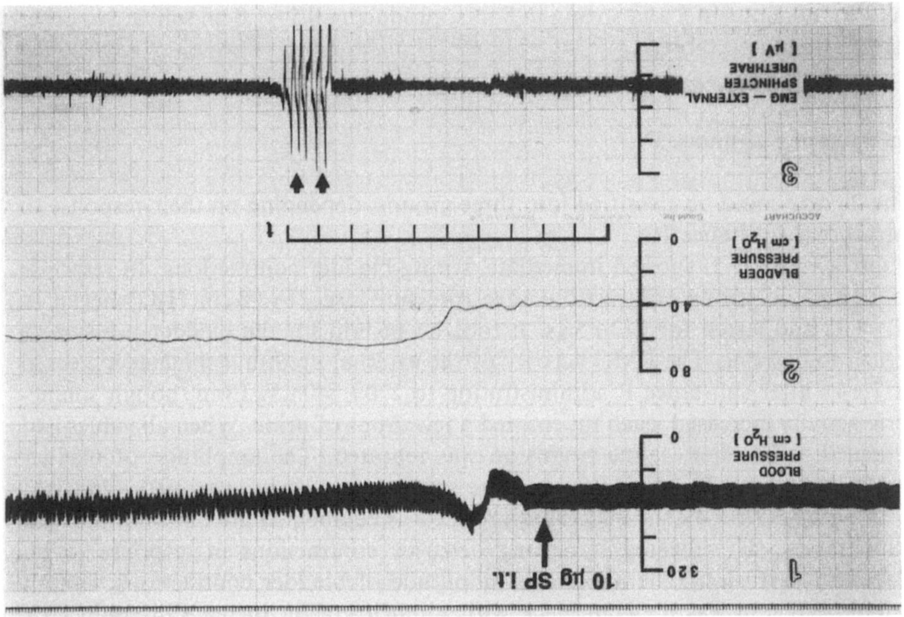

Fig. 2. One characteristic group C rat shows the tonic increase in bladder pressure to a high, steady peak starting 30 s after intrathecal administration of substance P. An artifact in the EMG tracing (*double arrows*) reflects pain-induced hindlimb movements (11 times) for scratching. The serrated blood pressure tracing reveals dyspnea due to bronchial constriction. (*t*, 1 unit = 10 s; EMG, 1 unit = 500 µV)

Hindlimb movement and tetanus were seen in nine rats from groups B and C (45%), occasionally with a delay of more than 1 min after intrathecal substance P administration. Hindlimb movements resembled scratching behavior in response to moderate pain stimuli such as may be evoked in conscious animals by pinching the prepuce, glans penis, or perineal skin. Frequently, the movements produced EMG artifacts, and thus each hindlimb movement appeared as a countable event on the EMG (Fig. 2).

Discussion

Substance P, when given intravenously or intra-arterially, exerted a powerful spasmogenic effect, eliciting strong bladder contractions. This effect was repeatable and limited only in some experiments by a pronounced fall in blood pressure. The spasmogenic and hypotensive properties of substance P have been shown to result from direct smooth muscle contraction (von Euler 1936) and peripheral vasodilation respectively (Pernow 1983).

Administration of substance P intrathecally did not give consistent results, even though it was verified at autopsy that the subdural tube was in the correct position. In the five group A rats many values were similar to those obtained with intravenous administration: bladder pressure before and after substance P; the form, duration, and maximum amplitude of substance P-generated bladder contractions, and the incidence of pronounced hypersalivation. It seems likely that, in group A, the intrathecal substance P spread into the systemic circulation to exert at least part of its action. A possible explanation may lie in the positioning of the subdural tube close to the posterior spinal vein.

In groups B and C, the bladder pressure responses after intrathecal substance P were different from that in the intravenous group. In group B only the sphincteric activity increased; bladder pressure remained nearly unaffected. During intravesical saline perfusion, strong rhythmic bladder contractions were recorded that had not been present before substance P and persisted for the duration of perfusion. All rats in group C showed a protracted, but still high increase in bladder pressure that peaked at about 3 min, remained for a few minutes at that plateau, and then fell. With additional intravesical perfusion, four rats displayed rhythmic detrusor contractions of high amplitude, which they had not demonstrated during perfusion before substance P. In nine animals (groups B and C) the increase in detrusor and sphincteric activity was accompanied by pain-induced hindlimb movements, which may have been generated by pathological intraspinal neural reflexes due to substance P.

Some of the effects of substance P given intrathecally probably result from direct motor neuron stimulation or a lessening of the threshold level of excitability of motor neurons in the lumbosacral spinal cord. This hypothesis is supported by several findings:

1. Substance P exerts a remarkably strong excitatory action on spinal motor neurons, characterized by a prolonged time course commencing after a delay of several seconds to minutes (Otsuka et al. 1972).
2. Substance P-like immunoreactive cell fibers end at the L6–S1 spinal cord level in the sacral parasympathetic nucleus – the origin of the pelvic nerve, which innervates the urinary bladder with parasympathetic efferents and afferents (Paxinos 1985).
3. Intrathecal administration of substance P antagonists effects profound flaccidity (Yaksh 1986).
4. The homovanillic derivative capsaicin, which produces a significant depletion of substance P immunoreactivity in the dorsal horn after systemic administration, causes, when given intrathecally in high doses, a profound, long-lasting motor weakness reminiscent of the effects produced by substance P antagonists (Yaksh 1986).

These data and our observations underline the probability that the substance P-like immunoreactive cell and cell fiber systems at the lumbosacral spinal cord level are not exclusively related to the afferent processing of pain; they also seem to be important in providing a tonic influence on motor horn cells.

The distribution of substance P immunoreactivity in the human spinal cord is very similar to the pattern found in rats. Based on our results obtained in rats, we conclude that substance P at the spinal cord level in man may influence neuronal circuits controlling bladder and sphincteric activity, and that afferent and efferent functions at spinal segment level are functionally closely intermingled.

These observations suggest that substance P, or other putative neuropeptides, if produced and synaptically released in abnormal amounts, could very well mediate spastic dysfunction either at the muscle cell level or via a spinal reflex, affecting the behaviour of the sphincter, bladder, rectum, or pelvic floor; this may be accompanied by discomfort and pain.

References

Applebaum AE, Vance WH, Coggeshall RE (1980) Segmental localization of sensory cells that innervate the bladder. J Comp Neurol 192:203

Euler US v (1936) Untersuchungen über Substanz P, die atropinfeste, darmerregende und gefässerweiternde Substanz aus Darm und Gehirn. Naunyn-Schmiedeberg's Arch Exp Pathol Pharmakol 181:181

Fields HL (1987) Pain. McGraw-Hill, New York, p 354

Hökfelt T, Vincent S, Dalsgaard C-J, Skirboll L, Johansson O, Schultzberg M, Lundberg JM, Rosell S, Pernow B, Jansco G (1982) Distribution of substance P in brain and periphery and its possible role as a co-transmitter. In: Ciba Foundation Symposium 91 Substance P in the Nervous System. Pitman, London, pp 84–100

Konishi S, Otsuka M (1974) Excitatory action of hypothalamic substance P on spinal motoneurons of newborn rats. Nature 252:734

Maggi CA, Santicioli P, Meli A (1986) The nonstop transvesical cystometrogram in urethane-anesthetized rats: a simple procedure for quantitative studies on the various phases of urinary bladder voiding cycle. J Pharmacol Methods 15:157

McKenna KE, Nadelhaft I (1986) The organization of the pudendal nerve in the male and female rat. Comp Neurol 248:532

Otsuka M, Konishi S, Takahashi T (1972) The presence of a motoneuron-depolarizing peptide in bovine dorsal roots of spinal nerves. Proc Jpn Acad 48:342

Paxinos G (1985) Hindbrain and spinal cord, vol 2. In: Paxinos G (ed) The rat nervous system. Academic Press, Sydney, p 362

Pernow B (1983) Substance P. Pharmacol Rev 35:85

Sasek CA, Seybold VS, Elde RP (1984) The immuno-histochemical localization of nine peptides in the sacral parasympathetic nucleus and the dorsal gray commissure in rat spinal cord. Neuroscience 12:855

Sharkey KA, Williams RG, Schultzberg M, Dockray GJ (1983) Sensory substance P-innervation of the urinary bladder: possible site of action of capsaicin in causing urine retention in rats. Neuroscience 10:861

Yaksh TL (1986) The central pharmacology of primary afferents with emphasis on the disposition and role of primary afferent substance P. In: Yaksh TL (ed) Spinal afferent processing. Plenum Press, New York, pp 165–195

Topographic-Anatomical Basis of the Sacral Application of Electro-Neurostimulation: Neuroanatomical Variations*

A. MERSDORF[1], T. MERSDORF[1], E. A. TANAGHO[1], and D. JONAS[2]

Introduction

Since 1971, the Department of Urology at the University of California, San Francisco, has been involved in the application of electrical neurostimulation to the human genitourinary tract (Schmidt and Tanagho 1979). Although the material and technique has been improved, the rates of success for intraspinal sacral root stimulation as well as for the sacral foramen electrode implants remained steady at about 75% (Schmidt 1988; Schmidt and Tanagho 1990). For a better understanding of the failure rate, we performed this supramicroscopic study of the human anatomy of the conus medullaris, the cauda equina, and the topography of the sacral spinal nerves in their relationship to the sacral foramina.

Materials and Methods

Dissection of human spinal cords and the corresponding spinal roots was accomplished in four male and five female glycerol/alcohol/formalin-fixed cadavers. The spinal cord, the cauda equina, and the spinal ganglia and nerves were exposed by dissecting away the muscles of the back and removing the spinous processes and arches including the vertebrae T7–S5. After describing the topographic-anatomical relationships, the spinal cords – including the caudae equinae and spinal ganglia – were removed, spread out on a foam plate, measured, and proved by photography. The following structural and topographic aspects were studied:

1. the conus medullaris;
2. the longitudinal extent of the spinal segment of origin of each root enclosing S1–S5;
3. the intradural length of the sacral roots;
4. the intradural anastomoses between adjacent sacral spinal roots (nerve bridging);
5. the topographic relationship between spinal ganglia/nerves and their sacral foramina. Although the anatomical features were grossly visible, measure-

* Supported by Grant ME 902/1-2 from the Deutsche Forschungsgemeinschaft, Federal Republic of Germany, Prize-winner 10th Symposium Experimental Urology, 1990, Munich, FRG.

[1] Department of Urology, University of California School of Medicine, San Francisco, CA 94143, USA.
[2] Abt. für Urologie der Universität, Theodor-Stern-Kai 7, W-6000 Frankfurt/Main 70, FRG.

ments and optical examination were executed by aid of a 30-magnification dissecting microscope and a micrometer.

Results

In seven cadavers the conus medullaris consisting of spinal segments S1–S5 was localized at the intervertebral disc level T12–L1; in two specimens it was at intervertebral disc level L1–L2. In male cadavers the mean of the dorsal ($\bar{X}$ 34±2.8 mm) and of the ventral ($\bar{X}$ 30.4±4.3 mm) dimensions of the conus medullaris was larger than in female cadavers (dorsal $\bar{X}$ 28.8±8.8 mm; ventral $\bar{X}$ 24.3±5.6 mm). In all instances the dorsal length of the conus was greater than its ventral extension.

The lengths of sacral spinal cord segments are shown in Table 1. The differences in length for the various sacral segments did not show the expected successive decrease in the lower-lying sacral segments; this was especially true for the dorsal segments in both genders (Table 1). A few increased values of standard deviation are explained by the fact that in some instances it was impossible to assign dorsal or ventral roots to a specific sacral spinal segment (see below).

Corresponding to the body length, the intradural path of the roots was longer in males (S5 = $\bar{X}$217±12 mm) than in females (S5 = $\bar{X}$184±21 mm). Intradural connections between adjacent ventral (Figs. 1, 3) or dorsal (Fig. 2) sacral roots were seen. These special kinds of nervous anastomoses are known as "bridging" and were noticed at various intradural levels (Fig. 1). Bridging was never seen *between dorsal and ventral roots.* In both sexes, bridging was more frequent between dorsal roots than between ventral roots, and, interestingly, more often on the left side than on the right side (Table 2). Ventral S5 roots were – with one exception – not seen (Fig. 3). Dorsal S5 roots were identified, but in three instances only

Table 1. Length of sacral spinal cord segments in male (n = 4) and female (n = 5) human cadavers. (Mean ± SD in millimeters)

	Dorsal segments		Ventral segments	
	Right	Left	Right	Left
Sacral segment lengths (males)				
S1	8.7±1.4	7.6±2.0	8.2±3.0	7.2±3.5
S2	6.9±0.8	7.8±1.0	6.9±0.9	7.2±2.4
S3	6.4±0.1	5.5±0.1	5.7±3.1	5.0±1.8
S4	7.4±2.0	5.5±1.2	3.6±3.0	2.5±0.8
S5	Missing	5.0±2.0	Missing	Missing
Sacral segment lengths (females)				
S1	6.3±1.0	6.6±1.2	6.4±1.6	6.6±0.8
S2	6.3±1.6	6.3±2.2	6.1±1.9	5.3±1.6
S3	5.7±2.0	6.2±1.7	4.6±1.7	5.4±2.1
S4	6.0±1.9	6.3±3.7	3.5±2.2	3.6±1.6
S5	3.5±1.0	2.6±0.9	Missing	Missing

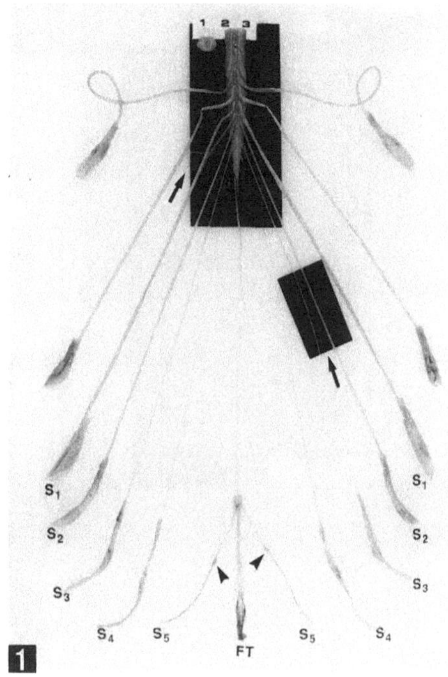

Fig. 1. Display of the *ventral* roots S1 – S4 after dissection of all dorsal roots for better visualization. The ganglia bearing spinal nerves S5 (*arrowheads*) on either side are lacking the ventral roots. Ventral nerve bridging is indicated by *arrows* and occurred proximal as well as distal to the conus medullaris. *FT*, filum terminale

Table 2. Occurrence of dorsal and ventral root nerve bridging in male ($n = 4$) and female ($n = 5$) human cadavers

	Dorsal roots		Ventral roots	
	Right	Left	Right	Left
Bridging (males)				
Mean ± SD	2.5 ± 0.6	5.0 ± 1.4	2.0 ± 1.0	1.7 ± 0.6
Minimum	2	3	1	1
Maximum	3	6	3	2
Bridging (females)				
Mean ± SD	2.8 ± 1.3	3.4 ± 2.9	1.0 ± 1.2	0.8 ± 0.5
Minimum	1	0	0	0
Maximum	4	7	2	1

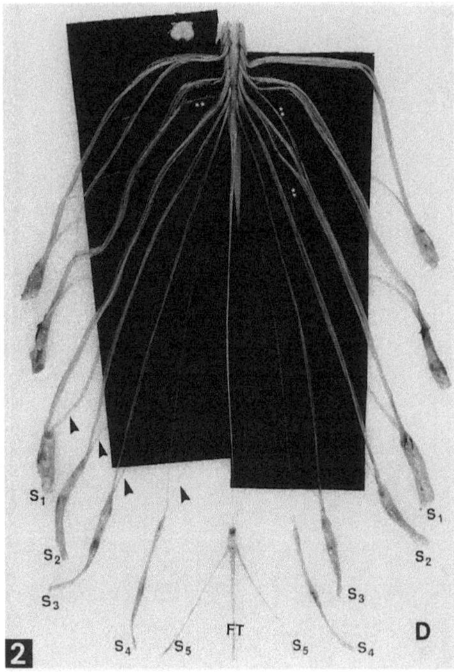

Fig. 2. In this preparation we see the *dorsal* roots S1 – S5. Dorsal and ventral roots are separated by black paper; this allows a rough estimation of the differences in thickness between dorsal and ventral roots. Four existing ventral roots on either side are indicated by *arrowheads* on the left side only. The ventral S5 roots are missing. **, dorsal nerve bridging; *FT*, filum terminale

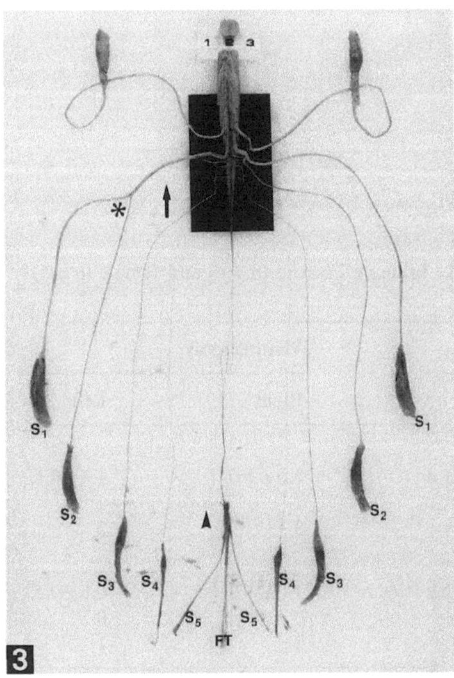

Fig. 3. Presentation of the *ventral* roots. The dorsal roots have been dissected. Only in this single preparation was one unilaterally localized, ventral S5 root found (*arrowhead*). It lacks its own spinal origin, deriving distally from the right ventral root S4. In a similar pattern S2 arises from S1 (*). *Arrow* indicates ventral nerve bridging. Note the outline of the perispinal plexus. *FT*, filum terminale

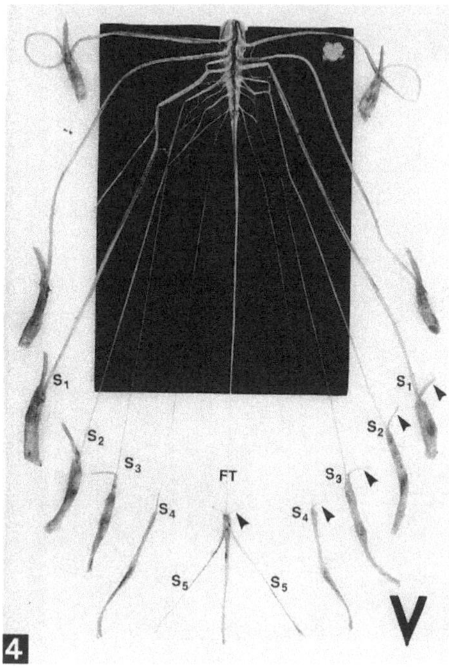

Fig. 4. The anatomy of a perispinal plexus, as it can be seen here, has not been described before (see also Fig. 3). This arrangement may be interpreted as an extreme occurrence of intradural anastomoses between adjacent sacral spinal roots, also known as nerve bridging. Thus, the reference of a specific ventral root to its own specific spinal segment seems difficult (S1, S4) or even impossible (S2, S3). *Arrowheads* indicate the remaining distal portion of the dorsal roots which were removed. This cadaver preparation displays five dorsal but only four ventral roots. *FT*, filum terminale

unilaterally, and in three other cases the S5 roots came from S4; Fig. 2 displays a specimen with two dorsal S5 roots. Ventral S4 roots were missing in two cadavers. Ventral and dorsal coccygeal roots were not seen at all.

The arrangement of a perispinal plexus, which is going to be described here for the first time, was found in two preparations (Figs. 3, 4). This pattern is interpreted as an extreme occurrence of intradural nerve bridging between ventral roots, which culminates in the anatomy of a plexus. In these cases the relating of a specific ventral root to a definite spinal segment seems difficult (S1, S4) or even impossible (S2, S3) (Figs. 3, 4).

The topography of the os sacrum and its nervous contents establishes the following: the best surgical approach for obtaining intradural access to the designated ventral and dorsal roots of urological interest – S2, S3, and S4 – is to perform a laminectomy of vertebra S1 (Fig. 5). Ventral and dorsal roots can be easily recognized by their own oblique-running blood vessels, which separate them from each other. Foramen S2 is completely filled by its ganglion, which prevents the approximation of a foramen electrode to the spinal nerve S2. In foramina S3 and S4 the corresponding spinal nerves will be met only in a very small medio caudal area of the lower medial quadrant. The bony sacral mass and the lipovascular, perineural wrapping structures of spinal nerves S3 and S4 hinder precise approximation of the foramen electrode which is applied blind. Furthermore, the insertion of the electrode through the foramen S3 or S4 will most likely cause a venous hemorrhage, since the spinal nerves are surrounded by a thick venous plexus. The outline of the hematoma will not be obstructed by the soft fatty tissue which en-

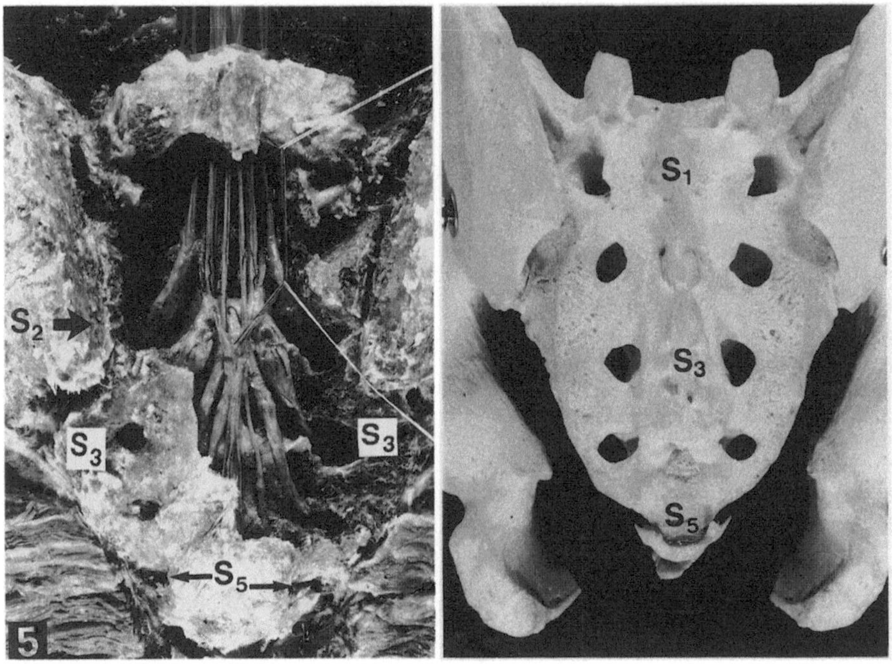

Fig. 5. The cadaver preparation reveals: (1) for applying electrodes intradurally to S2–S4, the best surgical approach is obtained by performing a laminectomy of S1. After pulling the filum terminale and the S5 roots laterally (as seen), the surgeon acquires free access to the ventral and dorsal roots of S2, S3, and S4. (2) The differences in size and position of the ganglia are obvious. Foramen S2 is completely filled by its ganglion. In foramina S3 and S4 the corresponding spinal nerves are localized; due to their oblique and medioventral path, spinal nerves S3 and S4 will be met only in a very small mediocaudal area of their respective foramina. Thus, approximation of a foramen electrode to spinal nerve S2 will be prevented by its ganglion. The bony sacral mass and the lipovascular, perineural wrapping structures of spinal nerves S3 and S4 hinder precise approximation of the blindly applied foramen electrode

closes the spinal nerves. Thus the electrode – probably isolated from the spinal nerve by hematoma – needs to provide higher current densities in order suitably to stimulate the nervous structures.

Discussion

The classical sacral neuroanatomy as still taught in anatomical or neurological textbooks is no longer valid. It seems that dorsal and ventral root organization according to the law of symmetry and metamery does not apply to the sacral spinal cord. Although it is known from the cervical region that anastomoses between adjacent dorsal roots do exist (Rickenbacher et al. 1985), among the ventral roots they are suspected to be very uncommon (Marzo et al. 1987; Rickenbacher et al. 1985). Like d'Avella and Mingrino (1979), we found intrathecal anastomoses (bridging) between adjacent dorsal and between juxtaposed ventral roots, but they were never seen *between dorsal and ventral roots*. Bridging between dorsal roots was more frequently observed than between neighboring ventral roots.

Ventral S4 roots were missing now and then, ventral S5 roots were mostly not found, and coccygeal roots were not seen at all. The formation of a ventral perispinal plexus is here reported for the first time; in these instances, association of a particular root to its spinal segment is difficult or even impossible; thus, stimulation of a particular spinal nerve does not necessarily permit a conclusion as to which spinal segment may be physiologically involved, because the electrical impulse has various neuroanatomical paths which terminate at different spinal segments.

References

d'Avella D, Mingrino S (1979) Microsurgical anatomy of lumbosacral spinal roots. J Neurosurg 51:819

Marzo JM, Simmons EH, Kallen F (1987) Intradural connections between adjacent cervical spinal roots. Spine 12:964

Rickenbacher J, Landolt AM, Theiler K (1985) Applied anatomy of the back. Springer, Berlin Heidelberg New York Tokyo

Schmidt RA (1988) Applications of neurostimulation in urology. Neurourol Urodynam 7:585

Schmidt RA, Tanagho EA (1990) Klinische Anwendung der Neurostimulation. Urologe [A]29:191

Schmidt RA, Tanagho EA (1979) Feasibility of controlled micturition through electric stimulation. Urol Int 34:199

Prostaglandin Production by Human Renal Pelvis and Ureter

U. ZWERGEL[1], T. ZWERGEL[1], S. ALLOUSSI[1], H. J. LEIS[2], and H. GLEISPACH[2]

Introduction

The metabolites of arachidonic acid (eicosanoids) such as prostaglandins and thromboxanes are potent tissue hormones. Each cell type is thought to produce its own pattern of arachidonic acid metabolites with a different biological action.

Several workers (Abrams et al. 1979; Brown et al. 1980; Jeremy et al. 1987) have demonstrated the ability of the bladder to synthesize various eicosanoids. The present study was designed to analyse the capacity of the human renal pelvis and ureter to produce prostaglandins. The inhibition of this synthesis was also investigated. Prostaglandins were measured by gas chromatography/mass spectrometry (Leis et al. 1987).

Materials and Methods

Tissue pieces of human renal pelvis and ureter (about 3×10 mm) were obtained from kidneys removed because of renal cell carcinoma. From one tissue piece at least eight discs of nearly the same size were cut out and each placed in 1 ml Krebs-Henseleit medium (113.8 mmol/l NaCl, 22 mmol/l $NaHCO_3$, 4.7 mmol/l KCl, 1.2 mmol/l KH_2PO_4, 1.1 mmol/l $MgSO_4 \times 7H_2O$, 2.5 mmol/l $CaCl_2 \times 2H_2O$ and 5.5 mmol/l glucose), pregassed with 95% O_2, 5% CO_2. The samples were then incubated at 37 °C in a shaking water bath. Two of the discs were incubated with the control medium alone. To the other discs arachidonic acid (200 mg/l) or indomethacin (10 mg/l) were added and incubated for 30 min. After the incubation reactions were stopped with formic acid, the tubes were centrifuged for 5 min and the supernatants removed for eicosanoid estimation. Figure 1 shows schematically the extraction and purification procedure for prostaglandins followed by their derivatization and detection with gas chromatography/mass spectrometry. A Finnigan 9610 gas chromatograph coupled to a Finnigan 4500 mass spectrometer with negative ion chemical ionization and an Incos data system were used.

Tissue pieces were always weighed after desiccation. Eicosanoid production was expressed in picograms per 10 mg dry tissue (mean ± standard error of the mean). Statistical differences were evaluated by the Wilcoxon test.

[1] Urologische Klinik der Universität des Saarlandes, W-6650 Homburg/Saar, FRG.
[2] Universitäts-Kinderklinik, Abt. f. Massenspektrometrie, 8036 Graz, Austria.

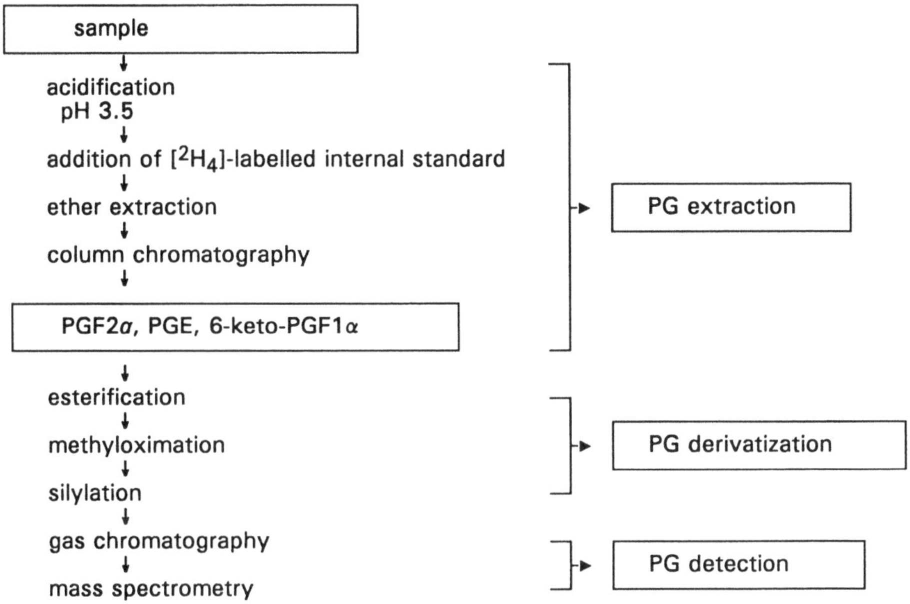

Fig. 1. Schematic illustration of the extraction, derivatization and detection procedure for prostaglandin (PG) estimation

Results

6-Keto-$PGF_{1\alpha}$ was released in the highest quantity, followed by $PGF_{2\alpha}$ (Table 1). PGE_2 synthesis was the lowest. Eicosanoid synthesis increased when the strips were incubated with arachidonic acid (Table 1).

After 30 min incubation with only 10 mg/l indomethacin there was a significant decrease in prostaglandin synthesis in vitro (Table 2). Larger amounts of indomethacin were shown to completely abolish prostaglandin synthesis.

Table 1. Prostaglandin synthesis of human renal pelvic and ureteric strips ($n = 9$) with and without incubation of the prostaglandin precursor, arachidonic acid (200 mg/l). (Mean ± SEM)

	Arachidonic acid	
	without (pg/10 mg tissue)	with (pg/10 mg tissue)
$PGF_{2\alpha}$	191 ± 80	2340 ± 350
PGE_2	114 ± 30	7980 ± 980
6-Keto-$PGF_{1\alpha}$	347 ± 120	6530 ± 330

Table 2. Prostaglandin synthesis of human renal pelvic strips ($n = 7$) with and without incubation of indomethacin (10 mg/l). (Mean ± SEM)

	Indomethacin	
	without (pg/10 mg tissue)	with (pg/10 mg tissue)
$PGF_{2\alpha}$	227 ± 90	33 ± 12*
PGE_2	121 ± 40	17 ± 8*
6-Keto-$PGF_{1\alpha}$	314 ± 140	90 ± 23*

* $p < 0.05$

Discussion

Gas chromatography/mass spectrometry with selected ion monitoring and labelled substances (stable isotopes) was used for qualitative and quantitative measurement of eicosanoid production (Leis et al. 1987). The labelled analogues are added to the biological sample immediately after collection and are detected simultaneously with the natural analogues. Since they behave in a very similar way to the natural substances, they act as ideal internal standards and allow an exact calculation of all losses.

The great number of chromatographic steps combined with the negative ion chemical ionization and the mass-specific detection renders the method highly specific for prostaglandin determination. Gas chromatography/mass spectrometry is probably the best method available for analyses of prostaglandins in biological fluids (Maier et al. 1986), superior to specific radioimmunoassays also used for prostaglandin determination.

The present study shows for the first time that the human renal pelvis and ureter are able to synthesize prostaglandins, as has been found in the bladder of man (Abrams et al. 1979; Jeremy et al. 1987) and of rabbit (Brown et al. 1980). These results give credence to the experiments of Al-Ugaily et al. (1986), who described a large number of lipophilic granules in the vicinity of ureteric smooth muscle cells on electron microscopy and suggested them to be prostaglandin precursors. Our findings also reinforce the results of Thulesius et al. (1987), who found eicosanoid release from sheep ureter into an organ bath.

The measured amounts of the eicosanoids released by the urinary tract in this study (114–347 pg/10 mg tissue) are lower than those measured by Jeremy et al. (1987) from bladder mucosa (0.9–58 ng/mg tissue). There are some procedural differences between our study and that of Jeremy et al. (1987). They used specific radioimmunoassays and the different results may be due to the different methods of prostaglandin estimation. Furthermore, Jeremy et al. (1987) only analysed mucosal biopsies, whereas we used complete bladder strips. The validity of the present study is also limited by the small number of samples. In addition, it is known that trauma during tissue preparation is a stimulus for eicosanoid release and that variations in the physiological environment (for instance pH) or pathological conditions may alter eicosanoid synthesis (Jeremy et al. 1987). Since prostaglandins are also produced by other tissue (fat, blood), great care must be taken to remove these tissues (Abrams et al. 1979).

Experiments in isolated ureteric and renal pelvic strips have shown that exogenous prostaglandins can alter the contractile response of these smooth muscle preparations. Indomethacin and other prostaglandin synthetase inhibitors are known to inhibit not only renal blood flow and diuresis but also contractions of smooth muscle from the upper urinary tract (Lundstam et al. 1985; Thulesius and Angelo-Khattar 1985; Cole et al. 1988; Zwergel et al. 1988). Furthermore, our results showed that the release of prostaglandins could be inhibited by indomethacin. In conclusion, indomethacin may directly change smooth muscle activity of the upper urinary tract, a mechanism which might be another contributing factor in pain relief during renal colic.

Acknowledgements. This work was sponsored by a grant of Fresenius AG, Oberursel, FRG. Dr. Leis and Dr. Gleispach received financial support through grants of the *Fonds zur Förderung der wissenschaftlichen Forschung*, Austria; project number 8013.

References

Abrams PH, Sykes JAC, Rose AJ, Rogers AF (1979) The synthesis and release of prostaglandins by human urinary bladder muscle in vitro. J Urol 16:346–348

Al-Ugaily L, Thulesius O, Angelo-Khattar M (1986) New evidence for prostaglandin induced motility of the ureter. Scand J Urol Nephrol 20:225–229

Brown WW, Zenser TV, Davis BB (1980) Prostaglandin E_2 production by rabbit urinary bladder. Am J Physiol 239:452–458

Cole RS, Fry CH, Shuttleworth KED (1988) The actions of the prostaglandins on isolated human ureteric smooth muscle. Br J Urol 61:19–26

Jeremy JY, Tsang V, Mikhailidis DP, Rogers H, Morgan RJ, Dandona P (1987) Eicosanoid synthesis by human urinary bladder mucosa: pathological implications. Br J Urol 59:36–39

Leis HJ, Hohenester E, Malle E, Mayer B, Gleispach H (1987) Measurement of prostaglandins, thromboxanes and hydroxy fatty acids by stable isotope dilution gas chromatography/mass spectrometry. Biomed Environ Mass Spectrom 14:617–621

Lundstam S, Jonsson O, Kihl B, Pettersson S (1985) Prostaglandin synthetase inhibition of renal pelvic smooth muscle in the rabbit. Br J Urol 57:390–393

Maier B, Moser R, Leis HJ, Gleispach H (1986) Rapid separation of arachidonic acid metabolites by silicic acid chromatography for subsequent quantitative analysis by gas chromatography-mass spectrometry. J Chromatogr 378:430–436

Thulesius O, Angelo-Khattar M (1985) The effect of indomethacin on the motility of isolated sheep ureters. Acta Pharmacol Toxicol 56:298–301

Thulesius O, Angelo-Khattar M, Ali M (1987) The effect of prostaglandin synthesis inhibition on motility of the sheep ureter. Acta Physiol Scand 131:51–54

Zwergel U, Zwergel T, Ziegler M (1988) Effects of indomethacin and metamizol on the upper urinary tract. Conference of the International Society for Dynamics of the Upper Urinary Tract (ISDU), Marlow, UK

VI. Urolithiasis, Lithotripsy, Kidney-Pathophysiology

Electrophoretic Studies on Proteinuria on Calcium Oxalate Stone Patients

O. SCHARREL and A. HESSE [1]

Introduction

Proteinuria is regarded as one of the main symptoms of renal disease. At the same time, temporary or permanent proteinuria may often occur without renal involvement.

Stone disease may be a consequence or cause of renal dysfunction. The subsequent proteinuria may play a role in stone formation. Above all, proteins are found in the stones themselves. Many other variables in the urine of calcium oxalate stone patients have been measured in order to calculate the risk of stone formation [2, 3], but examination of urinary proteins of these patients has so far been neglected. The reasons for the appearance of the proteins not only in the urine but also in the stones, as well as their role in the pathogenesis of urolithiasis, are still the subject of controversy. It therefore seems important to obtain more information about the origin of these proteins and the reasons for their extensive appearance in the urine of patients with calcium oxalate stones.

In the present study both quantitative and qualitative protein analysis were carried out and compared with measurements taken in healthy persons.

Material and Methods

Twenty-four-hour urine from 45 healthy persons and 45 calcium oxalate stone patients was analyzed. In the healthy group the average age of the 38 men was 27.3 years (range 22–32) and of the 7 women 30.6 years (range 20–47). The patient group was composed of 20 men averaging 47.3 years in age (range 33–57) and 25 women of an average age of 43.1 years (range 22–69). Only patients who formed only calcium oxalate stones and showed no other diseases accompanied by changes in protein excretion were included in the study. None suffered from urinary tract infection.

First, total urinary protein was measured according to the method of Iwata and Nishikaze [5]. Urinary protein excretion >150 mg/d was regarded as pathological. For the subsequent qualitative analysis, ultrathin SDS polyacrylamide gel gradient electrophoresis ($T = 4\% - 22.5\%$, $C = 4\%$) was used according to the method of Görg et al. [1]. This technique allows separation of the proteins according to their molecular weight. It helps in obtaining further information about the renal origin of the urinary protein fractions because the proteins are filtered in the

[1] Experimentelle Urologie, Urologische Universitätsklinik, Sigmund-Freud-Str. 25, W-5300 Bonn 1, FRG.

glomerulum according to their molecular weight too, small proteins being reabsorbed in the tubules. Visualization of the proteins after electrophoretic separation was achieved with Coomassie brilliant blue followed by silver stain according to the method described by Heukeshoven and Dernick [4].

For quality monitoring the migration distances of molecular marker proteins were plotted against their logarithms of molecular weight; standard deviation, variation coefficient, and the correlation coefficient were calculated. All electropherograms stained with Coomassie blue that showed more than the two protein bands of the healthy persons (albumin and transferrin) were regarded as pathological and classified as showing tubular, glomerular, or mixed proteinuria (Fig. 1). For assessing the urinary electropherograms stained with silver, the protein bands of the calcium oxalate stone patients were compared with those of the healthy persons. Quantitative analysis of the electropherograms was not possible because the proteins took up the stain differently.

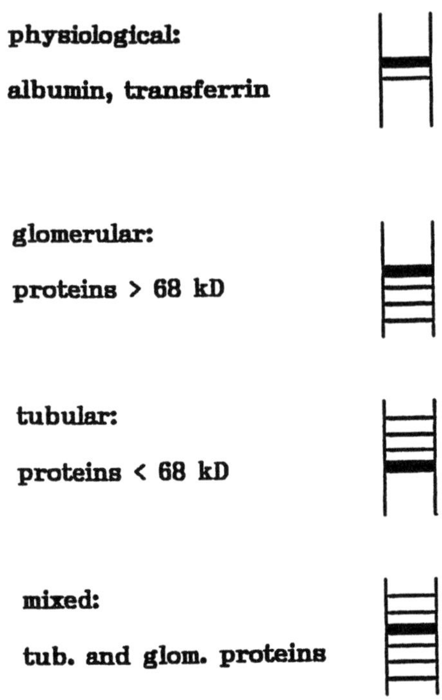

Fig. 1. Classification of urinary protein electropherograms (SDS-PAGE) stained with Coomassie brilliant blue

Results

The results of the analysis of total protein are shown in Fig. 2. In the urine of the calcium oxalate stone patients significantly higher amounts of protein were found than in the urine of the healthy persons: an average of 311 mg/24 h, against only 131 mg/24 h. As there were no differences in 24-h volume of urine, the high protein excretion by stone patients could only be explained by high urinary protein

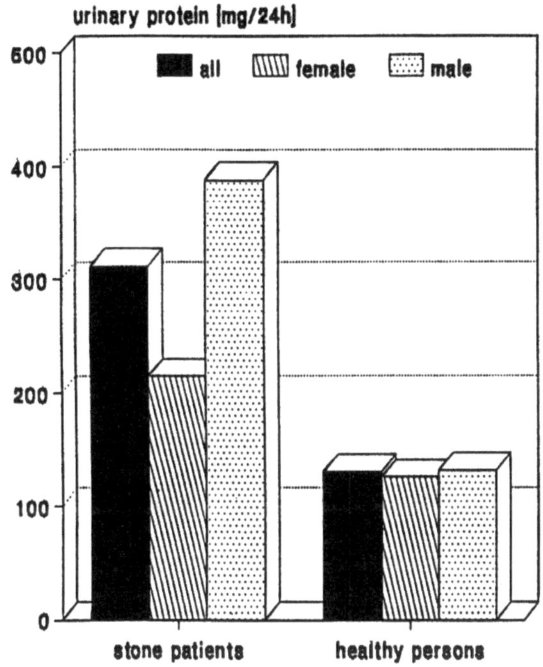

Fig. 2. Total urinary protein excretion in calcium oxalate stone patients and healthy persons

concentrations. A raised rate of protein excretion (> 150 mg/24 h) was thus diagnosed in only 8.9% of the healthy persons but in 44% of the calcium oxalate stone patients.

Before qualitative analysis of the urinary proteins, we checked the quality of the electrophoretic technique used. Verification of constant migration distances showed that the marker proteins differed only slightly in their mobility. Good correlation between molecular weight and migration distance confirmed the quality of the gels and justified their use for the determination of the molecular weight of unknown proteins (Fig. 3).

The results of the electrophoretic separation of the urinary proteins followed by Coomassie blue staining are shown in Table 1. Of the calcium oxalate stone patients 33.4% showed pathological protein bands in their urine. All forms of proteinuria could be observed: 6.7% of the patients had tubular proteinuria, 6.7% glomerular, and 20% mixed proteinuria. Surprisingly, 13.3% of this proteinuric group had normal total urinary protein values. No pathological protein bands were seen in the urine of the healthy control group.

For assessment of the urinary protein electropherograms stained with silver, the protein bands of the calcium oxalate stone patients were compared with those of the healthy control persons. Figure 4 shows the average number of protein bands for the various ranges of molecular weight in the calcium oxalate stone patients and the healthy persons. In the calcium oxalate stone patients we observed overall significantly more protein patterns in urine, but not over the entire range of molecular weight: in the range of low molecular weight range (< 20 kD) significantly

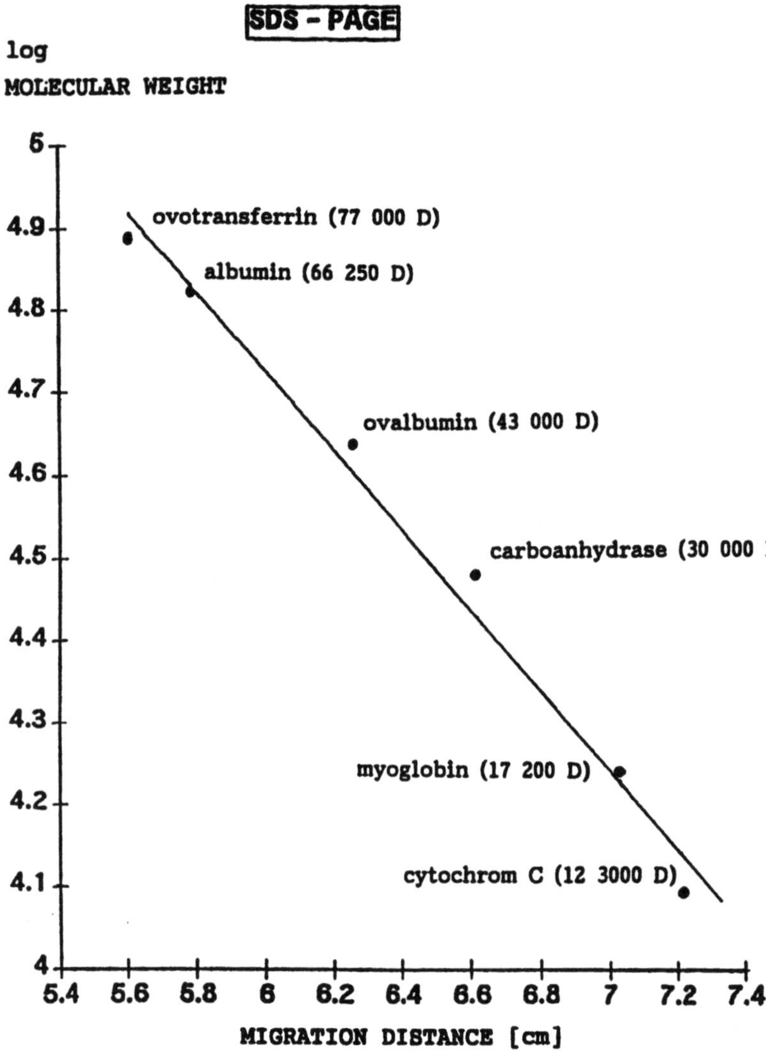

Fig. 3. Relationship between molecular weight of the marker proteins and their mobility in SDS-PAGE ($y = -0.49\,x + 7.65$; $r = 0.993$, $n = 30$)

Table 1. Results of SDS-PAGE with subsequent Coomassie blue staining

Proteins	Healthy persons (%)	Stone patients (%)
Physiological (albumin, transferrin)	100	66.7
Pathological	–	33.3
tubular (proteins < 68 kD)	–	6.7
glomerular (proteins > 68 kD)	–	6.7
mixed (tub. and glom. proteins)	–	20.0

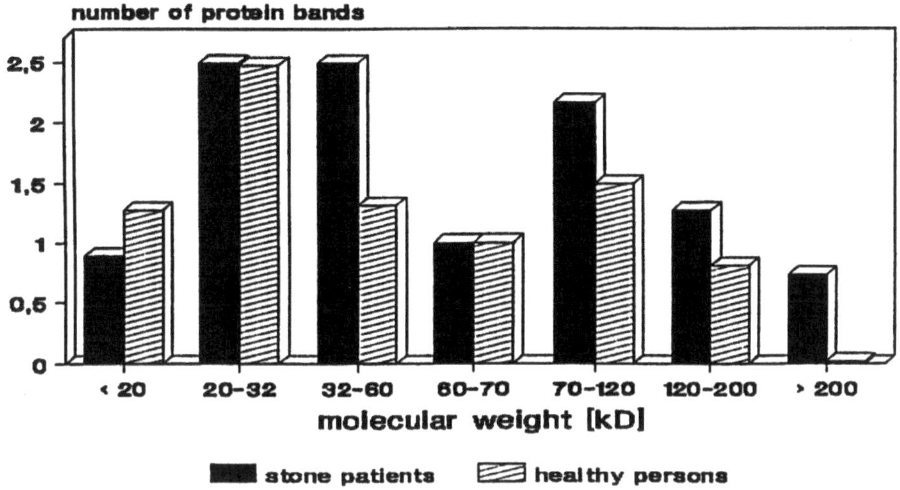

Fig. 4. Average number of urinary protein patterns of calcium oxalate stone patients and healthy persons in the different ranges of molecular weight (after SDS-PAGE; silver stain)

more protein fractions for the healthy persons were found compared to the stone patients. In regard to the protein fractions in the range 20–32 kD there was no difference between the two groups, but in the range of higher molecular weight the calcium oxalate stone patients had significantly more proteins.

Summary

Stone patients have significantly higher urinary total protein excretion than healthy persons, due to a higher urinary protein concentration. One third of the stone patients showed pathological protein patterns in the electrophoresis stained with Coomassie blue, but no homogeneous form of proteinuria and therefore no specific renal dysfunction could be diagnosed.

The results of the silver staining show significant differences in the molecular weight ranges of the urinary proteins of the two groups. The selective appearance or absence of some proteins probably indicates a special significance of these substances in urolithiasis. Some of the lower molecular weight proteins of healthy persons could be inhibitors of stone formation; the higher molecular weight substances of the patients could promote or accelerate urolithiasis, especially since proteins can be found in the concretions themselves.

Monitoring of proteinuria from calcium oxalate stone patients with SDS-PAGE should be integrated in laboratory program to obtain better knowledge of the onset and course of proteinuria and to gain the possibility of treating these symptoms. For effective treatment, the proteins involved need to be analyzed in greater detail.

References

1. Görg A, Postel W, Westermeier R, Gianazza E, Rhigetti PG (1980) Gel gradient electrophoresis, isoelectric focusing and two dimensional techniques in horzontal, ultrathin polyacrylamide layers. J Biochem Biophys Methods 3:273–284
2. Hesse A, Bach D (1982) Harnsteine. Thieme, Stuttgart
3. Hesse A, Schaefer RM (1987) Analyse von Harnsteinen und Charakterisierung der Bildungsursachen. Urologe [B]27:81–86
4. Heukeshoven J, Dernick R (1983) Simplified method for silver staining of proteins in polyacrylamide gels. In: Radola BJ (ed) Electrophoreses Forum '83, Munich
5. Iwata S, Nishikaze O (1979) New micro-turbidimetric method for determination of protein in cerebrospinal fluid and urine. Clin Chem 25:1317–1319

Creation of an Animal Model to Investigate the Bioeffects of Extracorporeal Shock Wave Lithotripsy and Alternative Treatment Techniques for Renal Stones

G. J. FUCHS, B. A. WOLFSON, R. D. DAVID, and Z. L. BARBARIC[1]

Introduction

Since its inception in 1980, extracorporeal shock wave lithotripsy (ESWL) has evolved to become the treatment of choice for urinary stones (Chaussy et al. 1986; Fuchs et al. 1985, 1990; Lingeman et al. 1986). There have been over two million treatments performed worldwide. The reasons for its dominant role in the management of urinary stone disease include a high rate of efficacy and a low rate of reported complications.

The side effects seen in the peri-treatment period with ESWL include transient macroscopic hematuria in over 90% of patients, and the rare complication of peri-renal bleeding, which occurs in less than 1% of treatments (Lingeman et al. 1988; Knapp et al. 1988). These short-term effects are similar to those seen in the initial animal trials performed by Chaussy et al. (1986). This led to the implication that because there were minimal acute clinical side effects there would also be minimal chronic effects.

However, recent reports in the literature have noted a significant incidence of new-onset hypertension within 2 years following ESWL treatment (Peterson and Finlayson 1986; Lingeman and Kulb 1987; Williams et al. 1988; Lingeman et al. 1990). These reports, along with their implications for future treatment planning for patients with urinary stone disease, prompted us to ask the question: is ESWL safe enough to remain the primary treatment for urinary stones?

Previous human studies have been complicated by the lack of an appropriate control group, retrospective analysis of data, and a myriad of other host factors which make human studies difficult to perform. Thus our goal in this pilot study was to create an animal model to investigate the bioeffects of ESWL and alternative treatment modalities for urinary stones, with specific emphasis on the physiologic parameter of blood pressure, the functional parameter of renal clearance, and the morphologic changes as assessed by magnetic resonance imaging (MRI). A well-defined animal model could then be utilized as a standard for investigating treatment-related effects of new stone treatment modalities, comparison of the bioeffects of various shock wave energy sources, and establishment of safety margins for the use of high energy shock waves.

[1] UCLA School of Medicine, Division of Urology, Dept. of Surgery, 10833 Le Conte Avenue, Los Angeles, CA 90024-1738, USA.

Materials and Methods

The animal selected was the house pig (*Suis scrafus*, 40–50 kg), because its renal anatomy and physiology, including a renin angiotensin system, is similar to that of the human (Tumbleson 1985). The swine has also been studied extensively as a model for hypertension, and demonstrates a stable blood pressure in historic controls.

Twelve animals were treated in the study groups. Four animals underwent open renal surgery via a flank incision, two had a pyelotomy, and two had a pyelotomy with radial nephrotomies. Four animals underwent percutaneous placement of a nephrostomy tube which was subsequently dilated to 24 French and left in place for 3 weeks. Two had a single tract placed, while two animals had two separate tracts placed. Four animals were treated with high energy shock waves (SW) in an unmodified Dornier HM3 Lithotripter at 18 kV. Cystoscopically placed ureteral catheters allowed visualization of the collecting system and focusing of the shock waves on the renal pelvis. One animal underwent 2000 SW, two animals underwent 2000 SW at two separate sessions, and one animal underwent a "supra-conventional" session of 4000 SW. The 4000 SW session was considered "supra-conventional" based on our previous studies in rabbits which showed renal morphologic changes to be dependent on the number of shock waves administered (Fuchs et al. 1988). At 6 months post-procedure, all pigs underwent removal of the treated kidney. During all procedures, anesthesia was induced with ketamine (10 mg/kg) and the animals were then intubated and maintained with suitable surgical anesthesia with inhaled halothane.

Each animal had blood pressures evaluated daily in the awake state via an indwelling arterial catheter (Terris et al. 1985). Before the start of the experiment, the animal had been conditioned to walk into a specially constructed box where the catheter was connected to a transducer and monitor. The electronically calculated systolic and diastolic blood pressures were recorded after stabilization of the readings (10–15 s). Blood pressure measurements were begun at least 2 weeks prior to the initiation of a treatment and continued until the animal was killed 2 weeks after removal of the treated kidney.

Renal function was measured using a technetium-99 DTPA (^{99}Tc DTPA) clearance assay. The animal was injected with 1 mCi ^{99}Tc DTPA intravenously into an ear vein. After 1 h equilibration, six serial serum samples were obtained at 20-min intervals from the indwelling arterial line. Serum samples were analyzed in a scintillation counter and the renal clearance was calculated. Renal clearance assays were performed pre-procedure as well as immediately, 1 day, 1 week, 1 month, and 6 months post-procedure.

Renal morphology was assessed using MRI scans (Fonar B3000, T1 sequence). All MRI scans were reviewed with specific emphasis on loss of corticomedullary differentiation and presence of peri-renal collections. MRI scans were performed immediately, 1 day, 1 week, 1 month, and 6 months post-procedure.

Statistical Analysis

Blood pressure readings prior to treatment, at peak systolic pressure, prior to nephrectomy, and after nephrectomy were compared. Five-day time periods at each of the points were compared. Analysis of variance was used to identify significant changes in each animal compared to its pretreatment control period.

Results

In the open surgical groups, three of four animals failed to show an elevation of blood pressure (Fig. 1), while one animal (pyelotomy plus radial nephrotomies) developed a statistically significant increase in blood pressure. This elevation of blood pressure was sustained at 6 months post-surgery and was reversed by nephrectomy. This animals also displayed a significant decrease in renal DTPA clearance post-surgery which returned to baseline by 1 week, while the remaining animals showed minimal changes in DTPA clearance. There were no significant changes noted on MRI scans in the open surgical groups (Table 1).

In the percutaneous groups, all animals developed a statistically significant elevation in blood pressure. The increase in blood pressure was transient in all ani-

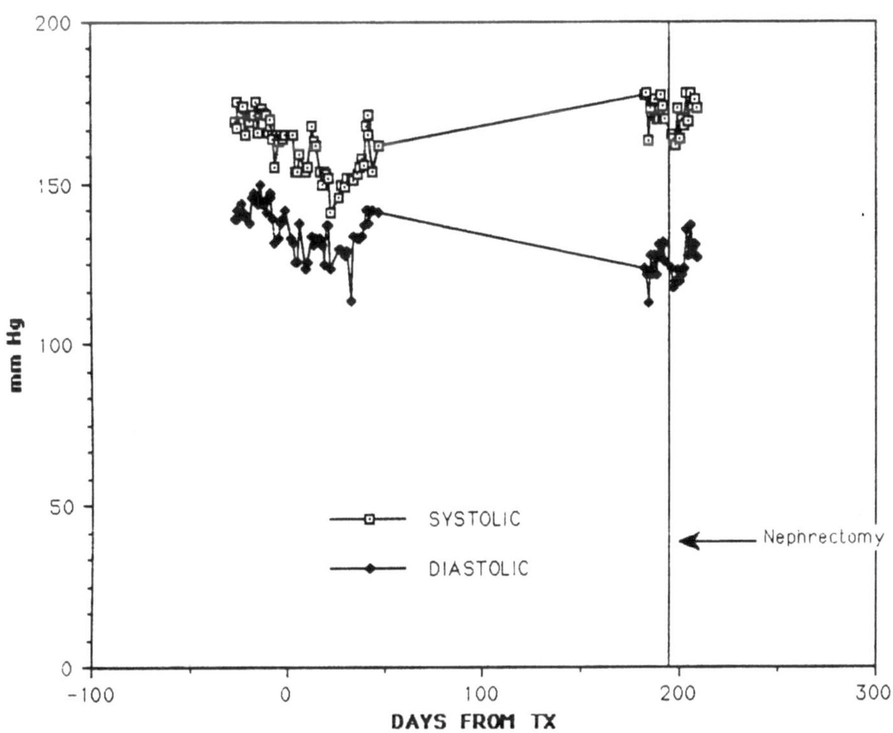

Fig. 1. Open surgery – long-term blood pressure

Table 1. Results (Summary)

	Open	Perc	ESWL
Elevated BP	1/4	4/4	2/4
Sustained ↑ BP	1/4	0	1/4
DTPA changes	1/4	2/4	4/4
MRI changes			
perirenal fluid	0	1/4	1/4
loss of CM diff.	0	4/4	4/4

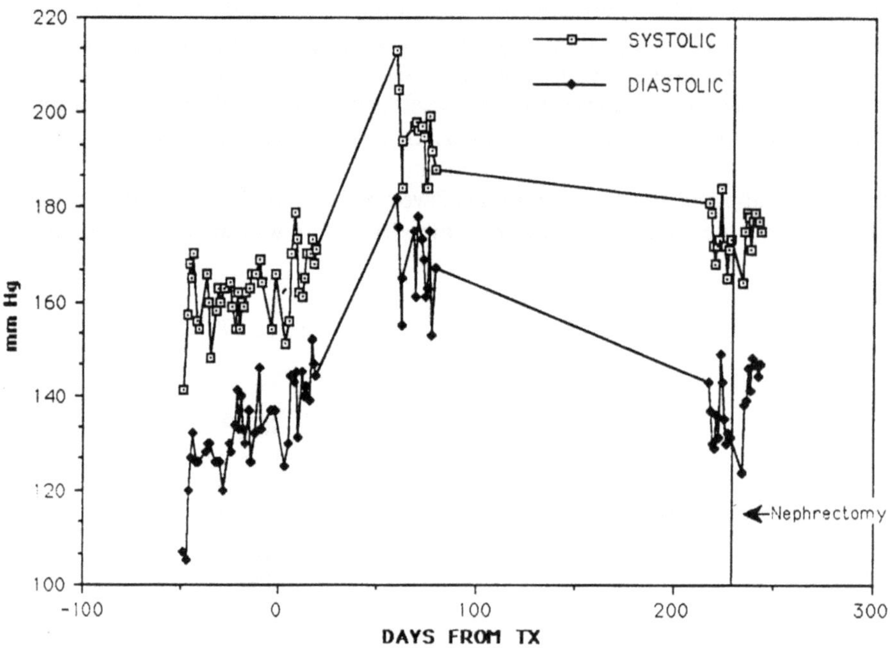

Fig. 2. Percutaneous – long-term blood pressure

mals, with the initiation of blood pressure elevation beginning at 3–6 weeks post-procedure and returning to baseline levels by 6 months (Fig. 2). One animal in each group (solitary or two separate nephrostomy tracts) developed a significant decrease in renal DTPA clearance post-procedure which returned to baseline by 1 week. On MRI scan, one animal developed a small peri-renal fluid collection which resolved by 1 week, and all animals showed loss of corticomedullary differentiation post-procedure which returned to normal by 1 week (Table 1).

In the extracorporeal shock wave (ESW) groups, two of four animals developed a statistically significant elevation of blood pressure. The blood pressure elevation was transient in the animal which received 2000 SW at two sessions, however in

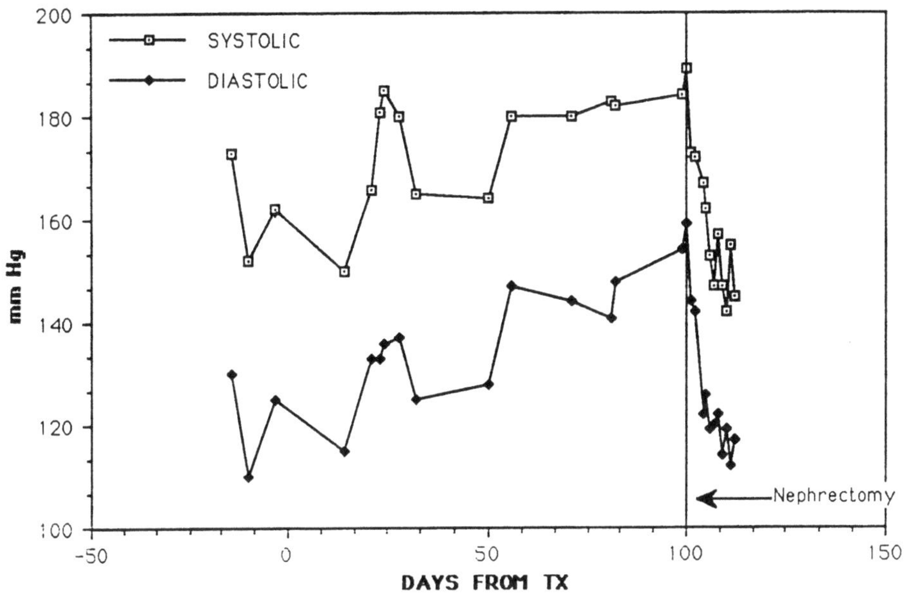

Fig. 3. ESWL 4000 SW – long-term blood pressure

the animal treated with the "supra-conventional" number of shock waves, the elevation of blood pressure was sustained and reversed by nephrectomy (Fig. 3). The remaining animals (2000 SW and 2000 SW at two sessions) displayed only mild transient elevations of blood pressure which were not statistically significant. All animals showed a decrease in DTPA clearance post-procedure which returned to baseline by 1 week. In addition, all animals showed loss of corticomedullary differentiation on MRI post-procedure which resolved by 1 week, and the animal treated with 4000 SW had a small peri-renal fluid collection (Table 1).

Discussion

ESWL has unquestionably revolutionized the treatment of stones in the upper urinary tract. The treatments are easily performed and the acute clinical side effects are generally well tolerated. What remains to be discerned are the possible long-term physiologic and clinical side effects of ESWL, including a potential for a decrease in renal function, an increased rate of stone recurrence, and an incidence of new-onset hypertension.

Peterson and Finlayson first reportet on three patients with new-onsed or accelerated hypertension following ESWL treatments (Peterson and Finlayson 1986). They suggested that ESWL caused focal areas of renal ischemia with subsequent alteration in systemic blood pressure such as is seen following renal trauma.

Lingeman and Kulb evaluated 900 patients treated with ESWL and found an annualized incidence of new-onset hypertension of 5.5% (Lingeman and Kulb

1987). Williams et al. (1988) similarly identified new-onset hypertension in 8.2%. Both of these studies were marred by a retrospective analysis of data, a lack of a non-ESWL control group, and an incomplete patient follow-up.

In a more recent report, Lingeman et al. (1990) evaluated over 900 patients treated with ESWL and alternative stone treatments. They did not find a significant difference in the annualized incidence of new-onset hypertension between the ESWL-treated and the non-ESWL-treated control group, despite a good match of patients for pre-treatment stone burden and blood pressure. However, they did observe a statistically significant increase in the diastolic blood pressure after ESWL treatment which was not seen in the control group, although the clinical significance and long-term effects of this change are unknown. This study was also marred by a lack of treatment and control group matching for other patient factors, especially pre-treatment renal function.

Because of the difficulties in performing a prospective, randomized, and well controlled human study of ESWL and alternative urinary stone treatments in the human, a well-defined animal model is important to allow investigation of the treatment effects and side effects of these procedures. Our previous pilot study showed the house pig to have potential as a suitable model (David et al. 1990). The swine were easily trainable, arterial catheters for blood pressure measurement were well tolerated, and the ESW, percutaneous, and surgical procedures were readily accomplished. In addition, when a "supra-conventional" number of shock waves were implemented, sustained elevation of blood pressure was identified which was reversed by nephrectomy.

The term "supra-conventional" applies for the following reasons. In his initial clinical trials, Chaussy arbitrarily limited the number of shock wave exposures to 1000 and the energy setting to 20 kV. These values were subsequently expanded to 2000 shock waves at 21 kV (FDA-IDE study) and eventually set at 2400 shock waves at 21 kV (Chaussy et al. 1986). Comparison of various clinical studies shows that adherence to these "guidelines" produces good clinical results with minimal side effects, while exposure to higher numbers of shock waves or higher energy settings results in an increased rate of energy-related complications (Fuchs et al. 1990). These clinical findings are corroborated by a number of animal studies, including a recent study performed at our institution which linked the occurrence of renal morphologic changes to the amount of shock wave energy delivered (Fuchs et al. 1988). In this rabbit model, the energy applied was adjusted according to the weight of the animal, and significant long-term renal morphologic changes were noted when more than 2000 SW were delivered to the kidney in a single session.

Our current additions to the swine pilot study have confirmed the advantages of the house pig model, and have identified some other interesting points. Animals treated with open surgery without invasion of the renal parenchyma (open pyelotomy) showed minimal functional and morphologic changes, while one of two animals which underwent associated radial nephrotomies displayed significant elevation of blood pressure which was sustained at 6 months and reversed by nephrectomy. Of note is that this kidney received 13 min warm ischemia during the surgical procedure. It is likely that the elevation of blood pressure was induced by renal tissue damage and renal ischemia at surgery, although the precise mechanism of this increase blood pressure is not evident.

All animals treated with percutaneous nephrostomies (single tract or two separate tracts) developed a statistically significant elevation of blood pressure post-procedure. The onset of the blood pressure elevation was 3 – 6 weeks post-procedure, and returned to baseline by 6 months. In addition, two of four animals treated with ESW developed an elevation in blood pressure at 3 – 6 weeks post-procedure. The blood pressure elevation was transient in the animal treated with a conventional number of shock waves (2000 SW at two separate sessions), but was sustained at 6 months post-treatment and reversed by nephrectomy in the animal treated with a "supra-conventional" number of shock waves (4000 SW at a single session).

Hypertension is recognized as a complication of traumatic renal injury, with a reported incidence between 0.7% and 33% (Cass et al. 1959; Knorring et al. 1981; Jameson 1978). The onset of the blood pressure elevation is usually within the first several weeks, but hypertension has been noted immediately or several years post-injury (Knorring et al. 1981). The hypertension may be transitory, with spontaneous resolution after periods of between 12 days and 9 months, or it may be sustained (Jameson 1978). The sustained hypertension has been documented to be reversed by nephrectomy (Freed and Tavel 1976). Possible etiologies of post-traumatic hypertension include renal ischemia and renal cicatrization by peri-renal collections (Page Kidney) (Jameson 1978; Page 1939; Carini et al. 1981).

The blood pressure elevations seen in our animals treated with ESW, percutaneous nephrostomy tracts, or open renal surgery are similar to those described following renal trauma. The delayed onset and transient nature of the blood pressure elevation could represent renal trauma from the shock waves or direct tissue injury from the percutaneous tubes which resolved over time. It is unknown whether the animals which had a sustained elevation of blood pressure at 6 months (open pyelotomy with radial nephrotomies, ESW 4000 SW) would have returned to baseline at a later time. Yet it is suggestive that the increase in blood pressure was of renal origin, since the blood pressure elevation reversed following nephrectomy. Perhaps the most important observation from this pilot study is not that sustained hypertension developed after these "unconventional" procedures, but that no animal treated with minimally invasive therapy in a conventional manner developed sustained elevation of blood pressure.

Decrease in renal clearance and loss of corticomedullary differentiation on MRI scan were documented on all ESW-treated animals, two of four percutaneously treated animals, and one open surgical animal. These changes were transient in all animals, with the renal clearance and MRI returning to baseline by 1 week post-treatment. The significance of these changes is uncertain, and further studies into the causative physiologic phenomenon are necessary.

In conclusion, this pilot study supports the role of the house pig as a model for comparing the bioeffects of ESWL and alternative treatment modalities for urinary stones. The physiologic parameter of blood pressure is easily monitored and the preliminary results suggest that using percutaneous techniques or conventional numbers of shock waves may not cause any permanent alteration in blood pressure. Likewise, when "supra-conventional" numbers of shock waves or open renal surgery are employed, sustained elevations of blood pressure may be encountered. The functional parameter of renal clearance and morphologic parameter of MRI showed specific changes in the peri-treatment period, although the significance of these changes still requires elucidation. With further studies, the house pig may provide a useful animal model to allow investigation of treatment-related bioeffects of various urinary stone treatments, comparison of the bioeffects of the diverse shock wave energy sources, and establishment of safety margins for the use of shock wave energy.

References

Carini M, Selli C, Trippitelli A et al. (1981) Surgical treatment of renovascular hypertension secondary to renal trauma. J Urol 126:101

Cass A, Luxenberg M et al. (1959) Long term results of conservative and surgical management of blunt renal lacerations. Br J Urol 59:17

Chaussy Ch, Schmiedt E, Jocham D, Fuchs G, Brendal W (1986) Extracorporeal shock wave lithotrips technical concept, experimental research, and clinical applications. Chaussy Ch (ed), Karger, Basel

David R, Fuchs G, Barbaric Z (1990) Comparison of bioeffects of open surgery, percutaneous surgery, and extracorporeal shock wave lithotripsy on renal function and morphology in the farm pig: creation of an animal model. J Endourol 4:27

Freed T, Tavel F (1976) Diagnosis and surgical treatment of Page kidney. Urol 7:330

Fuchs G, Miller K, Rassweiler J et al. (1985) Extracorporeal shock wave lithotripsy. Eur Urol 11:145

Fuchs A, Coulson W, Fuchs G (1988) Morphological effects of high energy shock waves on the rabbit kidney and ureter. J Endourol 2:341

Fuchs G, David R, Fuchs A, Chaussy Ch (1990) Complications of ESWL: detection, management and prevention. In: Ehrlich R, Smith R (eds) Complications in urologic surgery. Sanders, Philadelphia

Jameson R (1978) Transient hypertension associated with closed renal injury. Br J Urol 45:482

Knapp P, Kulb T, Lingeman J et al. (1988) Extracorporeal shock wave lithotripsy induced perirenal hematoma. J Urol 139:700

Knorring J v, Fyhrquist F, Ahonen J (1981) Varying causes of hypertension following renal trauma. J Urol 126:798

Lingeman J, Newman D, Mertz J et al. (1986) Extracorporeal shock wave lithotripsy. J Urol 135:1134

Lingeman J, Kulb T (1987) Hypertension following extracorporeal shock wave lithotripsy. J Urol 137:142A (abstract)

Lingeman J, McAteer J, Kempson S et al. (1988) Bioeffects of extracorporeal shock wave lithotripsy. Urol Clin North Am 15:507

Lingeman J, Woods J, Toth P (1990) Blood pressure changes following extracorporeal shock wave lithotripsy and other forms of treatment for nephrolithiasis. JAMA 263:1789

Page I (1939) The production of persistent hypertension by cellophane perinephritis. JAMA 113:2046

Peterson J, Finlayson B (1986) Effects of ESWL on blood pressure. In: Gravenstein J, Peter K (eds) Extracorporeal shock wave lithotripsy for renal stone disease. Butterworths, Stoneham, MA

Terris J, Martin T, Simmonds R (1985) Metabolism unit, confinement unit, and placement of indwelling catheters for use with swine. In: Tumbleson ME (ed) Swine in biomedical research. Plenum, New York, p 111

Tumbleson ME (ed) (1985) Swine in biomedical research. Plenum, New York

Williams C, Kaude J, Newman R et al. (1988) ESWL. AJR 150:311

The Value of Various In-Vitro Stone Models for Characterization of Different Shock Wave Sources

J. RASSWEILER[1], K. U. KÖHRMANN[1], E. MARLINGHAUS[2], St. FRÖHNER[1], M. RAAB[1], B. BERLE[1], and P. ALKEN[1]

Introduction

With the continuous development and introduction of new shock wave sources and modified shock wave generators, a simple and valid method for characterizing their efficacy in disintegrating stones becomes increasingly important. The main points here are

a) comparison of different shock wave sources and
b) evaluation of the efficacy of each particular generator.

Physical measurements are only of limited use for this purpose, as the various hydrophones are not standardized. Moreover, exactly which parameters describe the disintegrative efficacy of a shock wave source has not yet been completely defined (Coleman and Saunders 1990).

On the basis of our own previous studies (Rassweiler et al. 1990), we examined the newly developed electromagnetic lithotripter, Modulith (Storz-Medical), using three different in-vitro stone models. In addition, the electromagnetic shock wave source of the Lithostar (Siemens) was studied and previous results with different second generation lithotripters were noted. The main issues were:

1. How did the various stone models differ from one another?
2. What conclusions can be drawn from the different stone models
   a) in regard to the energy of the applied shock wave,
   b) in regard to the attenuation of shock wave energy by modification of the shock wave coupling, and
   c) in the comparison of different shock wave sources?
3. Can in-vitro stone models be utilized further?

Characteristics of the Shock Wave Generator

The shock wave source of the Modulith consists of an electromagnetic coil inducing repellment from a cylindrical membrane (Fig. 1). The radially propagating pressure waves are reflected and focussed by a metal paraboloid with an aperture of 40 cm, resulting in a bowl-shaped pressure wave with a pressure-free central ar-

[1] Urologische Klinik, Klinikum Mannheim der Universität Heidelberg, Theodor-Kutzer-Ufer, W-6800 Mannheim 1, FRG.
[2] Storz-Medical, Unterseestr. 80, 8280 Kreuzlingen, Switzerland.

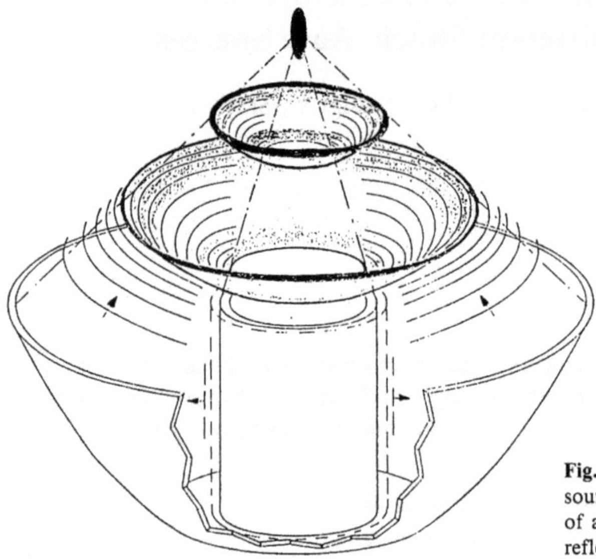

Fig. 1. Electromagnetic shock wave source of the Modulith, consisting of a cylinder and an parabolic reflector

ea converging towards the focal zone (28×6 mm at 15 kV). Shock wave coupling was by means of a waterbath in the laboratory lithotripter and by a water cushion in the clinical prototype.

The shock wave source of the Lithostar represents an electromagnetic element with a mental membrane inducing steepening of the shock wave front within a shock tube (aperture 12 cm). The shock waves are focussed by an acoustic lens (focal zone 95×10 mm) and coupled by means of a water cushion (Vergunst et al. 1989).

Physical Data

The acoustic data presented are based on our own assessment (E.M.), measurements published by Siemens physicists (Vergunst et al. 1990), and the comparative study by Coleman and Saunders (1989) (Table 1).

Table 1. Physical data of different shock wave sources (Coleman and Saunders 1989) compared to number of impulses required for complete disintegration of chalk cubes (model 3). Results at maximum energy setting

Lithotripter	Acoustic energy	Peak pressure	No. of shock waves
Storz Modulith	70 mJ	1300 bar	40 – 50
Dornier HM3	90 mJ	500 bar	80 – 100
Technomed Sonolith	30 mJ	780 bar	320 – 390
Siemens Lithostar	17 mJ	440 bar	420 – 470
Wolf Piezolith	8 mJ	1140 bar	830 – 850
Edap LT01	3 mJ	1050 bar	1500 – 3000

Modulith: The generator voltage ranges between 10 and 20 kV, resulting in peak pressures of 190–1200 bar (PVDF hydrophone, Imotec, Würselen).

Lithostar: The generator voltage can be set between 11 and 19 kV. However, data for pressure measurements exist only for 16.9–19 kV, ranging from 290 to 325 bar (PVDF hydrophone, Imotec, Würselen).

On reviewing the physical data assessed by Coleman and Saunders (1989, 1990), it must be noted that there is no correlation between the peak pressure and the amount of acoustic energy in each shock wave produced by the different lithotripters (Table 1).

In-Vitro Stone Models

Three different stone models were examined:

Model 1: Measurement of the cavity produced in a plaster cube (made of dental cement and provided by Dornier, Munich) after 100 shock waves. The results determined with the Modulith were compared to previous data relating to other lithotripters (Rassweiler et al. 1989).

Model 2: Calculation of the number of impulses necessary for disintegration of plaster balls (made of dental cement and provided by Storz-Medical, Kreuzlingen) in degassed water into fragments smaller than 2 mm which pass through a standard mesh.

Model 3: Calculation of the numbers of shock waves necessary for complete pulverization of chalk cubes (Drei Sterne-Kreide) in oil medium. The degree of pulverization was digitally controlled. This model was employed for the comparison of various coupling modalities and shock wave sources.

Results

Model 1: Table 2 summarizes the most important findings indicating the superior disintegrative efficacy of the Modulith compared to other lithotripters. However, this only applies to application of higher generator voltages: on the maximum setting (20 kV) only 50 shocks could be given because the plaster cube started to break. The significantly lower disintegrative efficacy of the piezoelectric systems must be noted.

Models 2 and 3: Plotting the applied shock wave numbers against generator voltage results in a characteristic curve for each stone model and each particular lithotripter (i.e., Modulith). The parallelism of the graphs of the two stone models demonstrates that these test models are equivalent (Fig. 2). Therefore, because of its simplicity and availability, model 3 was chosen for further comparative studies. Preliminary curve analysis has shown that both graphs represent a reciprocal qua-

Table 2. Model 1: volume of cavity produced after 100 impulses at minimum and maximum energy settings of each lithotripter tested

Lithotripter	Energy setting	Cavity (cm^3)	
		Minimum	Maximum
Storz Modulith	12–20 kV	10	450[a]
Dornier MPL 9000	14–24 kV	28	300
HM3+/HM4	16–28 kV	25	250
Technomed Sonolith	13–14 kV	120	135
Siemens Lithostar	12–19 kV	18	125
Wolf Piezolith	St. 3–4	13	85
Edap LT01	60–100%	13	23

[a] Only 50 impulses.

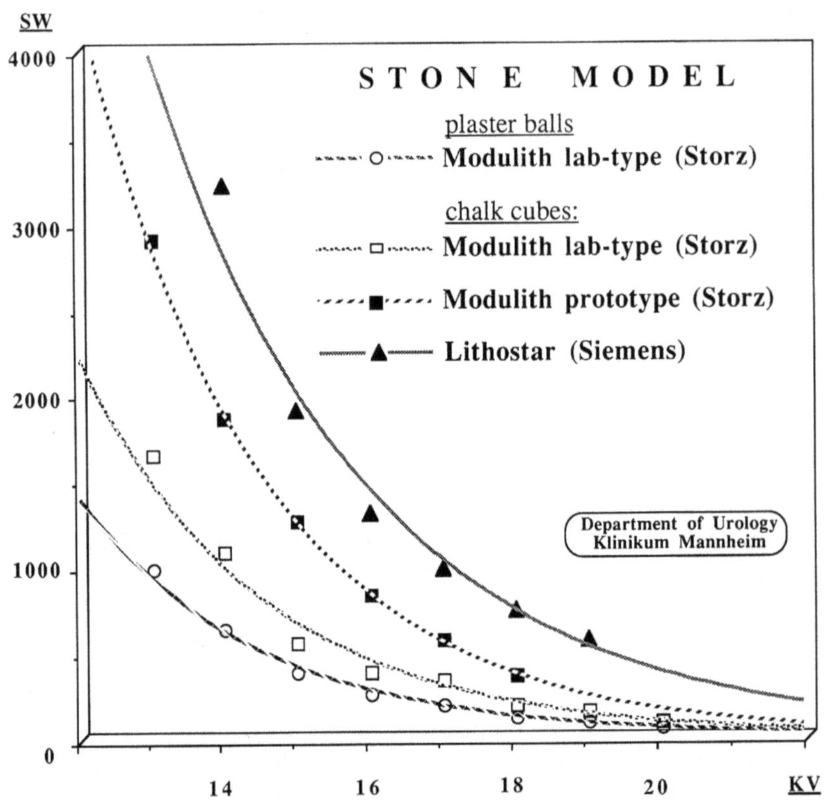

Fig. 2. Plotting of numbers of shock wave required for pulverization of plaster balls (model 2) and chalk cubes (model 3) against generator voltage, utilizing different shock wave sources and coupling modalities

dratic function of impulses versus generator voltage ($SW = a^{kV-2}$) analogous to the theoretically applied energy.

Model 3: Right deviation of the source-specific curve (i.e., Modulith prototype vs. laboratory lithotriptor) indicates the attenuation of the shock wave energy by changing the coupling modality (i.e., water cushion vs water bath): in our study a deviation of the prototype curve was found by about 2 kV (Fig. 2).

Left deviation of the curve demonstrates superior disintegrative capacity on examination of different shock wave sources. It should be noted that the values of generator voltage of the Modulith and Lithostar can only be taken as a scale for minimum to maximum shock wave pressure of each machine and not as absolute figures. According to our findings the disintegrative capacity of the Modulith is superior to that of the Lithostar on the basis of the energy setting of each lithotripter (Fig. 2).

Modified Model 1: To investigate the accuracy of the combined localization system of the Modulith, consisting of an integrated external C-arm and a coaxial ultrasound scanner, a modification of model 1 was used. A metal cross was placed on the plaster cube. The localization of the cavity produced after 50 shock waves (at 16 kV) showed a small deviation after primary installation of the fluoroscopic system which could be successfully corrected (Fig. 3).

Discussion

In addition to other technical details (e.g., localization system, handling of the lithotripter), the disintegrative efficacy is one of the main issues in comparison of new lithotripters. A well-defined standard of physical measurements using standardized hydrophones for classification of shock wave energy and efficacy should be aimed at, so that in-vitro studies or even animal experiments become practically unnecessary.

However, even nowadays, the exact influence of the various parameters of acoustic evaluation of shock waves (e.g., rise time, peak pressure, negative pressure, spectrum of frequencies) on the mechanism of stone disintegration and tissue traumatization is not completely understood (Coleman and Saunders 1989). Nevertheless, it could be demonstrated that the calculation of acoustic energy per impulse represents the disintegrative effect of the shock wave source better than the peak pressure (Table 1).

PVDF hydrophones have now attained a certain standard (Coleman and Saunders 1990; Vergunst et al. 1989; Eisenberger et al. 1990). They have replaced the PCB probes which proved to be ineffective; the calculated peak levels were too high owing to the inclusion of reflection (Rassweiler et al. 1988). However, Coleman and Saunders (1990) demonstrated that distinct differences may exist even between two PVDF hydrophones. Laser probes could solve these problems, but they are still at an early stage (Eisenmenger and Staudenraus 1988).

Utilization of standardized stone models is thus still of major importance. All three stone models used are easily reproduced and allow evaluation of the shock wave efficacy of various energy sources.

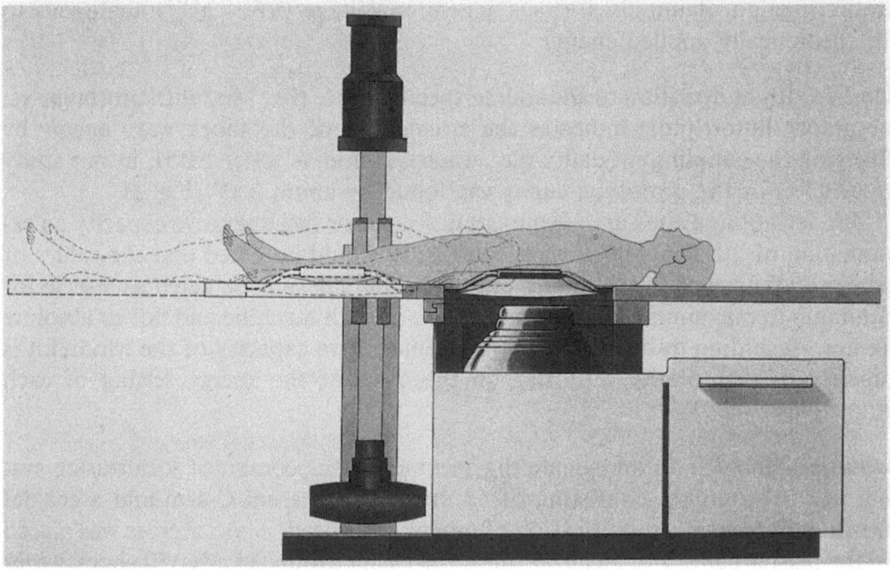

a

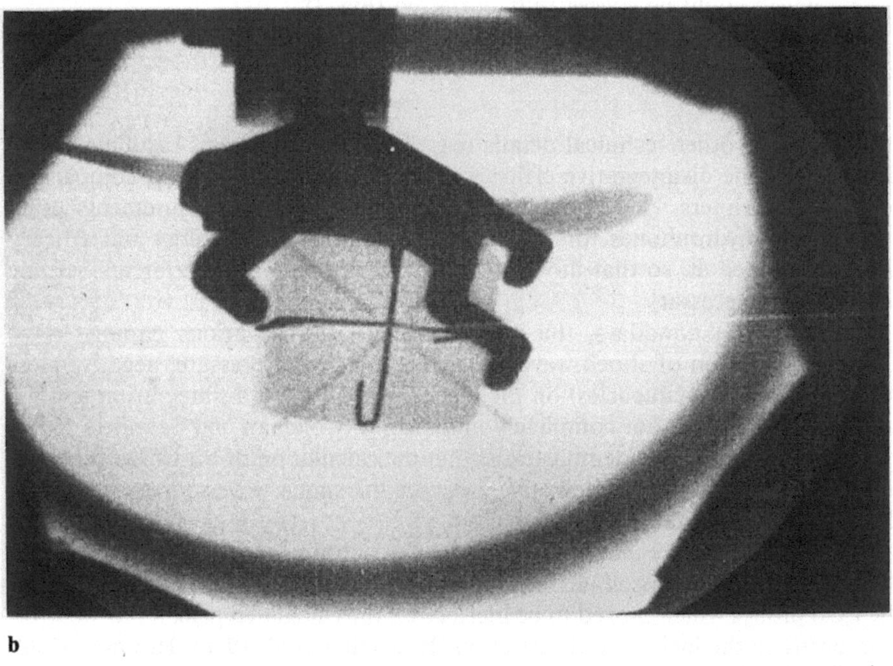

b

Fig. 3a–c. Use of modified model 1 for investigation of the accuracy of the combined localization systems of the Modulith. **a** Localization system of the Modulith SL 20, consisting of an integrated external fluoroscopic C-arm (with an isocenter = virtual focus) and a coaxial in-line ultrasound scanner; **b** A metal cross was placed on a plaster cube and it was focussed by use of the external C-arm. Thereafter, the fixed stone model was shifted back on the shock wave source and 50 impulses were applied at 16 kV; **c** After preliminary installation a slight deviation of the focal zone was observed (*left*), which was corrected by final adjustment (*right*)

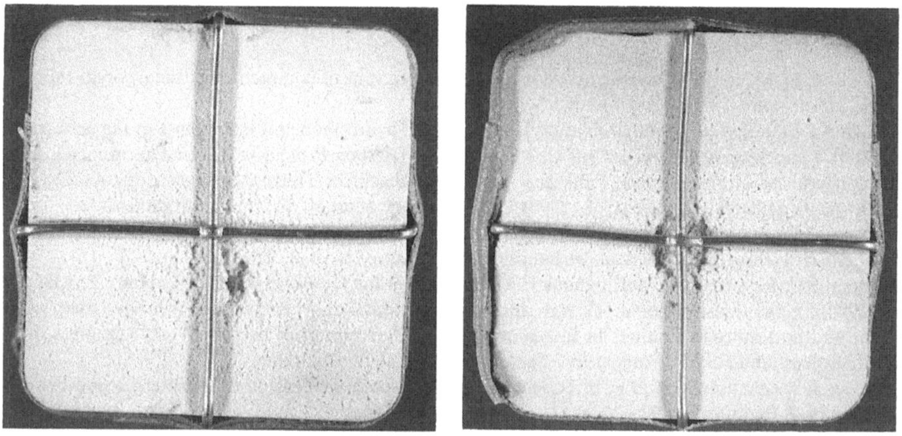

Fig. 3c

Model 1 proved to be particularly useful for rapid comparison of different shock wave sources. The cavity created illustrates the focal zone of the lithotripter and can thus be used, in a slightly modified version, for accurate real-time adjustment of the localization system (Fig. 3).

Models 2 and 3 both reveal a characteristic curve for each shock wave source with a reciprocal quadratic correlation between shock waves and generator voltage (Fig. 2). However, the two graphs cannot be compared directly, as there was a difference in the volume of the two models. However, since both curves displayed a similar correlation between impulses and voltage, we continued our studies with model 3 due to its simplicity. With this stone model a right curve deviation demonstrated the influence of shock wave attenuation by changing the coupling modality (water bath to cushion). Moreover, the disintegrative efficacy of different electromagnetic sources with similar shock wave coupling could be compared according to the energy output of each machine: left deviation indicates superior disintegrative capacity (Fig. 3).

Further improvement of stone models may lead to testing of stones of different geologically defined hardness, to evaluate the threshold of disintegrative capacity of each lithotripter (Hoffmann R. 1990, personal communication).

The correlation between in-vitro stone models and the renal trauma observed in animal models is of major interest. In preliminary studies, we compared the curve of model 3 to a graph plotting the number of sock waves required for induction of a grade 1 lesion (focal hemorrhage) in a canine kidney against the generator voltage applied. As observed in the in-vitro stone models, the threshold curve for a grade 1 lesion showed a reciprocal quadratic function analogous to the theoretically applied energy. Therefore, it may be possible to predict the renal trauma observed in the animal model using in-vitro stone models. However, further studies using different shock wave sources are necessary to determine the exact correlation factor between the two curves (Köhrmann et al. 1990).

References

Coleman AJ, Saunders JE (1989) A survey of the acoustic output of commercial extracorporeal shock wave lithotripters. Ultrasound Med Biol 15:213–227

Coleman AJ, Saunders JE (1990) A comparison of PVDF-hydrophone measurements in the acoustic field of a shock wave source. In: Ell C, Marberger M, Berlien P (eds) Extra- und Intrakorporale Lithotripsie bei Harn-, Gallen-, Pankreas- und Speichelsteinen. Thieme, Stuttgart, pp 14–22

Eisenberger F, Miller K, Rassweiler J (1990) Urologic stone therapy. Thieme, Stuttgart

Eisenmenger W, Staudenraus J (1988) Physikalisch-medizinische Aspekte selbstfokussierter elektromagnetisch erzeugter Stoßwellen. Verhandlungsber Dtsch Ges Urol 39:69–70

Köhrmann KU, Rassweiler J, Marlinghaus EH, Raab M, Fröner S, Berle B, Back W, Haux P, Alken P (1990) Energy threshold of shock wave-induced tissue damage – correlation of in vivo observations and post-mortem findings in the canine model. Proceedings of the 8th World Congress on Endourology and ESWL, August 29–September 2, 1990, Washington

Rassweiler J, Westhauser A, Bub P, Eisenberger F (1988) Second-generation lithotripters: a comparative study. J Endourol 2:193–203

Rassweiler J, Löbelenz M, Köhrmann U, Eisenberger F, Alken P (1990) In vitro comparison of second-generation lithotriptors using two stone models. In: Vahlensieck W, Gasser G, Hesse A, Schöneich G (eds) Proceedings of the 1st European Symposium on Urolithiasis, Bonn 1989. Excerpta Medica, Amsterdam, pp 133–136

Vergunst H, Terpstra OT, Schröder FH, Matura E (1989) Assessment of shock wave pressure profiles in vitro: clinical implications. J Lithotr Stone Dis 1:289–298

Evaluation of Ureteral Tissue Damage Caused by Laser-Induced Shock Waves: A Comparison of Laser Systems of Different Wavelengths

R. MUSCHTER [1], R. ENGELHARDT [2], R. BRINKMANN [2], M. SCHEU [2], P. RENNER [3], St. THOMAS [3], and G. BARETTON [4]

Introduction

Since patient positioning techniques have advanced and second- and third-generation lithotripters have been introduced, treatment of uretereal calculi by extracorporeal shock wave lithotripsy has become a more likely possibility. Although in certain cases relatively invasive endourological methods are still necessary, in most intracorporeal lithotripsy can be performed via ureteroscopy.

Laser lithotripsy, a method of intracorporeal fragmentation of urinary calculi by laser-induced shock waves, was developed to further reduce the invasiveness of endourological management of this condition (Hofstetter et al. 1985; Watson et al. 1987), e.g., the requirement of rigid ureteroscopes of large caliber in ultrasonic lithotripsy, or the potential hazards of energy sources used for intracorporeal stone disintegration, e.g., the high risk of ureteral perforation in electrohydraulic lithotripsy.

The real advantage of laser lithotripsy is the instrumentation used, which is of high flexibility and extremely small caliber, although it is dependent on combination with small-caliber ureteroscopes, which at first were unavailable, or must be used "blind" via stents, without a ureteroscope, under fluoroscopic guidance only. Especially with the latter method, but also when using a ureteroscope, it is possible for the distal end of the lithotripter to come into direct contact with the ureteral wall while the laser is on. In this case the laser-induced plasma and shock wave affect the tissue directly.

Since the introduction of laser lithotripsy the technique has advanced. Currently there are many different laser systems and application techniques with different physical and optical properties available for clinical and experimental use as well. To evaluate the type and quantity of effects of laser lithotripsy on tissue and their significance for clinical routine, it was necessary to compare all systems in one experimental set-up under standardized conditions.

[1] Urologische Klinik und Poliklinik der Universität, Klinikum Großhadern, Marchioninistr. 15, W-8000 München 70, FRG.
[2] Medizinisches Laser-Zentrum, Peter-Monnik-Weg 9, W-2400 Lübeck, FRG.
[3] Urologische Klinik; [4] Institut für Pathologie der Medizinischen Universität, Ratzeburger Allee 160, W-2400 Lübeck, FRG.

Material and Methods

All experiments were done in vivo under general anesthesia using young healthy female pigs of some 35 kg body weight. A total of 10 animals or 20 ureters were used in the study.

In 14 cases the retroperitoneal site was exposed by a subcostal incision. The preparation of the ureter was done without removing the adjacent tissue and blood supply. The ureter was incised longitudinally and held open by four sutures. All hemorrhages were coagulated. The site was kept completely covered by saline.

In a second series of 6 ureters a 9 F Wolf rigid ureteroscope was inserted into the ureter transurethrally via a 4 F ureteral catheter under visual and fluoroscopic guidance, using only a little irrigation and contrast medium. After removal of the ureteral catheter the laser fiber was inserted.

In both series the laser application instrument was abutted tangentially against the mucosa of the ureter. Using a repetition rate of 4 Hz, either 10 or 40 pulses at an energy of 45–50 mJ measured at the distal fiber tip were delivered to one precise point, representing the worst possible case where the laser was discharged accidentally while the fiber tip was touching the ureteral wall. A series of lesions were produced, starting proximally. The distance between any two lesions was 10 mm, to avoid confluence. There was continuous video recording to investigate the exact number of shock waves required until the first effect could be seen.

The histological appearance of the lesions was studied in HE-stained samples obtained from animals killed 1 h after the procedure and animals killed 3 weeks later (the latter relating to two ureters with lesions set by ureteroscopic access only).

Several different laser systems were employed.

The q-switched Nd:YAG laser (wavelength 1064 nm, pulse duration 12 ns) was used with two different application instruments, a 600-μm fiber with spherical polished tip and a 600-μm fiber with optomechanical ("slanted") coupler.

A flashlamp-pumped pulsed dye laser working with coumarin as active laser medium emitted light at a wavelength of 504 nm and a pulse duration of 2 μs. The application fiber had a core diameter of 200 μm.

A second type of flashlamp-pumped pulse dye laser used rhodamine 6G as active medium. The wavelength was 590 nm and the pulse duration 3 μs. The core diameter of the application fiber was 200 μm. This laser was used with and without the optional integrated stone detection and optical feedback system, which reduced the laser energy automatically to about 10% of the prechosen level in the case of "no-stone-contact", which meant in our series approximately 5 mJ while working properly.

The q-switched alexandrite laser (wavelength 755 nm) was used at a pulse duration of 250 ns, 750 ns and 1.5 μs. The application fiber had a core diameter of 200 μm in all cases.

Results

The effects of the laser energy delivered by all the systems investigated were nearly uniform in quality and quantity and occurred within the range of 1 – 12 pulses. The only exception was the dye laser with optical feedback system, where those effects were not seen until 35 pulses had been given to a single spot. The risk of causing damage rose with the number of laser pulses delivered, but in some cases severe damage could be observed after just one single pulse. This happened most often employing alexandrite laser at short pulse duration, especially in those cases where the analysis of the video recording showed plasma formation within the fiber. Once a lesion occurred, plasma and shock wave creation took place in each of the following pulses and the lesion increased in size and depth. Once a lesion was begun, the relationship between the number of pulses delivered and the extent of the effects was to some degree proportional when the Nd:YAG and dye lasers were used, the alexandrite laser had more of an all-or-nothing effect.

Histological examination showed thermal and mechanical tissue effects as well (Figs. 1 – 4). Thermal effects were frequent with both variants of the Nd:YAG laser system, but they were also observed with the dye and alexandrite laser systems.

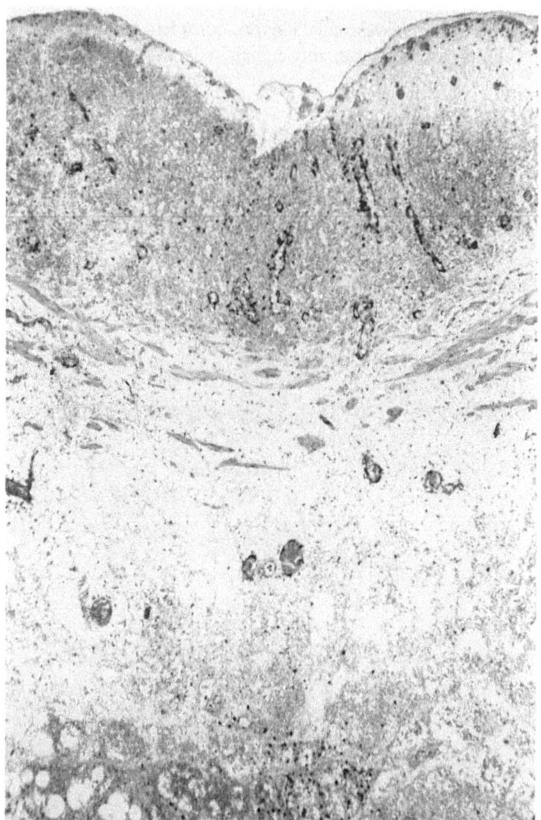

Fig. 1. Nd:YAG laser, spherical polished fiber tip: ablation of the urothelium, small coagulation zone in the stroma, exsudation and edema, bleeding throughout the wall. HE stain

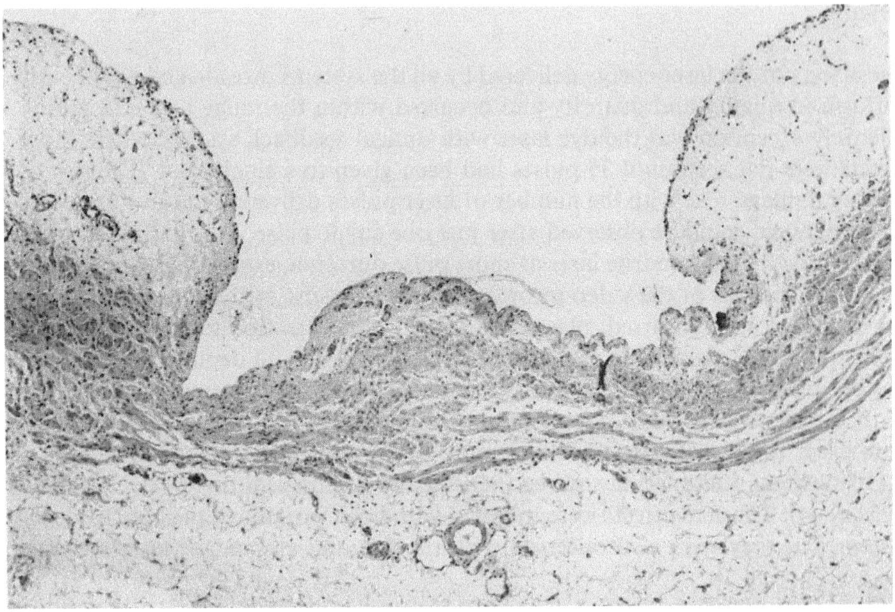

Fig. 2. Dye laser, wavelength 504 nm: complete ablation of the urothelium, small coagulation zone of the submucosa and inner muscularis, edema, bleeding throughout the wall. HE stain

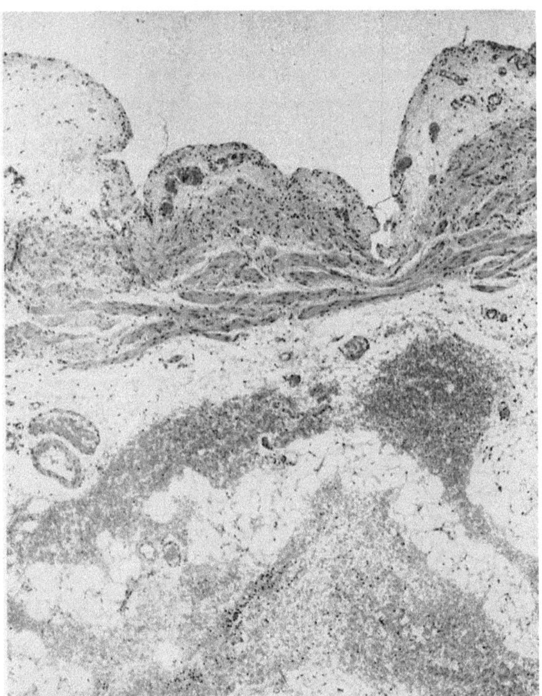

Fig. 3. Dye laser, wavelength 590 nm, without feedback system: complete ablation of the urothelium, edema, bleeding periureterally and throughout the wall. HE stain

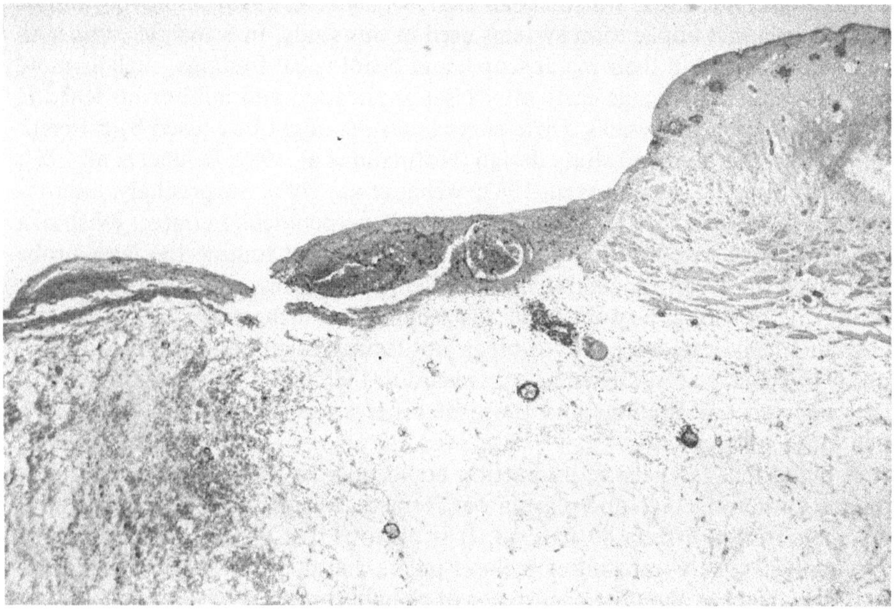

Fig. 4. Alexandrite laser, pulse duration 250 ns: complete perforation of the ureter and transmural defect, small coagulation zone at the edges, periureteral bleeding. HE stain

These effects were small coagulation zones in the submucosal stroma and the inner muscle layers (Figs. 1, 2). Mechanical effects were rupture and ablation of the mucosa and disintegration of deeper tissue layers such as submucosa, muscle, and even periureteral fat. Complete perforation of the ureter and a defect of the whole wall were also observed (Fig. 4). Bleeding and hematoma occurred in all parts of the wall of the ureter and in the adjacent periureteral tissue as well, mainly in the latter and the suburothelial stroma (Figs. 2, 3). Further effects were exsudation, edema, and scattered inflammatory cells.

The observed damages were relatively mild for the Nd:YAG laser with its different application systems (Fig. 1), medium for the dye lasers (Figs. 2, 3), and severe for the alexandrite laser, especially at short pulse duration (Fig. 4). Small pieces of glass identified as being parts of the application fiber were additionally found in the ureteral wall in this series.

The microscopical examination of the ureter 3 weeks later showed no evidence of scarring, but the reason for this might be that the spots treated could not be identified. Macroscopically neither strictures nor scars were found.

Discussion

The effects of laser-induced shock waves on the ureter have been investigated by several authors (Hofmann et al. 1987; Nishioka et al. 1988; Reichel et al. 1987;

Thomas et al. 1988, 1989; Watson et al. 1987; Weber et al. 1990) employing almost all of the laser and application systems used in this study. In principle, almost all investigators agreed in their macroscopic and histological findings, such as more or less severe tissue damage early after laser application and mild or no scarring and fibrosis after some weeks. Differences in results might be caused by different application techniques and study design (Hofmann et al. 1987; Reichel et al. 1987; Thomas et al. 1988; Watson et al. 1987; Weber et al. 1990). Surprisingly, laser-related injuries were less frequent and less severe in perpendicular contact (Nishioka et al. 1988) than in tangential contact. Since in clinical routine the laser probe might touch the ureter tangentially more often, experiments simulating the worst case in patients should be done using this technique. Furthermore, it is necessary, to use an energy level adequate to break up urinary calculi and not a too small number of shock waves. Differences in regard to the factors may explain discrepancies between our findings and those of other authors employing lasers at a much lower pulse energy.

The belief that laser-tissue interaction could only be harmful to the tissue if light absorption was high and plasma was formed (Watson et al. 1987) cannot explain the observed effects on its own. It is obvious that at least small amounts of thermal energy are transmitted by laser pulses that do not result in plasma creation. This might explain the occurrence of coagulation. In addition, these minor effects might change the tissue's absorptive capacity or blood content, so that plasma and shock wave formation took place with the next pulse. Furthermore, even in tissue with poor absorption of a certain wavelength, the "plasma threshold" could be reached at higher pulse energies, resulting in a laser-induced shock wave. This could be the explanation for the mechanical effects seen, such as ablation of the mucosa, disintegration and perforation of tissue, and hematoma.

In conclusion, therefore, laser lithotripsy performed in the ureter in clinical routine may possibly cause tissue damage. Even perforation may occur when pulses are delivered directly to the tissue while the fiber is in direct contact. The absorption of laser energy and the resulting creation of plasma and shock waves seems to depend not only on the laser wavelength and tissue color, but also on the pulse energy and other factors such as the degree of blood supply. The risk of severe effects which might force the urologist to stop the treatment before it was successfully finished increases with the number of laser pulses accidentally delivered to the ureter. Although all lesions seem to vanish with complete healing or little scarring, laser lithotripters should therefore not be used without constant visual monitoring or should be supplied with an automatic control and feedback system (Thomas et al. 1989).

References

Hofmann R, Hartung R, Geißdörfer K, Ascherl R, Erhardt W, Schmidt-Kloiber H, Reichel E (1987) Laser induced shock wave lithotripsy (LISL) – biologic effects and first clinical application. Laser 3:247–250

Hofstetter AG, Frank F, Keiditsch E, Wondrazek F (1985) Intracorporale, laserinduzierte Stoßwellen-Lithotripsie (ILISL). Laser 1:155–158

Nishioka NS, Kelsey PB, Kibbi AG, Delmonico F, Parrish JA, Anderson RR (1988) Laser lithotripsy: animal studies of safety and efficacy. Lasers Surg Med 8:357–362

Reichel E, Schmidt-Kloiber H, Schöffmann H, Dohr G, Eherer A (1987) Interaction of short laser pulses with biological structures. Optics Laser Technol 19:40–44

Thomas S, Pensel J, Engelhardt R, Meyer W, Hofstetter AG (1988) The pulsed dye laser versus the Q-switched Nd:YAG laser in laser-induced shock-wave lithotripsy. Lasers Surg Med 8:363–370

Thomas S, Engelhardt R, Meyer W, Pensel J (1989) Evaluation of optical feedback for preventing tissue damage in dye laser lithotripsy. In: Rübben H, Jocham D, Jacobi H (eds) Investigative urology, vol 3. Springer, Berlin Heidelberg New York Tokyo, pp 262–270

Watson G, Murray S, Dretler SP, Parrish JA (1987) An assessment of the pulsed dye laser for fragmenting calculi in the pig ureter. J Urol 138:199–202

Weber HM, Miller K, Rüschoff J, Gschwend J, Hautmann RE (1990) Experimentelle Ergebnisse und erste klinische Erfahrungen mit dem Alexandrit-Laserlithotripter. Urologe [A] 29:304–308

Zerbib M, Steg A, Moissonier P, Auvert V, Crespeau P, Cotard JP (1988) Effects of pulsed dye laser lithotripsy on tissues. Experimental study in the canine ureter. Urol Clin North Am 15:547–550

Stone Fragmentation Capacities of Different Lasers and EHL in Monohydrate, Cystine and Struvite Urinary Calculi

N. SCHMELLER [1]

Introduction

Laser lithotripsy of ureteral calculi is used in clinical practice with different laser systems. Not all calculi can be fragmented and different lasers have problems with different types of calculi due to the absorption and hardness of the stone. We therefore tested different lasers and electrohydraulic lithotripsy (EHL) on three urinary calculi to determine their fragmentation power on "problem stones".

Material and Methods

Three Calculi were Used

1. A large cystine staghorn stone, which was removed surgically.
2. A large complete staghorn stone consisting of pale struvite, excised in a specimen from nephrectomy for nonfunctioning kidney.
3. A large black stone with a smooth surface consisting of calcium oxalate monohydrate, which resisted fragmentation by sonotrode in percutaneous nephrolithotripsy, but had to be removed by EHL and forceps extraction.

Five Different Types of Lasers were Used

1. A flashlamp-pumped dye laser (Telemit) using rhodamine 6 G as dye, yielding a wavelength of 594 nm. The maximum head power is approximately 500 mJ. The maximum power output at the end of the quartz glass fibre with a core diameter of 200 µm is approximately 120 mJ and the maximum repeat frequency 10 Hz. For the in vitro experiments a power output of 100 mJ and maximum repeat frequency were chosen.
2. Two alexandrite lasers of different manufacturers (wavelength 755 nm). Fibres 200 µm in diameter were used with a power output of 70 mJ per pulse and repeat frequencies of 10 Hz (Dornier) and 6 Hz (MBB).
3. The same MBB alexandrite laser as in 2., but equipped with an optomechanical coupler which converts the laser energy into a shock-wave. This system consists

[1] Urologische Klinik und Poliklinik der Universität, Klinikum Großhadern, Marchioninistr. 15, W-8000 München 70, FRG.

of a small metal tip mounted onto the end of the quartz glass fibre (diameter 600 µm). The laser beam is directed onto an oblique metallic surface on which an optical breakdown is created at each laser pulse, resulting in a shock wave. This shock wave is emitted at right angles to the laser fibre. The coupler has a total diameter of 2 mm. Due to the larger fibre a power of 160 mJ per pulse could be used with a repeat frequency of 10 Hz.
4. The same optomechanical coupler as in 3., but driven by a neodymium: YAG laser (MBB, wavelength 1032 nm, 60 mJ per pulse, 10 Hz).
5. An excimer laser with a wavelength of 308 nm and maximum repeat frequency of 40 Hz (Technolas). A pulse power output of 18 mJ was used through a fibre of 600 µm core diameter.

All lasers were used at maximum repeat frequency and at the highest pulse power output that could be delivered through a flexible quartz glass fibre.

Lastly a normal *electrohydraulic lithotripsy unit* (Calcutript, Storz) was used with a newly developed 1.6-French probe at power settings 1 and 2 with a pulse frequency of 2 Hz.

The experiments were done in a bath of saline solution at room temperature. The calculi were first soaked for 10 min, then weighed with very sensitive electronic scales (±3 mg) after drying off with a paper towel. Laser or EHL treatment was done for exactly 1 min and residual calculi of more than 2 mm minimum diameter were dried and weighed thereafter. This treatment over 1 min was repeated twice and the average of stone material fragmented within this period was calculated as well as the average mass of stone material broken off per pulse.

Results

The stone mass broken off per minute or per pulse with different lasers and EHL is apparent from Figs. 1–3. To avoid advertising, the average of the two alexandrite lasers from different manufacturers was calculated (the difference was very small).

Discussion

It is obvious both from our results and from clinical practice that the *alexandrite laser* is significantly better for the fragmentation of monohydrate calculi, while calculi that are whitish or yellow in colour are difficult to treat with the alexandrite laser because of insufficient absorption of the laser radiation. The alexandrite laser does have some small action on cystine calculi.

The *dye laser* is preferable for treating light-coloured calculi and also works well in dihydrate stones, which are very common in clinical practice. It is available with an optical feed-back system which closes the shutter as soon as there is loss of contact with the stone. This system is very important as a protection device against ureteral laceration.

The *optoacoustic coupler* is very effective for light-coloured calculi and for cystine, if the shock wave is created by a powerful alexandrite laser. Unfortunately

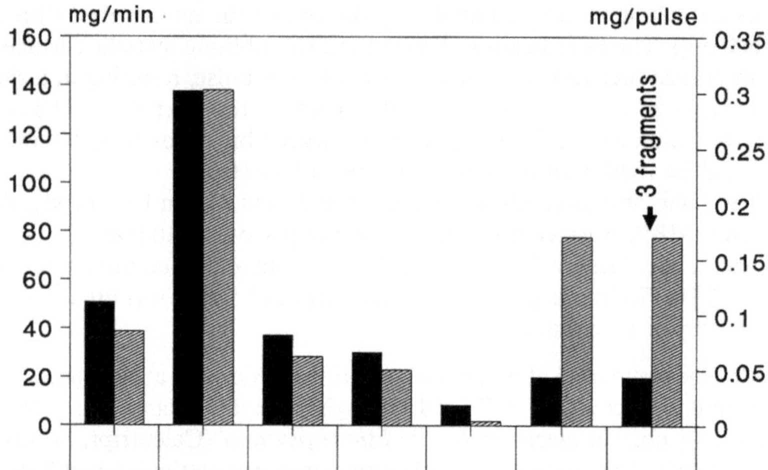

	Dye	Alexandrite	MBB Alex. coupler	Nd:YAG coupler	Excimer	EHL 1.6 Ch. Int.I	EHL 1.6 Charr. Int.II
mg/min	50.8	137.8	37	30	8.6	20	20
mg/pulse	0.085	0.302	0.062	0.05	0.004	0.17	0.17

Fig. 1. Calcium oxalate monohydrate fragmentation rates in vitro

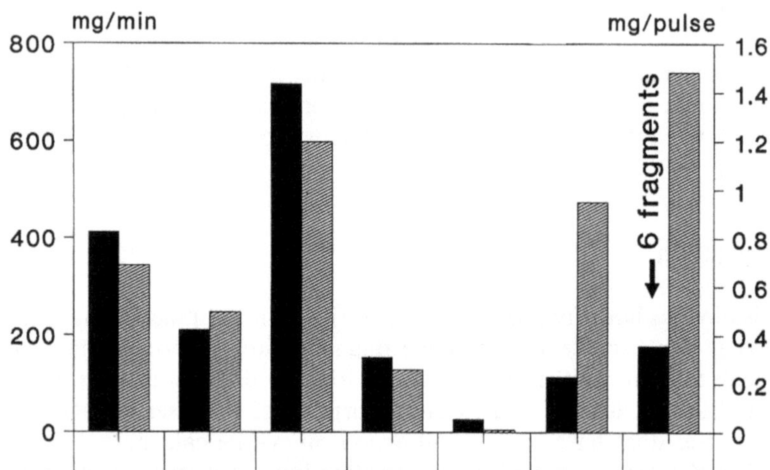

	dye	Alexandrite	MBB Alex. coupler	Nd:YAG coupler	Excimer	EHL 1.6 Ch. Int.I	EHL 1.6 Charr. Int.II
mg/min	412.4	210.3	718	154	26.9	114	178
mg/pulse	0.687	0.494	1.196	0.257	0.011	0.95	1.483

Fig. 2. Pale struvite fragmentation rate in vitro

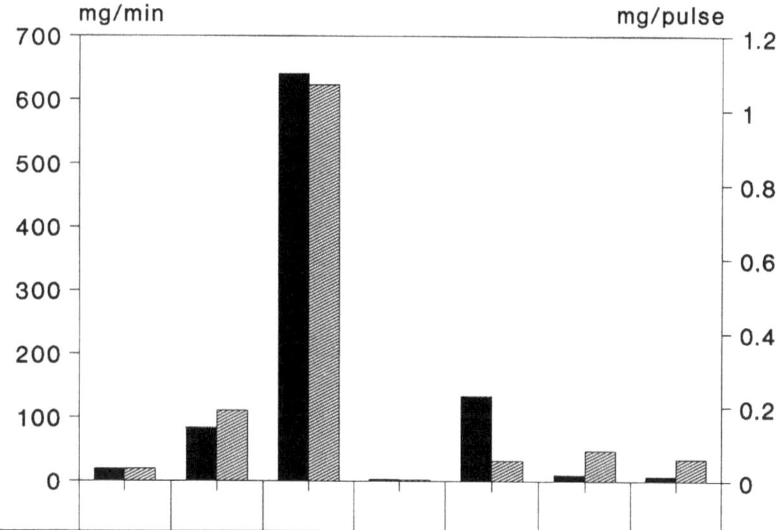

	Dye	Alexandrite	MBB Alex. coupler	Nd:YAG coupler	Excimer	EHL 1.6 Ch. Int.I	EHL 1.6 Charr. Int.II
mg/min	19.7	83.7	641	3	133.9	10	8
mg/pulse	0.033	0.19	1.068	0.005	0.056	0.083	0.06

Fig. 3. Cystine fragmentation rate in vitro

the coupler cannot be used through a small-caliber ureteroscope because of the 2-mm diameter. This is the greatest limitation of this device.

The *excimer laser* is of very limited use for stone fragmentation. It has some marginal action against cystine stones.

Electrohydraulic lithotripsy is now available with probes of less than 2 French. It can certainly effectively fragment most types of stones, including monohydrate. The effect in cystine is very limited, however. EHL usually breaks the stone up into several fragments which can be easily extracted, whereas laser lithotripsy leads to fine fragmentation into sand.

More studies are needed which would compare the potential for tissue laceration of EHL and the various lasers. Since both techniques are used in clinical practice, it seems necessary to compare them in a randomised fashion.

Experimental and First Clinical Results with the Alexandrite Laser Lithotripter

H. M. WEBER[1], K. MILLER[1], J. RÜSCHOFF[2], J. GSCHWEND[1], and R. E. HAUTMANN[1]

Introduction

Despite the ever increasing use of extracorporeal shock wave lithotripsy for the treatment of urolithiasis, there are still a limited number of stone patients who warrant a percutaneous or transurethral therapy. With the advent of flexible or semirigid ultrafine endoscopes, ultrasound lithotripsy with conventional sonotrodes is no longer possible, since they would require larger working channels. For this reason, laser lithotripsy has become increasingly important in endoscopic stone therapy (Drettler 1990). Since Nd : YAG and pulsed dye lasers that have been used so far each have their own disadvantages, there was a search for technical alternatives. The alexandrite laser being evaluated here represents a newly developed system for laser lithotripsy (Dornier Medizintechnik, Germering, FRG). The aim of this study was to evaluate the lithotriptic potential for different calculi as much as the biologic effects of this laser system. With the assumption that inadvertent exposure of the ureteric or bladder wall could not be entirely avoided, a worst case of laser radiation for an extended period of time had to be simulated.

Material and Methods

Laser System

The alexandrite laser is a flashlamp-pumped, solid-state laser whose active medium consists of an alexandrite monocrystal. With its Q-switch it generates highly energetic pulses with a pulse deviation between 150 and 800 ns. Pulse energy is set between 30 and 80 mJ but can theoretically be increased over 100 mJ. The wave length is 755 nm and the laser energy is delivered via flexible quartz fibers with a 200- and 300-μm core diameter respectively. The frequency is set at 1 and 10 Hz.

In Vitro Experiments

Preliminary information was gained with an experimental stone model that has been described previously (Hepp 1983). It consists of a plaster ball of 12 mm di-

[1] Urologische Universitätsklinik, Prittwitzstr. 43, W-7900 Ulm, FRG.
[2] Medizinisches Zentrum für Pathologie der Universität, Baldingerstraße, W-3550 Marburg, FRG.

Table 1. X-ray diffraction analysis of the calculi investigated

Whewellit I	Ca-Ox-1 H_2O 70% + calcium phosphate 30%
Whewellit II	Ca-Ox-1 H_2O 90% + calcium phosphate 10%
Whewellit III	Ca-Ox-1 H_2O 90% + calcium phosphate 10%
Whewellit IV	Ca-Ox-1 H_2O 100%
Cystine I	100%
Cystine II	100%
Phosphate I	Calcium phosphate 100%
Phosphate II	Calcium phosphate 80% + struvite 20%

ameter placed in a rigid net of 2-mm pore size. Plaster ball and net were then immersed in normal saline. Since fragments smaller than 2 mm would pass the ureter spontaneously, the time required to get the net "stone-free" was taken as a measure of the efficacy of the laser system. The time intervals were registered and stone and net were weighed at the same time. With the same setting, eight human calculi obtained during endoscopic or open surgery were then exposed to the alexandrite laser. All stones had been immersed in normal saline immediately after surgical removal. The size and weight of the different calculi were estimated at the beginning and at regular intervals during laser lithotripsy. The number of laser pulses and the energy required to break the stones were registered. The laser fiber with the 200-µm core diameter and a repetition frequency of 10 Hz was used routinely. Only if the lithotriptic results were insufficient was the 300-µm fiber employed and the system switched to a 1-Hz repetition rate. We investigated four calcium oxalate monohydrate, two cystine and two calcium phosphate stones. The average stone size was 13.6 (7.5 – 20) mm and all stones were derived from different patients. The stone analysis was performed after the lithotripsy study using X-ray diffraction (Table 1).

In Vivo Experiments

In 10 female pigs with an average age of 83.6 (69 – 97) days and an average weight of 21 (19 – 22.5) kg, bladder and/or ureteric wall were exposed to laser radiation after laparotomy under general anaesthesia. Laser exposure was performed with the 200-µm fiber within the bladder under cystoscopic guidance and within the ureter via a 5-F ureteric catheter in a retrograde or – after pyelotomy – in an orthograde fashion. Irrigation was performed with normal saline and in some animals the paraureteral space was also irrigated to simulate the normal retroperitoneal situation. Laser exposure was performed at 25, 40, 60 and 80 mJ with 1- and 10-Hz repetition rates and an average of 160 (1 – 1800) pulses. All laser exposure was undertaken with identical settings at two different locazations in the ureter and bladder. One group of those identical sets was removed intraoperatively to study early histological changes. At that stage the ipsilateral kidney was removed together with the upper half of the exposed ureter. In order to study the late histological changes, the second group of laser-exposed areas was left in situ for an average of 20.6 (5 – 35) days, until the animals were killed. All specimens were fixed in formalin, embedded in paraffin, cut, and stained with hematoxillin-eosin, trichrome (Masson/Goldner), or van Gieson's. During microscopy the pathological changes in the epithelium, submucosal layer, muscularis, and adventitia were assessed separately and classified into three different grades. Data analysis was computerized using a database program and plotted graphically with the help of a relative score. Because of the heterogeneity of the data in respect of localization, energy, and number of pulses, and because of the almost complete absence of late changes, no formal statistical analysis was performed.

Clinical Trial

In a preliminary series, 8 out of 12 patients were treated with the alexandrite laser lithotripter during ureteroscopy. In 4 patients the ureteral stone could not be reached with the ureteroscope or was inadvertently flushed back into the renal pelvis. All patients were treated via retrograde ureteroscopy with different instruments (Table 2). The patients (7 male and 1 female) had an average age of 55 (39–66) years. To assess possible laser-related damage, 4 (3–6) months postoperatively ultrasonography of the ipsilateral kidney was performed, and an additional intravenous pyelogram in 3 patients.

Table 2. Ureteroscopes used

	n
12.5F rigid (Wolf)	3
9.5F rigid (Wolf)	3
8.5F flexible (ACMI)	1
6F semirigid (Wolf)	1
Total	8

Results

In Vitro Experiments

Laser fragmentation of the plaster ball with the alexandrite laser was comparable to that obtained with the reference Nd:YAG system (Fig. 1). All stones investigated could be fragmented without any difficulty expect for one monohydrate stone (whewellit III). The average time required was 6.5 (5–11) min, with an average fragmentation rate of 2.1 (1.33–3) mm^3/min. The average energy was 50 (35–60) mJ. There was no consistent correlation between higher energy levels and pulse rates on the one hand and stone composition on the other. The stone that required the lowest energy (35 mJ and 1.33 mm^3/min) consisted of 100% calcium oxalate monohydrate. Even cystine stones did not cause any problems; their fragmentation rates were 1.8 and 2 mm^3/min with 55 and 65 mJ respectively. The on-

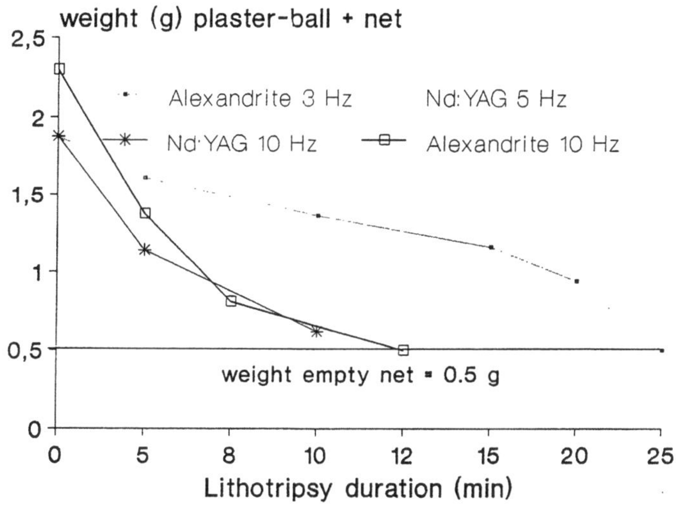

Fig. 1. Laser exposure in the stone model

ly laser-resistent stone consisted of 90% monohydrate and 10% calcium phosphate, was of very dark appearance, and had an extremely smooth surface. In this stone two ESWL treatments had been unsuccessful before ureteroscopic removal. Generally, stones with an irregular surface seem to respond better to laser lithotripsy than those with a smooth appearance.

In Vivo Experiments

Wherever a plasma formation occurred intraoperatively in the animal studies, a more or less pronounced hematoma could be observed in the bladder or ureter wall. The frequency of plasma formation was related to the amount of energy applied and the number of shockwaves. There was no correlation between the frequency and the amount of intramural hematoma and the angle between the fiber tip and the ureter wall. As to the filling of the retroperitoneum with normal saline, no differences were observed. Perforations of the bladder or ureter wall were repeatedly observed in connection with the abovementioned hematoma and plasma formations. It was, however, necessary to press the laser fiber against the organ wall to create such a perforation.

The histological slides showed, in addition to the expected hematoma-edema, capillary dilatation and ureteral abrasion due to the mechanical manipulation. Most of the slides showed mild to moderate changes; severe changes were rare overall.

In the secondary specimens practically no macroscopic changes could be shown. Even calibration and spatulation of the ureters showed no stricture formation where manipulation and laser exposure had been performed. Histologically, no pathological changes could be demonstrated in the epithelium. Scattered

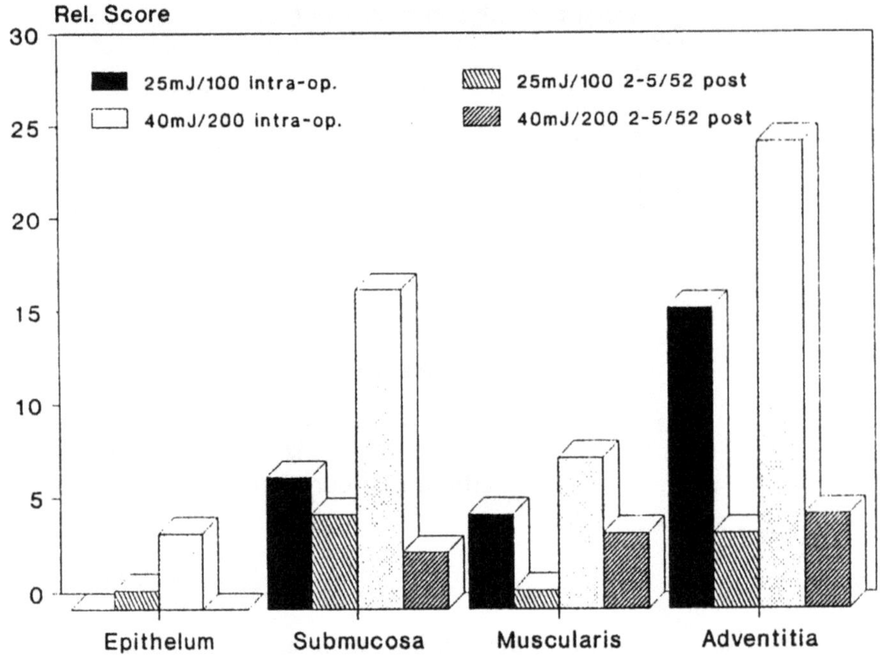

Fig. 2. Relative distribution of histological changes with different laser energy and at different time intervals

hemosiderin-deposits and vascular proliferation could be seen in the submucosa, muscularis, and adventitia, as an expected sign of normal tissue repair after the earlier trauma (Fig. 2). The longer the interval between laser exposure and removal of the secondary specimens, the less change could be found. After 30 days no changes whatsoever could be demonstrated histologically. Only one animal produced, in all specimens from bladder and ureter wall, a mild degree of fibrosis that did not lead to formation of stricture in the ureter.

Lost fiber tips due to technical problems with the quartz fiber at the beginning of the experiments led to foreign-body granulomas around the double refracting material. These were no longer seen after the breaking of fiber tips had been avoided in a technical modification.

Clinical Trial

All eight accessible stones were disintegrated without any difficulty. The average energy used was 37 (32–45) mJ, with 10 Hz and with 2047 (675–4326) pulses. Some stone fragments were extracted and others left in situ for spontaneous discharge. In four patients a double-J stent was placed that could be removed after the patients were completely stone-free. Sonographic and radiological follow-up did not reveal any ureteral stricture formation or secondary hydronephrosis.

Discussion

Extracorporeal shockwave lithotripsy is presently the standard therapy for urolithiasis of the kidney and the ureter. However, indications do still exist for percutaneous or transurethral techniques. With the increasing distribution of purely ultrasound-equipped lithotripters, these techniques may even increase in importance in the future. Endoscopic treatment via a small-sized fiber-endoscope has the advantage over the usual "push and smash" method that it is a monotherapy that can even be performed under analgosedation. So far, 15%–20% of ESWL-resistent ureteral stones have been treated ureteroscopically (Miller et al. 1989). The use of small-size fiber-endoscopes of 6–7 F permits only the use of small probes. The classical method of ultrasound lithotripsy therefore cannot be used with the currently available probes. During the last 3 years laser lithotripsy has been used in a few centers for this indication (Drettler 1990; Schmeller et al. 1987). Previously, the physical basics of laser lithotripsy had been investigated (Fair 1978; Reichel et al. 1983) and both the potential for lithotripsy and the biological side effects had been studied for the Nd: YAG and the pulsed dye laser (Hofmann et al. 1988; Watson et al. 1983, 1987). Because of their extremely short pulse duration of a few nanoseconds, and the resulting high energy density, most Nd: YAG lasers are dependent on relatively large-sized fibers of 600 µm; smaller fibers would be destroyed at this high density of energy. Moreover, a special coupling device or special treatment of the fiber tip is necessary to deliver the laser energy onto the stone. While the coupling device contributes further to an increase in fiber diameter, the treatment of the fiber tip decreases the life span of the fiber. The relatively large diameter makes the employment of this system via small, rigid fiberscopes with a narrow working channel impossible, while a 600-µm fiber would break in a flexible instrument once it is bent more than 90°. The pulsed dye laser, on the other hand, delivers its energy for endoscopic lithotripsy via an extremely flexible 200-µm fiber that does not have to be specially treated beforehand. A major drawback of this system, however, is its relatively high cost and the necessity of regular changes of the toxic cumarin laser dye.

These problems have led to the development of a new lithotripsy laser that should combine the advantages of a low-maintenance, low-priced solid state laser with the possibility of using very small-diameter fibers. The alexandrite laser evaluated here is an easy-to-use solid state system. Its lithotriptic potential and the effects on biological tissue were investigated with respect to the already existing systems. While the destruction of cystine stones seems to be problematic with the dye laser (Hofstetter et al. 1989), as does the fragmentation of oxalate monohydrate stones with the Nd: YAG laser (Hofmann et al. 1988), with the alexandrite laser only one monohydrate stone out of the eight investigated failed to be destroyed. The two cystine stones investigated did not present any problem for the alexandrite lithotripter; lithotripsy results for cystine stones with the Nd: YAG laser have not yet been reported.

Hoffmann et al. (1988) demonstrated only very superficial lesions in the ureter of the experimental animals exposed to the pulsed Nd: YAG laser. These experiments, however, were not performed under endoscopic conditions but in the open pig ureter. Watson et al. (1987), in their extensive experimental work, demonstrated pronounced early inflammatory reactions that agree well with the alexandrite laser data. They also were able to create perforations with the 200-µm fiber with laser exposure when the tip was pressed against the ureteral wall. The difference in intensity of primary trauma between Nd:YAG laser on the one hand and pulsed dye laser and alexandrite laser on the other might be related to the difference in pulse deviation, the smaller fiber diameter, or the shorter wavelength of pulsed dye and alexandrite laser, or could be seen in connection with the experimental set-up. Late changes could not be demonstrated for any of the systems with the maximum follow-up of 12 days for the Nd:YAG and about 4 weeks for the pulsed dye and alexandrite lasers. The results of Watson et al. show clearly that the most significant trauma for the ureter is caused by ureteroscopy with rigid, large-diameter endoscopes. This emphasizes further the necessity for the use of "miniscopes" in conjunction with very fine laser fibers of 200- to 300-µm core diameter.

In eight patients that have been treated with the alexandrite laser for ureteral stones, no adverse effects were observable at 4-month follow-up. Under therapeutic conditions no pronounced hematoma of the ureteral wall and no perforations occurred, since direct exposure of the ureteral wall to the laser beam could be avoided under endoscopic control. Similarly positive results have been reported by Schmeller et al. (1987) for the Nd:YAG and by Drettler (1990) for the pulsed dye laser in 225 patients.

Radiologically guided laser lithotripsy could represent an alternative to endoscopic treatment. In this technique, the laser fiber is brought through a ureteral catheter to the stone under X-ray guidance. To avoid inadvertent exposure of the ureteral wall, the laser system must have a feedback mechanism that interrupts the laser pulse whenever the fiber looses its contact with the stone. This principle has already been incorporated in one commercially available pulsed dye laser (Muschter et al. 1990). The concept has the disadvantage of increasing X-ray exposure and inadequate intraoperative monitoring of treatment results, especially in stones that are only slightly radiopaque or even radiolucent.

Finally, laser lithotripsy faces great competition from electrohydraulic lithotripsy, which can now be performed with probes of less than 2 F and from an alternative mechanical lithotripsy device, that is much cheaper than any laser lithotripter (Bhatta et al. 1989; Languetin et al. 1990). If Watson et al. (1987) are right in their assumption that not the lithotriptic technique is the crucial factor for ureteral trauma, but the diameter of the ureteroscope itself, these competing modalities will quickly gain ground against laser lithotripsy. Meanwhile, however, the alexandrite laser can, in regard to the experimental and first clinical results, be considered equivalent to the existing systems; in regard to its combination of their specific advantages, it may even be superior.

References

Bhatta KM, Rosen DI, Drettler SP (1989) Plasma shield lasertripsy: in vitro studies. J Urol 142:1110–1112

Drettler SP (1990) An evaluation of ureteral laser lithotripsy: 225 consecutive patients. J Urol 143:267–272
Fair HD (1978) In vitro destruction of urinary calculi by laser-induced stress waves. Med Instrum 12:100–105
Hepp W (1983) Zertrümmerungswirkung von Stoßwellen auf Nieren- und Gallensteine. Biomed Technik, Bd 33, Ergänzungsband 2, Stuttgart, S 15–16
Hofmann R, Hartung R, Geissdörfer K, Ascherl R, Erhardt W, Schmidt-Kloiber H, Reichel E (1988) Laser induced shock wave lithotripsy – biologic effects of nanosecond pulses. J Urol 139:1077–1079
Hofstetter AG, Thomas St (1989) Intrakorporale, laserinduzierte Stoßwellenapplikation zur Zerstörung von Harnsteinen, Urologe [A] 28:145–147
Languetin JM, Jichlinski P, Favre R, Niederhäusern W v (1990) The Swiss lithoclast. J Urol [Suppl] 143:179 A
Miller K, Bachor R, Sauter T, Hautmann R (1989) Aktuelle Therapie des Harnleitersteins. Urologe [A] 28:148–151
Muschter R, Thomas S, Knipper A, Maghraby H (1990) Intrakorporale laserinduzierte Lithotripsie. In: Ell C, Marberger M, Berlien P (eds) Extra- und Intrakorporale Lithotripsie. Thieme, Stuttgart
Reichel E, Schmidt-Kloiber H (1983) Die Anwendung laserinduzierter Stoßwellen am Beispiel der Zerstörung von Harnwegskonkrementen. Med Phys 197–201
Schmeller N, Hofstetter AG, Pensel J, Thomas S, Frank F, Wondrazek F (1987) Laserinduzierte Stoßwellenlithotripsie (LISL). Laser Med Surg 3:184–193
Watson G, Murray S, Drettler SP, Parrish JA (1987) An assessment of the pulsed dye laser for fragmenting calculi in the pig ureter. J Urol 138:199–202
Watson GM, Wickham JEA, Mills TN, Brown SG, Swain P, Salmon PR (1983) Laser fragmentation of renal calculi. Br J Urol 55:613–616

Effects of Extracorporeal Shock Wave Lithotripsy on the Female Reproduction Tract

F. RECKER[1], P. JAEGER[1], P. DIENER[2], and H. KNOENAGEL[1]

Introduction

The treatment of kidney stones with ESWL was at first directed at concretions in the upper urinary tract. Now, however, its use has been successfully extended to include the area of the distal ureter (Miller et al. 1986; McCullough et al. 1986). It has been established both clinically and experimentally that ESWL can be followed by renal parenchymal damage such as intra- or perirenal hematomas (Kaude et al. 1985; Jaeger et al. 1988; Recker et al. 1989). Short-term hematuria can be seen in all patients. The question whether ESWL in the small pelvis also leads to traumatisation of the female adnexae is of particular importance to female patients. In animal experiments we aimed to establish the short- and the long-term effect of shock waves on the morphology of the ovary, both by conventional light microscopy and by scanning electron microscopy (SEM).

Materials and Methods

Twenty-eight Siv Zur rats with body weights ranging from 200 to 250 g were treated with the modified Dornier HM3 system (SG40, E. 1.68), receiving either 600 or 1200 single shock waves with a generator voltage of 16 kV. The kidneys were located by pyelography (0.2 – 0.3 ml 30% Solutrast) under nembutal anaesthesia. The shock wave treatment was focused (focal point F2) on the right side, between the lower renal pole and the small pelvis. The thoracic region was protected by an aluminium sleeve. After 24 h or 35 days respectively, the animals were killed and the female reproduction tract examined by light microscopy and SEM. Four Wistar rats were killed as control animals, undergoing the same treatment as above, but without the shock wave therapy.

Results

Light Microscopy

Of the animals killed 24 h after ESWL, only one in seven showed minimal subcapsular hematoma, regardless of the number of shock waves received (Fig. 1, Table 2).

[1] Urologische Klinik des Universitätsspitals Zürich.
[2] Abt. für Pathologie des Universitätsspitals Zürich, 8000 Zürich, Switzerland.

Table 1. Numbers of healthy and atresic follicles per ovary

	600 SW		1200 SW		Control	
	24 h	35 days	24 h	35 days	24 h	35 days
Healthy	5.9	6.5	7.4	6.0	5.1	7.9
Atresic	12.4	15.8	17.5	13.0	17.1	14.2

SW, Shock waves.

The volume was smaller than the size of a corpus rubrum. No vasodilation occurred, neither arterial nor venous. In the 35-day group no histological changes in the ovary were seen in comparison with the control animals. The proportion of healthy to atresic follicles in each ovary, as a measure of possible damage after ESWL, is shown in Table 1. There was no difference between animals treated with shock waves and animals not treated, either immediately or 35 days later. The morphological examinations of the uteri bicorni in all six groups produced no remarkable findings.

Scanning Electron Microscopy

Immediately after ESWL, detachment of polygonal epithelial cells from the surface occurred, as did loss of cellular microvilli (Table 2, Fig. 1). In the 24-h groups

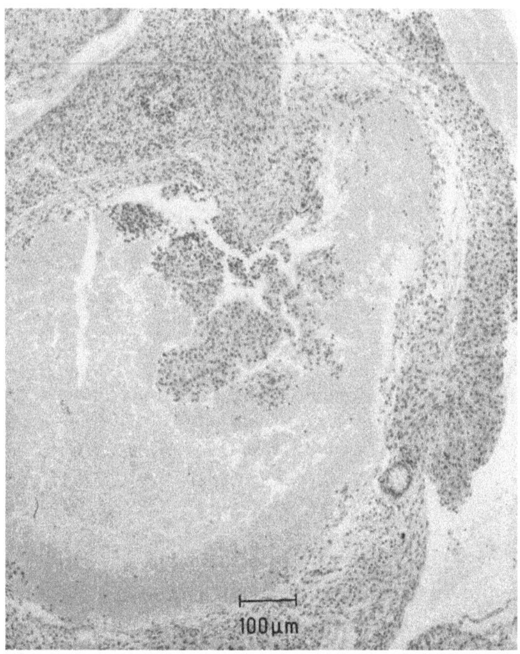

Fig. 1. Histology showed 24 h after ESWL a minimal subcapsular hematoma

Table 2. Histological changes in the ovary after ESWL

	600 SW		1200 SW		Control	
	24 h	35 days	24 h	35 days	24 h	35 days
Subcaps. bleeding	1/7	0	1/7	0	0	0
Venous dilation	0	0	0	0	0	0
Arterial lesions	0	0	0	0	0	0

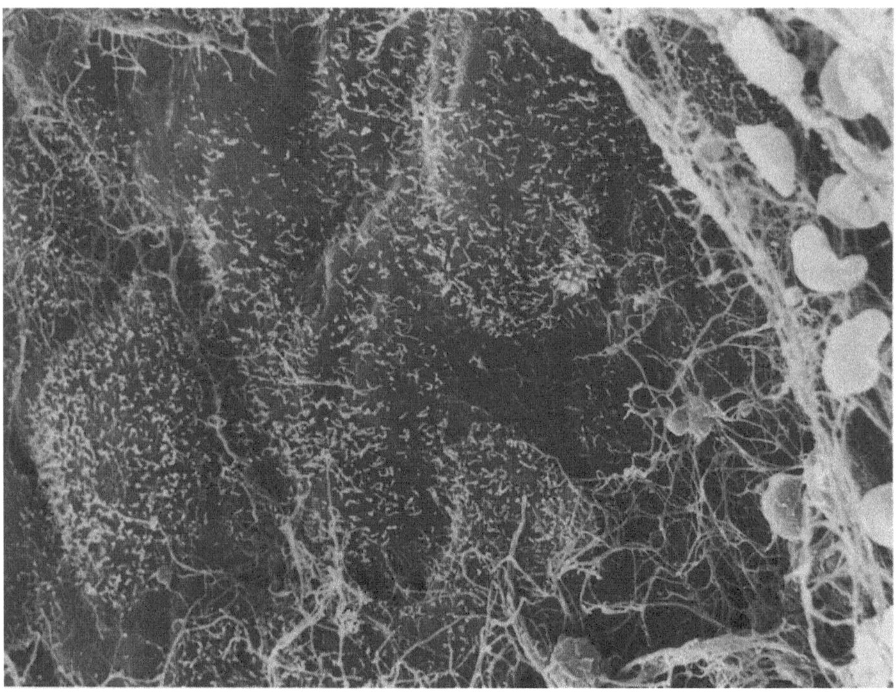

Fig. 2. Scanning electron microscopy (2600×) of polygonal epithelial cells from the ovary surface. At the right side fibrionous layers demonstrated minimal bleeding

isolated fibrinous layers on the ovary surface showed slight evidence of lesions (Fig. 2). The uterus area showed slight detachment of cells, loss of microvilli, and blebs immediately after treatment with 600 and 1200 shock waves. These changes did not occur in the 35-day groups.

Discussion

Traumatisation of the uterus and ovary by ESWL was found only immediately after treatment. The minor subcapsular bleeding registered in two cases was the only histological change. No changes were seen in the 35-day groups; more precisely, the proportion of normal to atresic follicles did not change. SEM showed only lesions in the ovarian epithelium and a detachment of the uterine mucus, both of which were fully restored after 35 days. The 16 kV used in the animal experiment is lower than the 18–23 kV used in clinics; however, the effective pressure of 680 bar is within an equivalent range.

Compared to relevant experimental results on the extent of kidney traumatisation after ESWL, the lesions reported here in the female reproductive tract are infinitesimal (Recker et al. 1988). This is partly due to the higher vulnerability of the renal vascular walls. Thus, the rupture of the thin-walled venae arcutae in the kidney (water reabsorption) and the exposure to the shock waves throughout their circular path parallel to the renal outline are the main causes of renal hematomas. Vulnerability seems to be a questions of vessel architecture. There is no morphological or functional equivalent in the ovary. It further remains to be discussed whether eruption of cavitation blisters as a cause of the lesions in the ovary and uterus is smaller, partly because of lack of a difference in acoustic impedance compared to the differences between cortex and medulla of the kidney.

Clinically it is of interest that in animal experiments ESWL did not cause traumatisation of the ovary or uterus that would lead to distinct morphological changes in the small pelvis. In particular, no long-term damage occurred. A teratogenic effect of ESWL cannot ruled out on the basis of this type of experiment, but to date no evidence to the contrary exists, despite the large number of cellular in vitro experiments performed in relation to ESWL. Certainly shock wave treatment should not be given during pregnancy.

References

Miller K, Bubeck JR, Hautmann R (1986) Extracorporeal shock wave lithotripsy of distal ureteral calculi. Eur Urol 12:305

McCullough DL (1986) Report of the American Urological Association Ad Hoc Committee to study the safety and efficacy of current technology of percutaneous lithotripsy and non invasive lithotripsy. May 22, 1986

Jaeger P, Redha F, Uhlschmid G, Hauri D (1988) Urol Res 16:161

Kaude J, Williams C, Millner MR (1985) Renal morphology and function immediately after ESWL. AJR 145:305

Recker F, Rübben H, Bex A, Constantinides C (1989) Morphological changes following ESWL in the rat kidney. Urol Res 17:229

Recker F, Hofstädter F, Daus HJ, Rübben H, Lutzeyer W (1988) Morphological pathomechanism following extracorporeal shock wave lithotripsy. In: Lingeman JE (ed) Shock wave lithotripsy: state of the art. Plenum, New York

Antitumor Effects of High-Energy Shock Waves are Potentiated by Doxorubicin and Biological Response Modifiers

G. A. H. J. SMITS, G. O. N. OOSTERHOF, A. E. DE RUYTER, J. A. SCHALKEN, and F. M. J. DEBRUYNE[1]

Introduction

High-energy shock waves (HESW) can alter the growth characteristics of tumor cells in vitro, depending on the experimental set-up (Brümmer et al. 1989). Furthermore, treatment with HESW can provoke suppression of tumor growth in vivo (Holmes et al. 1990; Randazzo et al. 1988; Russo et al. 1985, 1986). Our own experiments with several tumor model systems have confirmed this observation. The in vivo antitumor effect of HESW depends on the number of shock waves, the number of shock wave sessions, the initial tumor burden, and the tumor model used (Oosterhof et al. 1990). The observed tumor growth suppression in vivo is temporary and results rather in an elongated lag phase than in a permanent effect. This indicates that HESW treatment is not likely to be useful as monotherapy, and in order to obtain a longer and more definite suppression of tumor growth HESW should be combined with other treatment modalities. We therefore decided to treat the xenograft tumors with additional therapies which are known to be suboptimal. In this study we tested established tumors, known to be partially or completely insensitive to monotherapies (Beniers et al. 1988), with a combination of HEWS and either the chemotherapeutic drug doxorubicin or biological response modifier (BRM) therapy with TNFα/IFNα.

Materials and Methods

Animals

Xenografts were transplanted in 6- to 8-week old male Balb C nu/nu mice (Bornholt Gårt, Rye, Denmark). The mice were kept in groups of five in PAG type 2 cages (IFFA Credo) covered with an isocap for sterile conditions. The mice were fed ad libitum with irradiated (0.9 MR) SRM-A MM food (Hope Farms, Woerden, The Netherlands) and drinking water was acidified with 0.7 ml concentrated HCl/ml.

[1] Department of Urology, University Hospital, Geert Grooteplein Zuid 16, 6500 HB Nijmegen, The Netherlands.

Tumors

Human renal cell carcinoma NU-1 and NU-3 xenografts were used. These tumors were established in our laboratory by serial subcutaneous transplantation of tumor pieces after original subcutaneous transplantation of small primary tumor pieces directly after nephrectomy. The tumors were transplanted subcutaneously as trocar pieces in the hind limb of the animals, under ether anesthesia. The NU-1 renal adenocarcinoma is well vascularized and grows with a doubling time of 3–4 days. Histologically the tumor is characterized as sarcomatous and shows spontaneous hemorrhagic necrosis. The NU-3 has the same doubling time and consists of spindle cells of different sizes in a trabecular and acinar pattern and shows ischemic and hemorrhagic necrosis.

HESW Treatment

The shock waves were generated electromagnetcially by a commerically available lithotriptor (Lithostar Siemens) used clinically in the treatment of urolithiasis. The experimental set-up and way of administration of the shock waves have been described earlier in detail (Oosterhof et al. 1989). In brief, the shock wave tube of the lithotriptor was in contact with a water-filled plexiglass container via a silicon membrane in its lateral side. Optimal contact was ensured by a gel placket and lubricating gel. The characteristics of the shock waves and the focal area [area delimited by pressures which are half of the maximum pressure ($P_{max,50}$)] in our experimental set-up were determined, at an 18.4 kV energy level, as used in all experiments, with a polyvinylidene difluoride (PVDF) needle hydrophone (Imotect) connected with an oscilloscope (Gould, DSO, 4072). This needle transducer has a broad spectrum and an effective area of 0.5 m^2 with a constant sensitivity of up to 5 MHz. Measurements are possible up to the focal point with a measuring range from 0 to 200 MPa. The focal area is 6 mm in the lateral plane and approximately 8 cm in the transverse plane. The maximum pressure (P_{max}) is 37.5 MPa and the negative pressure (P_{min}) 5.0 MPa. Pressure rise time (t_r) is defined as the time for the pressure to rise from 10% to 90% of the value of P_{max} and is 30–120 nsec. The half width time (t_w) is defined as the half amplitude width of the initial positive pressure half cycle and is about 340 nsec. The pulse-to-pulse variation is about 3%. The shock waves were applied with a frequency of 1.25 Hz.

For HESW exposure the animals were placed in the water-filled container and kept in fixed position by a plastic cocoon. The temperature of the water was maintained at 37 °C. At the site of the limb of the animal a 1.5×1.5-cm hole in the tube allowed the shock waves to reach the tumor while the animal was protected by the tube against exposure to shock wave at other sites. The tumors were positioned in the center of the focal area (fluoroscopically guided).

The nude mice were anesthetized with ketamine hydrochloride (Ketalar, Parke-Davis) 150 mg/kg body weight and received 3 (or 4) sessions of 800 HESW on days 0, 2, 4 (and 6).

Additional Treatment

Doxorubicin (Adriablastine, Pharmitalia) 5 mg/kg was administered once on day 0, intraperitoneally, just before (20–30 min) the first HESW exposure. As BRM we used human interferon-α (IFN-α) and human tumor necrosis factor-α (TNF-α), which were kindly supplied by Boehringer Ingelheim, Alkmaar, The Netherlands. The specific activity of IFN-α was 3.2×10E8 units/mg protein. The specific activity of TNF-α was 6×10E7 units/mg protein. IFN-α was given 3 times a week 5.0 ng/g body weight and TNF-α 5 times a week 500 ng/g body weight subcutaneously around the tumor.

Evaluation of Tumor Growth

Tumor volume was determined every other day by measuring with a precision sliding caliper the three dimensions maximum diameter (length, L) and the diameters perpendicular to it (width, W, and height, H) and expressed as the tumor size index (TSI), calculated by the equation $L \times W \times H \times 0.52$. Tumor growth patterns were evaluated by calculating the mean tumor volume of the tumors in each group.

Statistical Analysis

When the tumor had reached the desired volume of 60–80 mm^3, the tumor-bearing animals were randomly divided into the different treatment groups. Each treatment group consisted of at least six animals. For each animal, log linear regression over the first 2 weeks was used to estimate the growth rate (α), i.e., the number of times the tumor volume doubled per day (the doubling time equals $1/\alpha$). Differences in treatment versus control growth rates were then analyzed by two-sided *t*-tests. For combined treatments, two treatments were considered partly additive if the decrease in growth rate resulting from the combined treatment was larger than the decreases resulting from each of the single treatments. They were considered synergistic if the decrease for the combined treatment was larger than the sum of the decreases for the single treatments (one-sided *t*-tests, $p < 0.05$).

Results

In Vivo Antitumor Effect of HESW

Exposure to HESW usually results in temporary delay of tumor growth. After cessation of therapy the tumor starts growing again with the same doubling time. From earlier studies we know that the in vivo antitumor effect depends not only on the number of shock waves administered, but also on the number of shock wave sessions, the initial tumor burden, and the tumor model used (Oosterhof et al. 1990).

Table 1. Estimated growth rates in NU-1 tumors

Tumor model	Treatment	First 14 days after treatment			Result
		α	SEM	P	
NU-1	Control	0.28	0.01	–	
	4×800 HESW	0.21	0.03	0.01	
	Doxorubicin	0.21	0.01	0.002	
	Combination	0.15	0.01	0.0001	Additive
	TNF/IFN	0.20	0.03	0.01	
	Combination	−0.02	0.03	0.0001	Synergistic

α, Estimated growth rates; *SEM*, standard error of the mean. Log linear regression calculation after treatment with HESW, doxorubicin, BRMs or combinations of these. Results of combined treatment were synergetic, additive, or not significant.

Repeated sessions of 800 HESW (18.4 kV), every 48 h on the human kidney tumors NU-1 and NU-3 subcutaneously implanted in the nude mouse caused a significant decrease in tumor growth. Four sessions of 800 shock waves to the NU-1 caused a suppression of tumor growth for 4 doubling times (Fig. 1). The growth rate of the NU-1 tumor ($\alpha = 0.28$) temporarily decreased to 0.21 after 4 sessions of 800 shock waves (Table 1) and that of the NU-3 from 0.29 to 0.19. Fourteen days after the first HESW exposure the tumors regained their original growth rate. In these experiments there was no animal mortality, either in the HESW treatment group or in the combined treatment groups.

In Vivo Effect of HESW Combined Treatment Modalities

In vitro and in vivo studies have shown an additional cytotoxic effect when HESW was combined with cytotoxic drugs (Berens et al. 1989; Holmes et al. 1990; Oosterhof et al. 1989, 1990a, b; Randazzo et al. 1988). Since HESW alone can only cause a temporary growth delay, additional treatment is needed for longer and more definitive suppression of tumor growth. Combination with another suboptimal treatment or a drug given in a suboptimal dose might thus result in a more complete effect. Therefor, we tested the combination of HESW and doxorubicin or BRMs (TNFα/IFNα) in the NU-1 xenograft.

Effect of Combination of HESW and Doxorubicin

Combination of 4 sessions of HESW with a single administration of 5 mg/kg doxorubicin intraperitoneally on day 0 just before shock wave exposure led to an additive decrease in tumor growth, resulting in a growth rate of 0.15 (Fig. 1, Table 1). The combination treatment was not only more effective ($\alpha = 0.15$), but the effect was permanent. The tumor did not regain its original growth rate after 14 days, as was the case after monotherapy (HESW or doxorubicin).

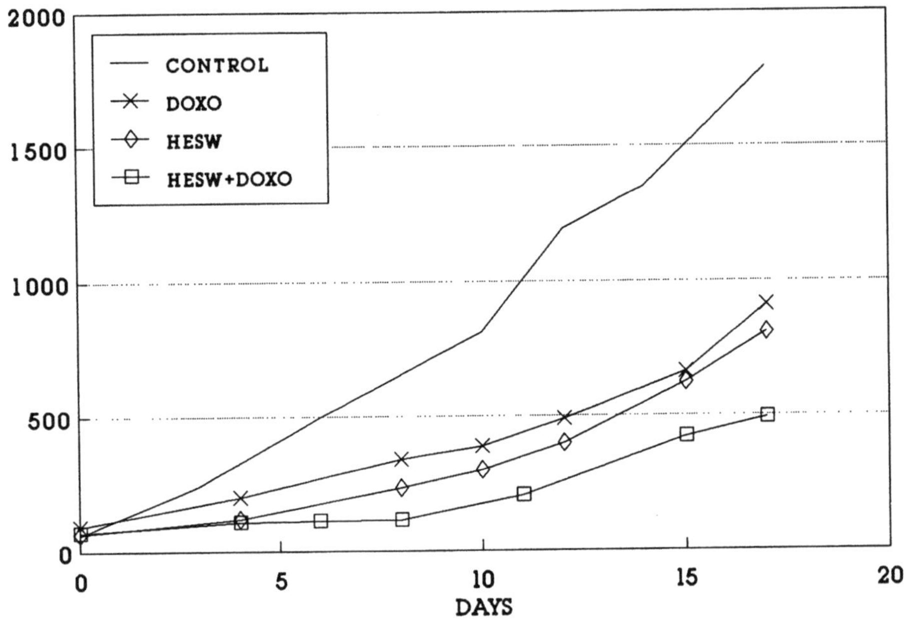

Fig. 1. Tumor volume after 4 exposures (every 48 h) to 800 HESW combined with doxorubic 5 mg/kg in the NU-1 human kidney tumor

Combination of HESW with TNFα and IFNα

When the NU-1 tumor was exposed to IFN-α and TNF-α alone the growth rate (α) decreased to 0.20 (Table 1). Combination of 4 sessions of HESW and BRM treatment resulted in a prolonged decrease in tumor growth (Fig. 2); in fact, there was a complete cessation (and even slight regression) of tumor growth in the 7 animals exposed to this combined treatment, resulting in a growth rate of -0.02 (Table 1). Thus, this combination proved to have a highly synergistic antitumor effect. Further studies revealed a dose-response relation after exposing tumors to increasing numbers of shock wave sessions together with TNFα/IFNα. No complete regression of tumor was seen after combined treatment with less than 4 sessions of HESW.

Combination of Three Sessions of HESW and TNFα or IFNα Alone

The highly synergistic antiproliferative effect of the combination of shock waves and TNFα/IFNα treatment incited us to study this antitumor effect more in detail. Therefore, in order to gain more insight into the effects of IFNα, TNFα, or combination of these, we exposed the NU-1 and the NU-3 tumors to 3 sessions of 800 shock waves combined with these three different BRM treatments.

In the NU-1 xenograft the same synergistic antitumor effect could be obtained by exposing the tumor to the combination of 3 sessions of HESW and TNFα, suggesting that TNFα is the active agent responsible for the synergism. This was confirmed by the fact that IFNα had no potentiating antitumor effect when it was combined with HESW, although IFNα alone had a clear effect on tumor growth (Table 2). In the NU-3 kidney tumor too a synergistic antitumor effect was obtained with the combination of HESW and TNFα. IFNα alone had no effect on tumor growth and the antiproliferative effect of HESW alone was even slightly suppressed when it was combined with IFNα. The combination of shock waves with TNFα plus IFNα was also less effective than the combination of shock waves and TNF-α: while the first was synergistic, the latter only had an additive antitumor effect (Table 2).

Table 2. Estimated growth rates in NU-1 and NU-3 tumors

Tumor model	Treatment	First 14 days after treatment			Result
		α	SEM	*P*	
NU-1	Control	0.29	0.01	–	
	TNF/IFN	0.20	0.03	0.01	
	3×800 HESW	0.17	0.01	0.01	
	Combined	0.04	0.03	0.01	Synergistic
	Control	0.28	0.01	–	
	TNF	0.23	0.02	0.0001	
	3×800 HESW	0.17	0.01	0.0001	
	Combined	0.023	0.02	0.0122	Synergistic
	Control	0.22	0.02	–	
	IFN	0.18	0.03	0.2967	
	3×800 HESW	0.17	0.01	0.1239	
	Combined	0.17	0.01	0.2709	Not significant
NU-3	Control	0.29	0.02	–	
	TNF/IFN	0.23	0.01	0.0023	
	3×800 HESW	0.18	0.01	0.0001	
	Combined	0.09	0.03	0.0785	Additive
	Control	0.23	0.01	–	
	TNF	0.19	0.01	0.0001	
	3×800 HESW	0.19	0.02	0.0001	
	Combined	0.04	0.03	0.0051	Synergistic
	Control	0.26	0.01	–	
	IFN	0.25	0.02	0.3383	
	3×800 HESW	0.18	0.01	0.0002	
	Combined	0.21	0.01	0.1182	Not significant

α, Estimated growth rates; *SEM*, standard error of the mean. Log linear regression calculation after treatment with HESW, doxorubicin, BRMs, or combinations of these. Results of combined treatments were synergistic, additive or not significant.

Discussion

In several in vivo experiments, a delay in tumor growth rate was seen after exposure to HESW. This effect was temporary and depended on the number of HESW.

From our studies we concluded that the effects of in vivo HESW also depend largely on the tumor line used and on the initial tumor volume. Repeated HESW can suppress tumor growth as long as shock waves continue to be administered.

Little is still known about the exact mode of action of shock waves on tumor cells. In vitro no cell-cycle-specific effect could be found. In vivo, different ways of action can be considered. There is probably direct nonspecific damage to the cells, since tumor necrosis and hemorrhage are the main microscopic findings; histologic examination of the tumors after shock wave administration alone shows shock-wave-induced tissue damage with subsequent inflammation reactions and a wound healing process (Oosterhof et al. 1990). In this respect HESW can cause "debulking" of the viable tumor load. In addition, damage to the vasculature of the tumor, especially the small capillaries, and subsequent impairment of tumor bloodflow, may explain the growth delay after HESW. Indeed, it is known that shock waves have a major impact on the vasculature (Brendel et al. 1987; Goetz et al. 1988). Microscopical studies of the NU-1 xenograft immediately after shock wave exposure showed small petechial and peritumoral bleedings, which were seen after only 20 HESW. Disruption of capillaries within the tumor also became evident. Intact capillaries became distended and were tightly packed with erythrocytes. These events were accompanied by focal thrombosis and evidence of focal necrosis.

Since we failed to obtain complete destruction of even a small tumor through serial exposure of shock waves every 48 h, we studied the combination of two treatment modalities that might have a potentiating antitumor effect. Combined treatment of shock waves and doxorubicin is more effective (Table 1, Fig. 1). No histologic explanation for the additional antitumor effect can be seen. This additional antiproliferative effect is intriguing and several explanations (like changes in cell membrane properties) have been postulated. In vitro studies show that HESW can cause dose-dependent direct cytotoxicity, impairment of the proliferative capacity, and increased drug cytotoxicity (Berens et al. 1989; Oosterhof et al. 1989; Russo et al. 1985). However, the results of in vitro studies of shock-wave-induced bioeffects depend mainly on the way how cells are exposed to the shock waves and need careful interpretation. It is therefore difficult to extrapolate to the in vivo situation.

Recent ^{31}P magnetic resonance spectroscopy studies in vivo show that shock wave treatment of the NU-1 xenograft results in immediate, temporary acidosis and impairment of tumor cell metabolism, resembling an acute impairment of oxygenation such as can be seen in acute ischemia (Smits et al. 1990). Besides direct intrinsic cellular effects, shock waves affect tumor vasculature with subsequent changes in bloodflow and tumor cell metabolism. The temporarily metabolically disturbed (inactivated) tumor cells may become more susceptible to different types of chemotherapeutic drugs. In addition, changes in tumor perfusion can lead to altered local concentrations of drugs.

In the 7 NU-1 tumor-bearing animals given the combined treatment of 4 sessions of HESW and BRMs (TNFα and IFNα) we observed complete regression of the tumor in two (Table 1, Fig. 2). The disappearance of the tumors was seen on day 10 and 15 respectively after the start of the treatment. The other animals were killed for histologic tumor examination while the tumor was in partial re-

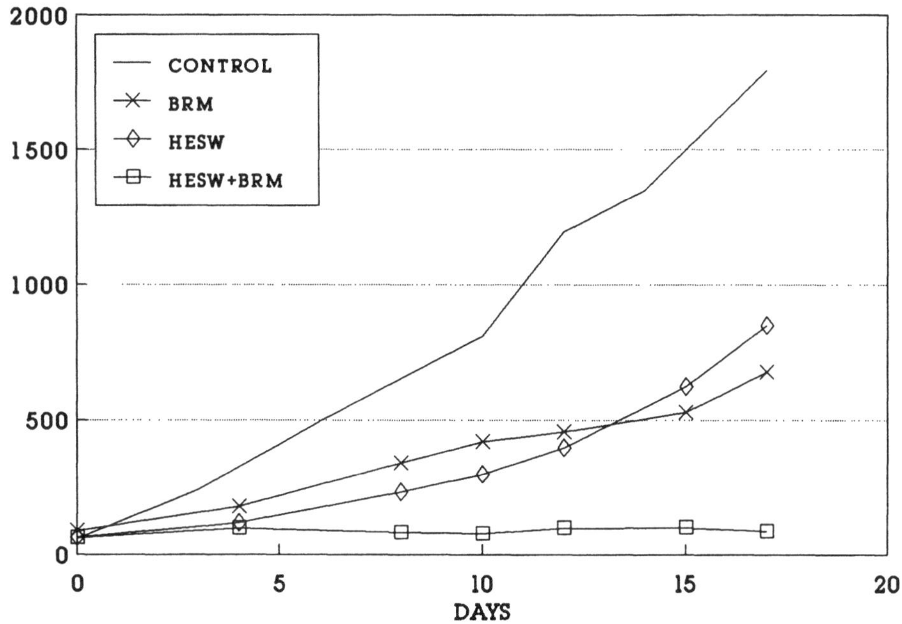

Fig. 2. Tumor volume after 4 exposures (every 48 h) to 800 HESW combined with interferon-α and tumor necrosis factor-α in the NU-1 kidney tumor

gression or stabilized. In the animals treated by the combination of HESW and doxorubicin, no complete disappearance of the tumor was seen.

Tumors treated with the combination of HESW and BRMs showed extensive necrotic parts, surrounded by areas with marked vasodilatation, leukocyte migration and infiltration, and fibrin clots within the capillaries, suggesting that the tissue damage with subsequent inflammation reactions induced by the shock waves is modulated by the BRMs resulting in a necrotic tumor (Oosterhof et al. 1990).

Further investigation of the synergistic antitumor effect of combined BRM and HESW treatment revealed that only TNFα is potentiated by HESW (Table 2). One of the explanations for the synergism of the combination of HESW and TNFα is that both act on the microcirculation (Shine et al. 1989; Smits et al. 1990). Combination of these actions results in an enhanced disturbance of tumor vasculature and blood flow and may thus explain the potentiated antitumor effect. Further studies in five different human kidney cancer xenografts indicate that this synergistic effect is mainly related to the vascularization of the tumor (Oosterhof et al. 1990).

In conclusion, exposure of the NU-1 and NU-3 human kidney tumors to shock waves leads to a growth delay. A potentiating antitumor effect can be obtained when the shock wave treatment is combined with another suboptimal treatment. Further fundamental research is necessary to elucidate the exact mode of action of shock waves on tumors and tumor cells in order to come to a better understanding of how to improve the effectiveness of HESW and develop new (combined) treatment modalities. It remains an exciting and challenging idea that HESW, generated outside a target location and focussed onto a limited area, can be used to alter tumor growth and response to therapy in vivo.

Acknowledgments. This work was supported by: The Dutch Kidney Foundation (grant no C87.699), the Siemens Company, and the Maurits and Anna de Kock Foundation. We would like to acknowledge Drs. H. E. Schaafsma (Department of Pathology, University Hospital, Nijmegen, The Netherlands) for the histological examinations, Dr. G. Borm (Department of Statistics of the University of Nijmegen) for the statistical analysis, and J. Koedam and M. Derks animal Laboratory Department, University of Nijmegen) for their excellent technical assistance with the in vivo experiments.

References

Beniers AJMC, van Moorselaar RJA, Peelen WP, Debruyne FMJ, Schalken JA (1988) Differential sensitivity of renal xenografts towards therapy with interferon-α, interferon-γ, tumor necrosis factor and their combinations; possible implications for clinical studies. Urol Res (in press)

Berens ME, Welander CE, Griffin AS, McCullough DL (1989) Effect of acoustic shock waves on clonogenic growth and drug sensitivity of human tumor cells in vitro. J Urol 142:1090–1094

Brendel W, Delius M, Goetz A (1987) Effect of shock waves on microvasculature. Prog Appl Microcirc 12:41–50

Brümmer F, Brenner J, Bräuner T, Hülser DF (1989) Effects of shock waves on suspended and immobilized L1210 cells. Ultrasound Med Biol 15:229–329

Goetz AE, Konigsberger R, Hammersen F, Conzen P, Delius M, Brendel W (1988) Acute shock wave induced effects on the microcirculation. In: Steiner R (ed) Laser lithotripsy. Springer, Berlin Heidelberg New York Tokyo

Holmes RP, Yeaman LI, Li W, Hart LJ, Wallen CA, Woodruff RD, McCullough DL (1990) The combined effects of shock waves and cisplatin therapy on rat prostate tumors. J Urol 144:159–163

Laudone VP, Morgan TR, Huryk RF, Heston WDW, Fair WR (1989) Cytotoxicity of high energy shock waves: methodologic considerations. J Urol 141:965–968

Oosterhof GON, Smits GAHJ, de Ruyter JE, van Moorsealaar RJA, Schalken JA, Debruyne FMJ (1989) The in vitro effect of electromagnetically generated shock waves (Lithostar) on the Dunning R3327 PAT-2 rat prostatic cancer cell line. Urol Res 17:13–19

Oosterhof GON, Smits GAHJ, de Ruyter JE, Schalken JA, Debruyne FMJ (1990) In vivo effects of high energy shock waves on urological tumors; an evaluation of treatment modalities. J Urol 144:785–789

Oosterhof GON, Smits GAHJ, de Ruyter JE, Schalken JA, Debruyne FMJ (1990) Effects of high energy shock waves combined with biological response modifiers or adriamycin on a human kidney cancer xenograft. Urol Res (in press)

Oosterhof GON, Smits GAHJ, de Ruyter JE, Schalken JA, Debruyne FMJ (1990) Effects of high energy shock waves combined with biological response modifiers in different human kidney cancer xenografts. Ultrasound Med Biol (in press)

Randazzo RF, Chaussy CG, Fuchs GJ, Bhuta SM, Lovrekovich H, de Kernion JB (1988) The in vitro and in vivo effects of extracorporal shock waves on malignant cells. Urol Res 16:419–424

Russo P, Heston WDW, Fair WR (1985) Suppression of in vitro and in vivo tumor growth by high energy shock waves. Surg Forum 36:645–648

Russo P, Stephenson RA, Mies C, Huryk R, Heston WDW, Melamed MR, Fair WR (1986) High energy shock waves suppress tumor growth in vitro and in vivo. J Urol 135:626–628

Shine N, Palladipp MA, Patton JS, Deisseroth A, Karczmar GB, Matson GB, Weiner MW (1989) Early metabolic response to tumor necrosis factor in mouse sarcoma: a phosphorus-31 nuclear magnetic resonance study. Cancer Res 49:2123–2127

Smits GAHJ, Oosterhof GON, de Ruyter JE, Schalken JA, Debruyne FMJ (1990) Cytotoxic effects of high energy shock waves in different model systems: influence of the experimental set-up. J Urol 144 (in press)

Smits GAHJ, Heerschap A, Oosterhof GON, Debruyne FMJ, Ruys JHJ, Hilbers CW, Schalken JA (1990) Early metabolic response to high energy shock waves in a human tumor kidney xenograft monitored by ^{31}magnetic resonance spectroscopy (submitted).

A New Method for Renal Perfusion Fixation

M. KALLERHOFF[1], H. J. GRÖNE[2], G. KEHRER[3], T. KNIESS[4], U. HELMCHEN[5], H. J. BRETSCHNEIDER[3], and R. H. RINGERT[1]

Introduction

Kidneys can tolerate ischemia lasting up to 2 h at a temperature of about 30 °C when protected by HTK (histidine trytophane ketoglutarate) (Groenewoud et al. 1989; Gubernatis et al. 1990; Isemer et al. 1988; Kallerhoff 1989; Kehrer et al. 1989; Pichlmayr et al. 1990; Preusse et al. 1987; Schnabel et al. 1987). Structural recovery after such ischemic stress as examined by light microscopy on immersion-fixed sections – is completed after 2–3 h reperfusion. There are no visible structural differences to normal kidney tissue. This was the reason for also testing this solution for improvement of renal perfusion fixation.

Perfusion fixation of kidneys is difficult, as complete, homogeneous washout of blood may be prevented by the immediate onset of fixation (Pfaller 1982; Sakai and Kriz 1987). Postcapillary arteriolar beds as they occur in the kidney are fixated later. It may thus be difficult to differentiate between ischemic insult and fixation artefacts.

Materials and Methods

For our experiments we used eight kidneys from German Shepherd cross-breed dogs of both sexes, the average animal weight being 32 kg. Thirty minutes following premedication with 90 mg Dipidolor (piritramide) and 0.5 mg atropine, the animals were anesthesized with thiopental. Anesthesia was maintained with a combination of fentanyl, halothane, and a 3 : 1 mixture of N_2O and oxygen (for further details see Kallerhoff et al. 1987 and Kallerhoff 1989). Following median laparotomy, the kidneys were isolated from the surrounding tissue with ligation of all capsule vessels; then the renal artery, the renal vein, and the ureter were dissected. For perfusion of the kidneys with the HTK solution, the renal perfusion catheter with its terminal pressure lead and four lateral openings was inserted into the abdominal aorta distal to the branching of the external iliac artery. To avoid any preperfusion ischemia, the flow of HTK solution (Custodiol, Dr. Franz Köhler Chemie GmbH, D-6141 Alsbach-Hähnlein 1, FRG; Table 1) cooled to 4 °C, was initiated at a flow rate of 100 ml/min while the catheter was advanced into the renal artery, where it was fixed by means of a tourniquet string. After

* Supported by the Deutsche Forschungsgemeinschaft – SFB 330 Organprotektion.

[1] Klinik und Poliklinik für Urologie; [2] Zentrum Pathologie; [3] Zentrum Physiologie; [4] Zentrum Chirurgie, Abt. Allgemeinchirurgie der Universität, Robert-Koch-Str. 40, W-3400 Göttingen, FRG.
[5] Institut für Pathologie der Universität, Martinistr. 52, W-2000 Hamburg 20, FRG.

Table 1. HTK solution of Bretschneider (Custodiol)

NaCl	15 m*M*
KCl	9 m*M*
$MgCl_2$	4 m*M*
K-α-Ketoglutarate	1 m*M*
Tryptophane	2 m*M*
Histidine	180 m*M*
Histidine-HCl	18 m*M*
Mannite	30 m*M*
pH at 8 °C	7.3
pO_2 at 37 °C	200 mmHg
Osmolarity	310 mosmol/l

Table 2. Fixation solution

Glutaraldehyde	150 m*M*
Na^+-Dimethylarsenic acid	94 m*M*
Osmolarity (calculated)	338 mosmol/l
(measured)	314 mosmol/l
pH (37 °C)	7.4

6 min HTK perfusion the perfusion fixation started. Via a Y-piece, the perfusion with the fixation solution (Table 2) started without any interruption of flow. Perfusion with the warm (37 °C) fixation solution also lasted 6 min. Afterwards the kidneys were excised and were prepared for morphological examinations.

Furthermore, we perfused rat kidney in situ via an 18-Charrière venule, which was placed in the aorta distal to the origin of the renal artery, according to the following perfusion procedure: first 6 min perfusion with the HTK solution (4 °–6 °C) at a flow of about 5 ml/min, then 6 min perfusion with glutaraldehyde/ Na^+-dimethylarsenic acid (37 °C), also at a flow of 5 ml/min by a perfusion pump (Infusomat, Braun Melsungen, FRG).

Results

The perfusion pressure should be kept between 80 and 100 mmHg during the 6-min HTK perfusion to equilibrate the extracellular space of the kidney as fast as possible to the electrolyte composition of the HTK solution. During the first 2 min the temperature of the kidney drops from body temperature to below 10 °C (Fig. 1). At the end of protective perfusion the switch to perfusion fixation is made without interruption of flow. The perfusion pressure is also kept at 80–100 mmHg. During this perfusion the temperature of the kidney rises to 37 °C again, as this is the temperature of the solution (Fig. 1).

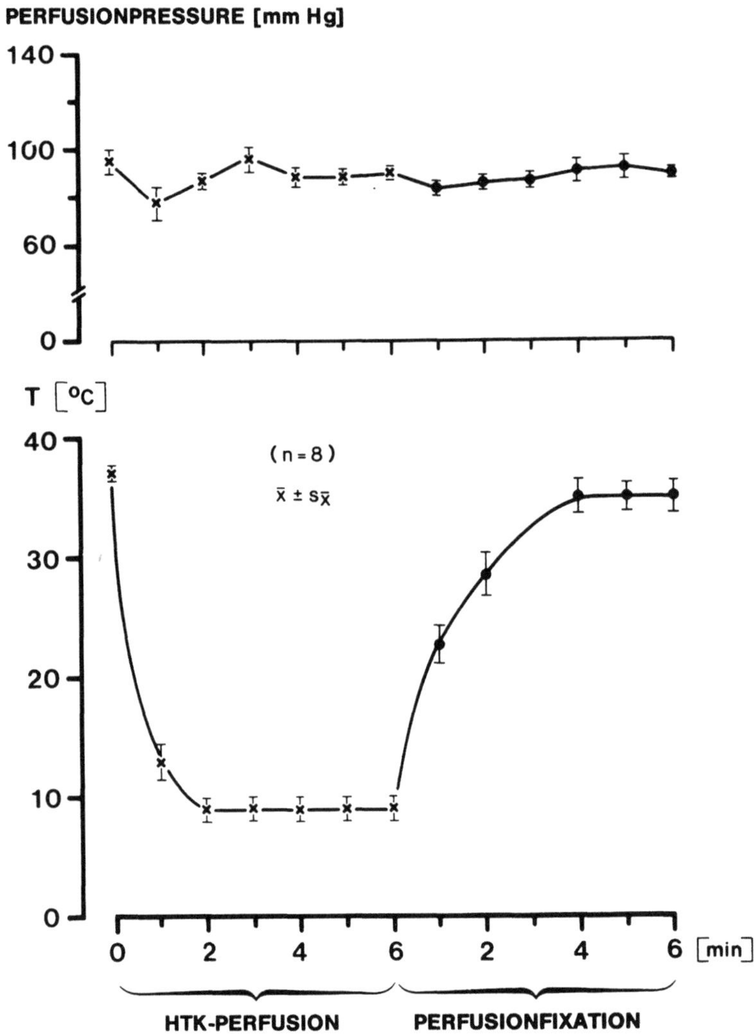

Fig. 1. Perfusion pressure (*top*) and temperature (*bottom*) during HTK perfusion and perfusion fixation

A perfusion pressure of 80–100 mmHg can be achieved with the HTK solution at a flow of 450 ml/min with kidneys weighing about 100 g. Then about 30 ml/6 min come out of the tubular and collecting duct system as "perfusion urine". This leads to equilibration of these compartments of the kidney with the electrolyte composition of the HTK solution (Fig. 2). After the change to perfusion fixation, the flow is reduced to 400–450 ml/min in order to keep the perfusion pressure below 100 mmHg. The "perfusion diuresis" is constant.

By light microscopy, the renal cortex shows a dilated vas afferens and vas efferens, totally unfolded capillary tuft and open tubuli with well-preserved brush

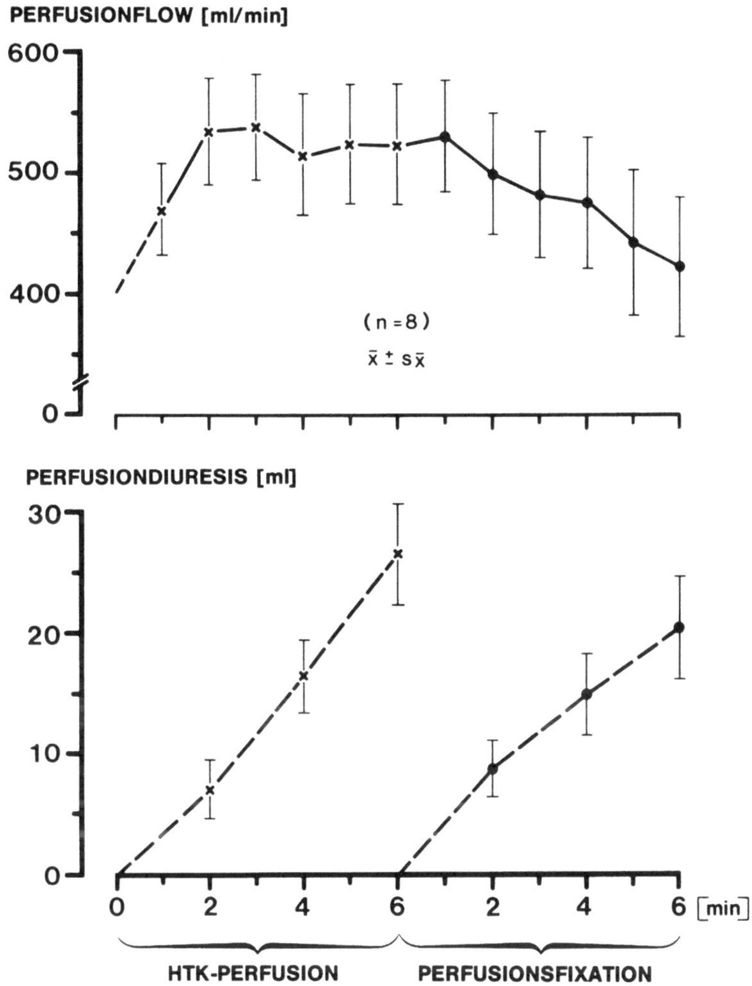

Fig. 2. Perfusion flow (*top*) and perfusion diuresis (*bottom*) during HTK perfusion and perfusion fixation

border membrane (Fig. 3). The outer and inner medulla including the papilla also demonstrate open tubuli and collecting duct systems.

The good, in-vivo-equivalent conditions can also be seen by electron microscopy for the glomerular capillary wall with endothelium, basement membrane, and podocytes (Fig. 4).

Figure 5 shows homogeneously perfusion-fixed open vascular and tubular parts of the rat kidney. Endothelia cover a stretched lamina elastica interna in preglomerular vessels. Proximal tubules show open lumina with brush borders of normal height. Glomeruli are almost free of erythrocytes with a nonedematous mesangium and regularly attached visceral epithelial cells.

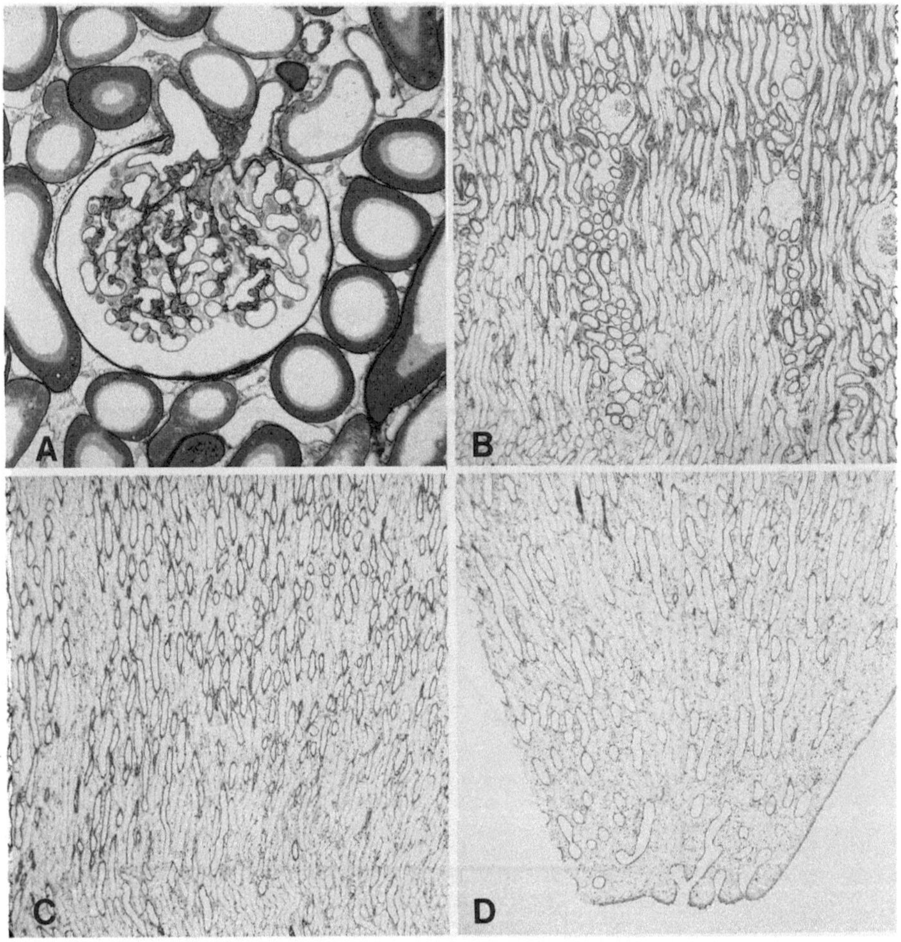

Fig. 3a–d. Experiment 320, dog, left kidney. **a** Silver impregnation (MOVAT), renal cortex, glomerulus with unfolded tuft of capillary, open and dilated proximal tubuli with well-preserved brush border membrane, distal tubuli with regular structure; **b–d** (Goldner-Masson) outer stripe of medulla of the same kidney; **c** inner stripe; **d** papilla, dilated tubuli, and collecting duct system

Fig. 4. Experiment 320, dog, left kidney. Electron microscopy of the glomerular loops: typical mesangial and endothelial cells, basement membrane of normal width, podocytes with regular foot processes

Fig. 5a–d. Rat kidney; **a, b** cortex with stretched preglomerular vessel, interlobular artery, well-perfused glomeruli, and open tubules. **c** Straight segments of proximal tubules in outer stripe of outer medulla with clearly visible and preserved brush border. **d** Inner medulla with open vessels of vascular bundle and surrounding well-preserved distal tubules

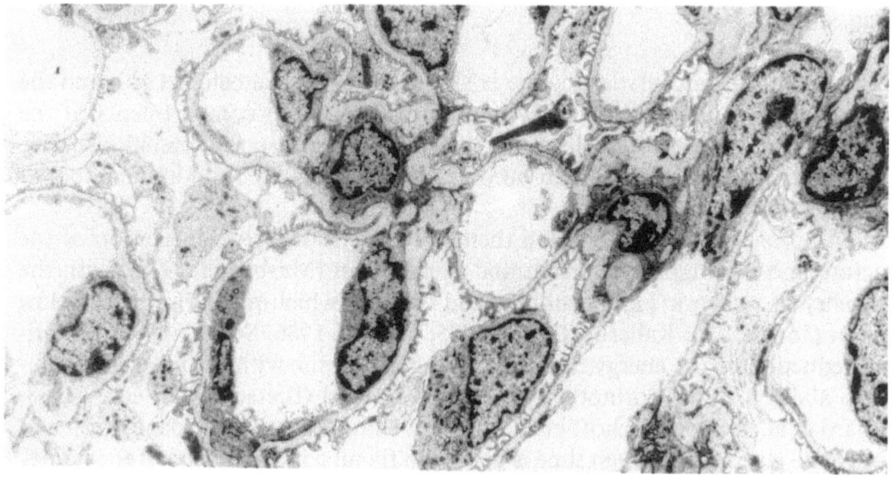

Fig. 4

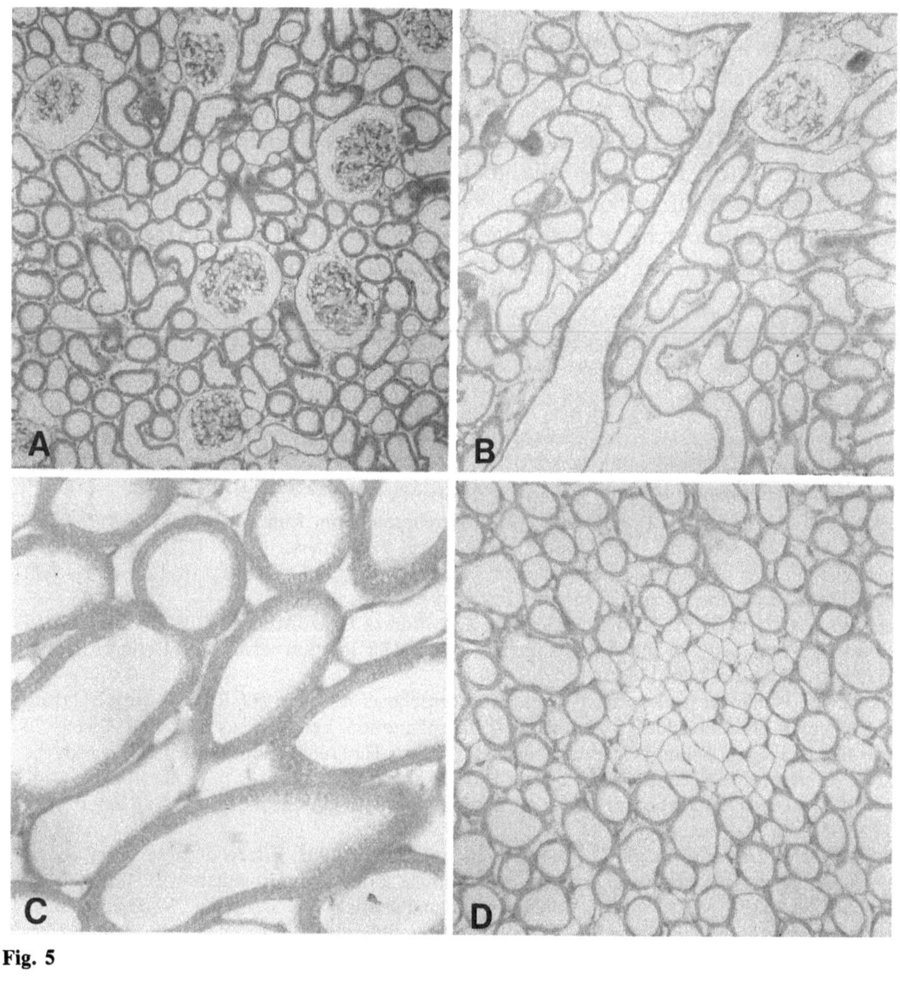

Fig. 5

Discussion

As a result of the vasodilation by the HTK solution (Bretschneider 1980) and the washout of the tubuli, the fixation solution can reach all compartments of the kidney – the intravasal and intratubular space as well as the interstitial space (Sakai and Kriz 1987). The organ becomes homogeneously solid and can be excised after 12 min in toto.

At an optimal perfusion fixation there is competition between fixation of the structure and its ongoing function and metabolism (Marberger 1978), with the possibility of ischemic induced injury and changes which may arise by too slow fixation (Jones 1986; Kallerhoff et al. 1985; Mandel 1986; Soltoff 1986). By primary reduction of the energy demand of the renal tissue with the protective solution to about 1/30 of normothermic energy demand (Bretschneider et al. 1988; Gebhard et al. 1987; Kallerhoff et al. 1989), in eliminating blood coagulation and vasospastic reactions, enough time is gained to fix all compartments of the kidney – including the postglomerular parts of the vascular system – without regressive or ischemic injury.

The medulla and the papilla are difficult to perfuse homogeneously by perfusion fixation (Pfaller 1982). As Fig. 3b–d demonstrates, with preperfusion of the HTK solution it is possible to achieve homogeneous fixation of all parts of the kidney, as after HTK perfusion the same osmolarity is reached in the extracellular space, in the cortex, in the medulla, and even in the papilla.

The concentrating ability of rat kidneys is up to 2000 mosmol and it is therefore even more difficult to achieve homogeneous washout of all compartments. In this species too, however, this new method of perfusion fixation leads to homogeneous fixation of tissue.

References

Bretschneider HJ (1980) Myocardial protection. Thorac Cardiovasc Surg 28:295–302

Bretschneider HJ, Helmchen U, Kehrer G (1988) Nierenprotektion. Klin Wochenschr 66:817–827

Gebhard MM, Bretschneider HJ, Gersing E, Schnabel PA, Preusse CJ (1987) Bretschneider's histidine-buffered cardioplegic solution: concept, application, and efficiency. In: Roberts AJ (ed) Myocardial protection in cardiac surgery. Dekker, New York, pp 95–119

Groenewoud AF, Isemer FE, Stadler J, Heideche CD, Florack G, Hölscher M (1989) A comparison of early function between kidney grafts protected with HTK solution versus Euro-Collins solution. Transplant Proc 21:1243–1244

Gubernatis G, Pichlmayr R, Lamesch P, Grosse H, Bornscheuer A, Meyer HJ, Ringe B, Farle M (1990) HTK-solution (Bretschneider) for human liver transplantation. Langenbecks Arch Chir 375:66–70

Isemer FE, Ludwig A, Schunk O, Bretschneider HJ, Peiper HJ (1988) Kidney procurement with the HTK solution of Bretschneider. Transplant Proc 20:885–886

Jones DP (1986) Renal metabolism during normoxia, hypoxia, and ischemic injury. Ann Rev Physiol 48:33–50

Kallerhoff M, Hölscher M, Kehrer G, Kläß G, Bretschneider HJ (1985) Effects of preservation conditions and temperature on tissue acidification in canine kidneys. Transplantation 39:485–489

Kallerhoff M, Blech M, Kehrer G, Kleinert H, Langheinrich M, Siekmann W, Helmchen U, Bretschneider HJ (1987) Short-term perfusion and "equilibration" of canine-kidneys with protective solutions. Urol Res 15:5–12

Kallerhoff M (1989) Nierenprotektion in Anlehnung an das Verfahren zur Myokardprotektion nach Bretschneider im Vergleich zum Euro-Collins Verfahren. Z Tx Med 1:15–33

Kallerhoff M, Blech M, Kehrer G, Langheinrich M, Helmchen U, Bretschneider HJ, Ringert RH (1989) Improvement of in situ renal protection against complete ischemia through the replacement of chloride by aspartate in the HTK solution of Bretschneider. In: Rübben H et al. (eds) Investigative urology, vol 3. Springer, Berlin Heidelberg New York Tokyo, pp 197–208

Kallerhoff M, Blech M, Götz L, Kehrer G, Bretschneider HJ, Helmchen U, Ringert RH (1990) A new method for conservative renal surgery – experimental and first clinical results. Langenbecks Arch Chir 375:340–346

Kehrer G, Blech M, Kallerhoff M, Langheinrich M, Bretschneider HJ (1989) Postischemic interrelations between energy metabolism and functional recovery of protected canine kidneys. Eur J Clin Invest 19:328–336

Mandel LJ (1986) Primary active sodium transport, oxygen consumption and ATP: coupling and regulation. Kidney Int 29:3–9

Marberger M (1978) Ischämie und regionale Hypothermie bei Operationen am Nierenparenchym. Steinkopff, Darmstadt

Pfaller W (1982) Structure function correlation on rat kidney. Springer, Berlin Heidelberg New York

Pichlmayr R, Grosse H, Hauss J, Gubernatis G, Lamesch P, Bretschneider HJ (1990) Technique and preliminary results of extracorporal liver surgery (bench procedure) and of surgery on the in situ-preserved liver. Br J Surg 77:21–26

Preusse CJ, Schulte HD, Bircks W (1987) High volume cardioplegia. Ann Chir Gynaecol 76:39–45

Sakai T, Kriz W (1987) The structural relationship between mesangial cells and basement membrane of the renal glomerulus. Anat Embryol 176:373–386

Schnabel PA, Gebhard MM, Pomikay Th, Preusse CJ, Schmiedl A, Richter J, Bretschneider HJ (1987) Myocardial protection: left ventricular ultrastructure after different forms of cardiac arrest. Thorac Cardiovasc Surg 35:148–156

Soltoff ST P (1986) ATP and the regulation of renal cell function. Ann Rev Physiol 48:9–31

Investigations into the Medicinal Protection from Acute Kidney Failure of Ischemic Origin in Animal Experiments

B. Langkopf, U. Rebmann, H.-J. Forth, and J. Schabel[1]

Introduction

Successful kidney transplantations essentially depend on the vitality of the organs donated. Warm and cold ischemic times (WIT/CIT) during harvesting, storage, and transplantation damage the transplant, so that in 20% – 60% of cases acute kidney failure must be anticipated.

Although the influence of acute kidney failure on long-term survival of transplanted kidneys is a subject of controversy, there is no doubt about the advantages of immediate function in regard to diagnosis of rejection, access to dialysis, and period of hospitalization. Despite keeping to the limits fixed in the East German (GDR) guideline for kidney transplantation, the incidence of actue kidney failure at our institute was about 50%.

The following are regarded as potential risk factors for acute kidney failure:

1. The hemodynamic condition of the kidney donor at the moment of harvesting;
2. The method of kidney preservation and
3. The hemodynamic condition of the recipient during transplantation.

We investigated the effect of four selected drugs in improving the ischemic tolerance of the kidney (Table 1):

1. The prostacyclin analogue Iloprost (Schering, Berlin), the marked vasodilatatory and cytoprotective properties of which should be utilized as well as its inhibitory effect on the aggregation of thrombocytes.
2. The coronary drug trapidil, which has a direct influence on the metabolism of prostaglandins, produced by the pharmaceutical industry as Rocornal (by the Deutsches Hydrierwerk, Rodleben).
3. A trapidil derivative 12463 (Deutsches Hydrierwerk, Rodleben).

Table 1. Test drugs and dosages

Drug	Dose/min	Total dose[a]
Iloprost (ZK 36374)	1 µg/kg min	15 µg/kg
Trapidil	1.334 mg/kg min	20 mg/kg
Trapidil derivative 12463	0.667 mg/kg min	10 mg/kg
Dimethylsulfoxide (DMSO)	166.7 mg/kg min	2.5 g/kg

[a] Total dose administered via perfusor at 1 ml/min for 15 min.

[1] Klinik und Poliklinik für Urologie der Martin-Luther-Universität Halle, Leninallee 16, O-4010 Halle, FRG.

4. The cryoprotective DMSO (dimethylsulfoxide), which is also reported to improve ischemic tolerance.

Material and Methods

The experiments were conducted on 86 rabbits with an average weight of 3.0 kg in five test groups as follows:

1. Drug only
2. Sham operation
3. 60 min warm ischemic time, drug pretreatment
4. 120 min warm ischemic time, drug pretreatment
5. 120 min warm ischemic time, drug pre- and post-treatment.

Under pentobarbital narcosis (40 – 60 mg/kg) the abdomen was opened along the median line. Each animal was administered heparin at a dose of 350 IU/kg. The preparation of the vessels of the kidney hilus was followed by administration of the preischemic drug with subsequent renal artery clamping of the vessels of the kidney hilus for 60 or 120 min (warm ischemia time, WIT). Administration of the postischemic drug followed immediately after release of the blood stream through the kidneys. The interruption of the blood stream and its reperfusion were monitored by Doppler ultrasonographic probes. The abdomen was then closed. Drugs were administered intravenously via a perfusor at a rate of 1 ml/min for 15 min. Each test group was compared with control animals, who instead of a drug received physiological sodium chloride solution to the same volume. Blood samples were carried out daily up to the 17th day after operation. Survival rates and the evolution of serum creatinine levels were evaluated.

Results

In the first group, in which a direct pharmacological effect on renal function was to be examined, the survival rate was 100%. The serum creatinine stayed within the range 90 – 120 µmol/l at all times during the experiment. As expected, the same held true for the sham-operated animals, in whom no effect on survival rate and renal function was seen either (Table 2). A marked increase in serum

Table 2. Survival rates (number of survivors/number of animals)

Group	Iloprost	Trapidil	Trapidil derivate	DMSO	No drug
1 Drug only	4/4	4/4	4/4	4/4	2/2
2 Shamoperation					3/3
3 60 min WIT, drug pretreatment	3/3	3/3	3/3	3/3	2/2
4 120 min WIT, drug pretreatment	5/8	3/4	2/6	1/5	7/13
5 120 min WIT, drug pre- and posttreatment	10/11	7/8	6/8	0/4	3/6

WIT, warm ischemic time.

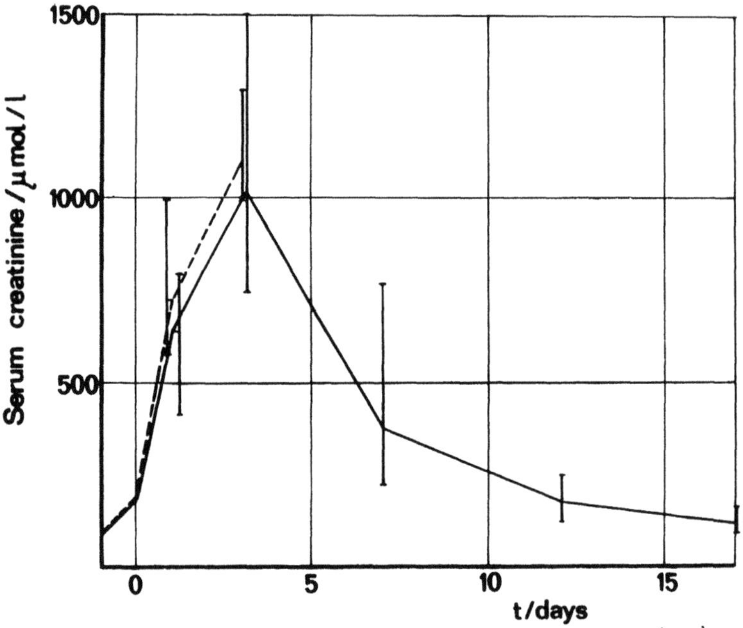

Fig. 1. Serum creatinine levels after 120 min WIT: control group

eatinine was found in those test animals who were exposed to warm ischemia for 60 min (group 3), with maximum values on the 1st day after operation. In the Iloprost, trapidil, and trapidil derivative groups these values amounted on average to about 350 µmol/l. In the control animals they reached about 430 µmol/l and in animals that received DMSO about 640 µmol/l. After 3 days the values were again within 90–120 µmol/l. All test animals of group 3 survived. The best survival rates were found after a warm ischemic time of 120 min after pre- and postischemic medication with Iloprost, trapidil, and trapidil derivative: 10 out of 11, 7 out of 8, and 6 out of 8 animals, which is 85.2% of the test animals. Of the animals given medication only prior to ischemia, only 55.5% survived, while out of 19 control animals just 10 survived. The administration of DMSO after 2 h ischemia resulted in death in 8 out of 9 test animals in groups 4 and 5. In the animals that survived, serum creatinine levels reached their highest values on the 3rd day after operation. In the control animals they amounted to about 1000 µmol/l (Fig. 1) and in the groups treated with Iloprost, Trapidil and trapidil derivative approximately 700 µmol/l (Fig. 2). Normal values in the treated animals returned between the 7th and the 12th day.

Discussion

By clamping the renal artery at the kidney hilus for 60 or 120 min, acute kidney failure of varying severity was caused. The results show especially pre- and post-

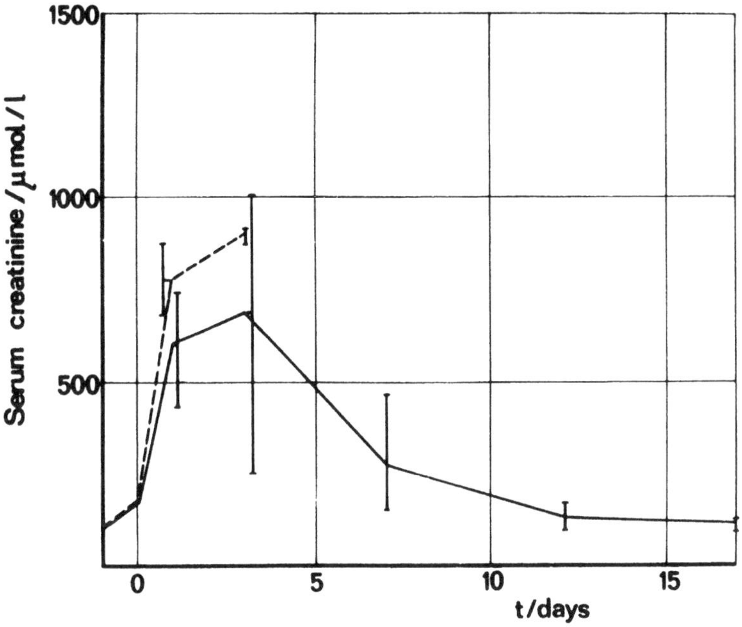

Fig. 2. Serum creatinine levels after 120 min WIT: iloprost group

ischemic administration of Iloprost, trapidil, and trapidil derviative to have a favorable influence on the severity and course of acute kidney failure. The positive effect of Iloprost is explained by its hemodynamic and cytoprotective characteristics and its ability to inhibit the aggregation of thrombocytes. Whether the effect of trapidil and trapidil derivative is via direct stimulation of prostacyclin synthesis or thromboxane-antagonistic properties cannot be decided on the basis of these investigations. Krause and Karczewski (1976) were able to prove that trapidil brings about an accumulation of cyclic adenosine-monophosphate with considerable vasodilatory potency by inhibiting phosphodiesterase. Last but not least, we also have to consider direct cardiac and diuretic characteristics.

For administration as cryoprotective we considered the examination of DMSO to be of particular interest, especially since improvement of ischemic tolerance through postischemic medication with DMSO has been observed by several investigators, such as Le Hann and Horita (1975) and Ketar et al. (1981). However, neither with pre- nor postischemic administration did we find a positive effect on the course of acute kidney failure. As the application of DMSO alone, without ischemic stress on the kidneys did not result in any observable impairment of kidney function, it can be concluded from our experiments that DMSO aggravates ischemic damage to the kidney. By contrast, Iloprost, trapidil, and trapidil derivative clearly improve the ischemic tolerance of the kidneys.

References

Kedar I, Cohen J, Jacob ET, Ravid M (1981) Alleviation of experimental ischemic acute renal failure by dimethyl sulfoxide. Nephron 29:55–58

Krause H-G, Karczewski P (1976) Hemmung der cyclo-MAP spaltenden Nukleotidhydrolyse des Herzens durch 5-Methyl-7-diethylamino-*S*-triazolo-(1,5-*a*)-pyrimidin (Rocornal). Acta Biol Med Germ 35:167–173

Le Hann TR, Horita A (1975) Effects of dimethyl sulfoxide (DMSO) on prostaglandin synthetase. Proc West Pharmacol Soc 18:81–82

MIX
Papier aus verantwortungsvollen Quellen
Paper from responsible sources
FSC® C105338

If you have any concerns about our products,
you can contact us on
ProductSafety@springernature.com

In case Publisher is established outside the EU,
the EU authorized representative is:
Springer Nature Customer Service Center GmbH
Europaplatz 3, 69115 Heidelberg, Germany

Printed by Libri Plureos GmbH
in Hamburg, Germany